H. Peter Chase, M.D.
Barbara Davis Center for Childhood Diabetes
Department of Pediatrics
University of Colorado Health Sciences Center

9th Edition, 2000

UNDERSTANDING INSULIN-DEPENDENT DIABETES

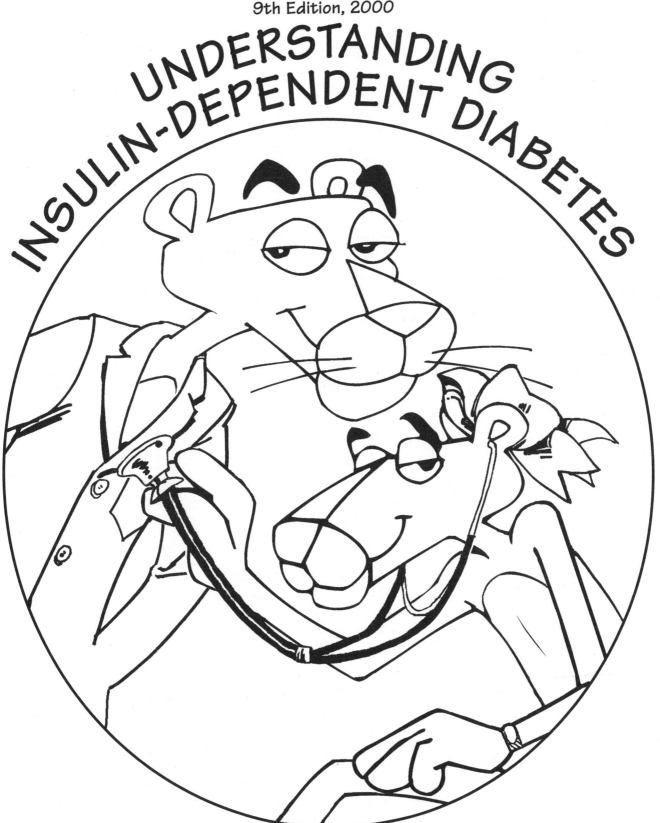

i

Barbara Davis Center
www.uchsc.edu/misc/diabetes/bdc.html

Children With Diabetes
www.childrenwithdiabetes.com

Juvenile Diabetes Foundation
www.jdfcure.org

American Diabetes Association
www.diabetes.org

This edition of the Pink Panther book
is dedicated to my wife, Virginia Carey Chase.
Her love, help, and support through the years
have helped to make my career an enjoyable one.

TABLE OF CONTENTS

Please note: Many parts of this book have been written at a 10th to 12th grade level and may be too complex for younger children. The coloring book follows the same outline and may be more appropriate for them. A parent working with a child in reading and understanding parts of this book may also be helpful.

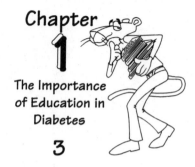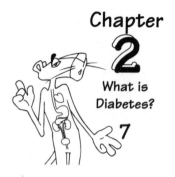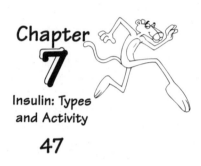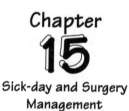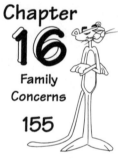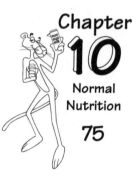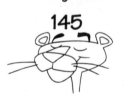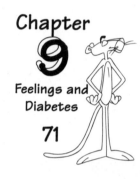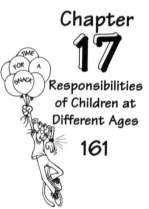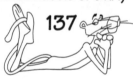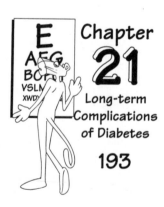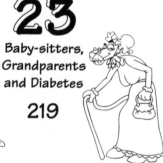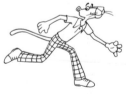
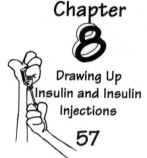

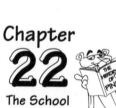

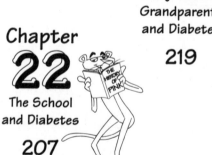

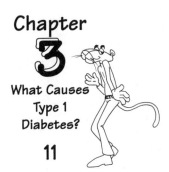
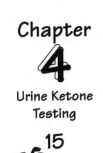
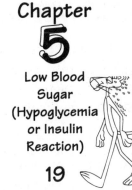
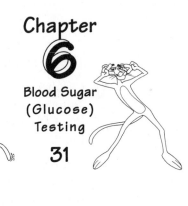
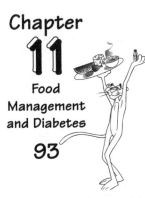
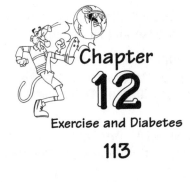
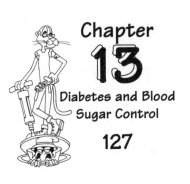
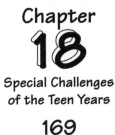
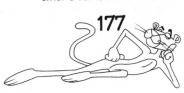
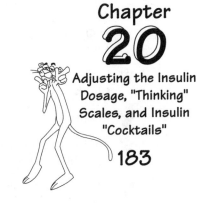
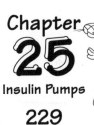
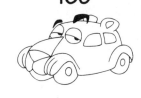

ACKNOWLEDGMENTS

The assistance of the following is greatly appreciated:

- Carolyn Banion, RN, MN, PNP, CDE, Paul Jensen, RN, ND, CDE, Cathy Johnson, RN, MS, CPNP, CDE, DeAnn Johnson, RN, BSN, and Susie Owen, RN, CDE, for their assistance on Chapter 8 (Drawing Up Insulin and Insulin Injections)

- Jana Gaston, MS, RD, CDE, Michelle Hansen, MS, RD, CDE, Darcy Owen, MS, RD, Gail Spiegel, MS, RD, CDE, Markey Swanson, RD, CDE, for editing Chapters 10 (Normal Nutrition) and Chapter 11 (Food Management and Diabetes)

- Carey and Jessie LeJeune, and Michelle Hansen, MS, RD, CDE, for their comments on Chapter 12 (Exercise and Diabetes)

- Ellen Fay, MSW, and Rita Temple-Trujillo, MSW, LCSW for their suggestions relating to Chapters 16 (Family Concerns), 17 (Responsibilities of Children at Different Ages) and 18 (Special Challenges of the Teen Years)

- Cathy Johnson, RN, MS, CPNP, CDE, DeAnn Johnson RN, BSN and Susie Owen, RN, CDE, for their help with Chapter 22 (The School and Diabetes)

- Peter Gottlieb, MD, Georgeanna Klingensmith, MD, Rob Slover, MD, Carolyn Banion, RN, MN, PNP, CDE, Michelle Hansen, MS, RD, CDE, Paul Jensen, RN, ND, CDE, Susie Owen, RN, CDE, Gail Spiegel, MS, RD, CDE, Dan Baxter and Ray Palandri for their comments on Chapter 25 (Insulin Pumps)

- Cathy Woodward, Tai Lockspeiser, Laura Kim and the staff of the Children's Diabetes Foundation for their help with proofreading.

- Regina Reece for editing and manuscript preparation.

- Finally, appreciation is expressed to Sue Palandri and the entire staff of the Children's Diabetes Foundation for their continued support.

- Book Design, Graphics, and Illustrations: Cindy Barton

- Printing: FGI Print Management

- The author wishes to thank the United Artists Corporation for allowing me to use the Pink Panther character (©1999 United Artists Pictures, Inc. All Rights reserved) in this publication.

- Additional copies of this book may be purchased for $15.00 from The Guild of The Children's Diabetes Foundation at Denver. See order form on the last page of this book.

Table 1

TOPICS COVERED IN A THREE-DAY DIABETES TREATMENT PLAN*

1st Day in Hospital or Clinic (often the day of diagnosis)

Explore family concerns, questions, and begin treatment of the diabetes. Treatment on the first day includes: blood sugar testing (Chapter 6); learning to do urine ketone measurements (Chapter 4); learning to recognize the signs of low blood sugar and how to treat it (Chapter 5). We write hour-by-hour instructions (see Table 2) for the family (meals, snacks, when to test blood or urine and how to record results, and when to phone us) for the period until returning to clinic. The solid protein/carbohydrate bedtime snack is emphasized.

Day Two: a.m. (usually first day of education)

The Importance of Education in Diabetes (Chapter 1)
What is Diabetes? (Chapter 2)
What Causes Diabetes? (Chapter 3)
Urine Ketone Testing (Chapter 4)
Ketoacidosis (Chapter 14)
Low Blood Sugar (Chapter 5)
Blood Sugar Testing (Chapter 6)
Insulin (Chapter 7)
Insulin Injections (Chapter 8)

Day Two: p.m.

Review previous chapters and answer questions
Feelings and Diabetes (Chapter 9)
Normal Nutrition (Chapter 10) and meet dietitian
Food Management and Diabetes (Chapter 11)
Prescriptions for supplies

Day Three: a.m.

Review previous chapters and answer questions
Review Low Blood Sugar (Chapter 5)
Exercise and Diabetes (Chapter 12)
Diabetes and Blood Sugar Control (Chapter 13)
School and Diabetes (Chapter 22): Watch school videotape
"Thinking" Scales (Chapter 20)

Day Three: p.m.

Review previous chapters and answer questions
Family Concerns (Chapter 16) and meet social worker
The Outpatient Management of Diabetes (Chapter 19)
Long-Term Complications of Diabetes (Chapter 21)
Baby-Sitters and Diabetes (Chapter 23)
Vacations and Camp (Chapter 24)

At One-Week Visit (or Day Four)

Review all of the above
Review Ketonuria and Acidosis (Ketoacidosis) (Chapter 14)
Sick-Day Management (Chapter 15)
Research and Diabetes (Chapter 26)
Problem solving and/or quiz

This is a general plan. The timing is varied from family to family. Also, the plan may change if the person is hospitalized versus when treated only in the clinic. A trend in recent years has been to teach survival skills in the first two days, and to make the visit at one week (when stress is lower) a longer and more in-depth visit.

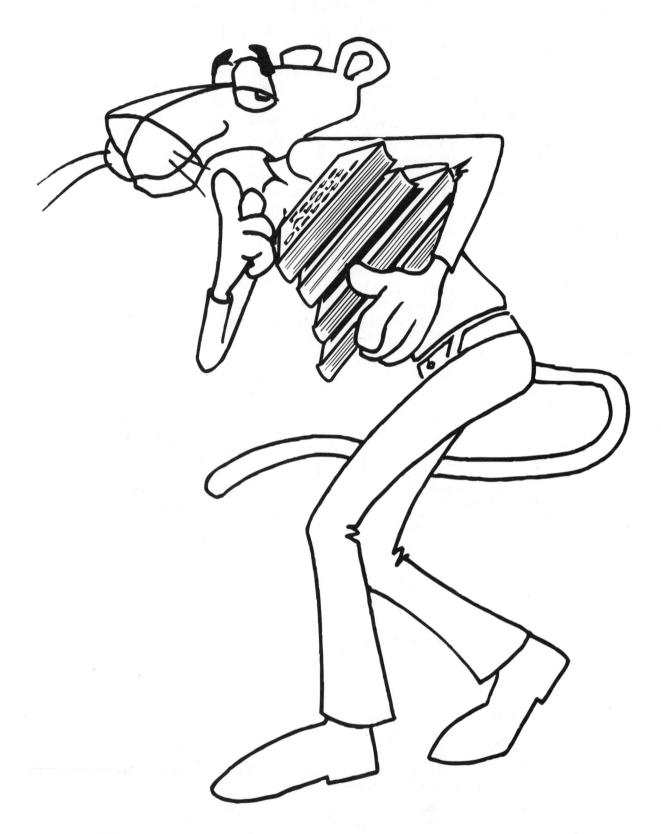

The Importance of Education in Diabetes

Chapter 1 THE IMPORTANCE OF EDUCATION IN DIABETES

Key ideas of this chapter:

🐾 Appreciate the importance of education in relation to diabetes.

🐾 Develop a care plan (for the newly diagnosed).

Families need to understand as much as possible about diabetes. This knowledge will help them feel more secure about the diabetes, help them manage problems when no doctor is available, and help them avoid hospitalizations for diabetes problems. Knowledge helps families feel they control the diabetes rather than the diabetes controls them.

This book is written both for families whose diabetes is new to them and for those families who have had the condition for a long time. This book can be used with the doctor and the diabetes team, or alone as a "refresher" course once the basic ideas are understood. Some of the chapters are written to provide very basic information. Other chapters (as indicated) are for the more advanced readers. Advances are taking place at such a rapid rate that new editions are needed about every three years. Many families bring this book to all clinic appointments so that they may continue their education.

OUTLINE FOR INITIAL EDUCATION

Day One (Table 1) is used to help the newly diagnosed person feel better, explore family concerns, answer questions, and learn the skills needed until returning to the clinic. As there is often much stress and uncertainty at this stage, the nurse or doctor can outline a suggested schedule to follow between the first- and second-day visits (Table 2). Education will continue on Day Two, which is often the first full day of education, as shown in Table 1 of this chapter. The chapters in this book generally follow the order in which the material is presented. Most families initially come to the clinic for six to eight hours per day for two to four days. We do not expect families to remember all the information the first time, so they must review the information often, over and over. Please write down questions and make notes. Video tapes, library books, parent and child educational group meetings, and our Pink Panther coloring book, which presents a synopsis of each of the chapters in this book, are other ways to continue learning.

CONTINUING EDUCATION

After the initial education, the family usually returns to the clinic in one week, then after two weeks, four weeks, eight weeks, and eventually every three months. This may vary for different families and different clinics. Clinic visits every three months allow for updating of information and, eventually, education of children who were too young to learn much at the time of the onset of their diabetes.

When children develop diabetes very early in life, it is difficult for them to learn specifics about the disease. It is important that these children develop an understanding of their condition as they reach ages 10-13 years. Parents may encourage their child to do a science report on diabetes, which would require reading this book. The diabetes nurse educator may start working on chapters in the book with the child alone to encourage the child to ask and answer questions. If families cannot attend a clinic every three months, it may be helpful to attend an in-depth education course on diabetes as the child reaches the adolescent years. It is our belief that good education will help the person to stay in good diabetes control throughout life and will help to prevent the need for later diabetes-related hospitalizations.

FAMILY RESPONSIBILITIES

Diabetes is a unique disease because the patient and/or family does almost all of the day-to-day care. Families must assume responsibility for consistency in meals, snacks, shots, doing blood sugar and urine ketone checks, and other tasks. A knowledgeable family is very important for good diabetes care. This is discussed in more detail in Chapter 16, Family Concerns.

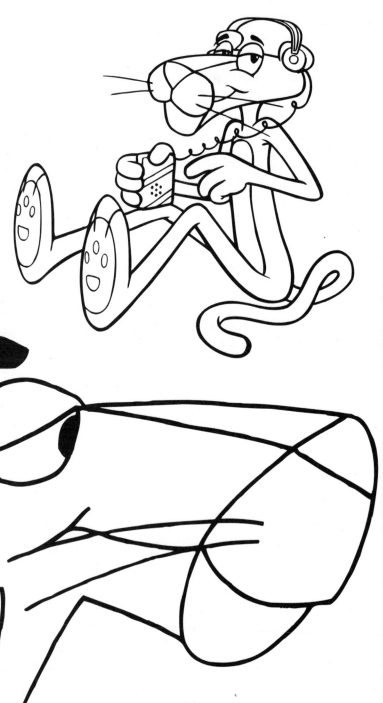

NEW PATIENT FIRST-NIGHT INSTRUCTIONS FOR _____

The diabetes supplies that you will need the first night include:
__ Syringes   __ Alcohol swabs   __ Meter test strips   __ Phone contact card
__ Log book   __ Glucose gel   __ Ketone check strips   __ Glucose tablets
__ Insulin   __ Blood sugar (glucose) meter

If you receive the insulin at the clinic:

1. If you receive Regular insulin, try to eat dinner within 30 minutes of receiving the insulin dose, or have a carbohydrate snack on the way home.

2. If you receive Humalog® insulin, you will need to eat in 10-15 minutes.

3. Allow your child to eat until his/her appetite is satisfied, avoiding high-sugar foods.

If you give the insulin at home:

1. Check your child's blood sugar before dinner. Enter result into log book.

2. Check for urine ketones. Enter result into log book.

3. Call Dr. _____ at _____ or page him/her at _____ for an insulin dose. Write the insulin dose here:_____ and in the log book.

4. Draw up and give the insulin injection containing Humalog insulin just before dinner (for a young child, you can wait to see how much has been eaten and give the shot after dinner).

5. Eat dinner, allowing your child to eat until his/her appetite is satisfied, avoiding high-sugar foods.

Before bed:

1. Check your child's blood sugar. Enter result into log book.

2. Check for urine ketones. Enter result into log book.

3. Call your doctor at the numbers listed above if your child's blood sugar is below _____ or above _____, or if urine ketones are "moderate" or "large." If urine ketones are "trace" or "small," have your child drink 8-12 oz of water.

4. Give an insulin injection if your doctor instructs you to do so. Write the type and amount of insulin here: _____ and into log book.

5. Have your child eat a bedtime snack. Some ideas for this snack include: cereal with milk, toast or crackers with peanut butter or cheese, a slice of pizza, or yogurt and graham crackers.

The second morning before coming to the clinic:

1. Some doctors prefer to have you do the morning blood sugar and urine ketone tests at home and, then, have you go ahead and eat breakfast, waiting to take the insulin shot at the clinic. (We generally want to observe both parents giving a shot, even if one has given shots previously, so that we can teach our techniques.)

2. Other physicians prefer that you do the morning blood sugar and urine ketones at home, but wait to eat breakfast until after the shot is given at the clinic (either bring breakfast [to save 1-2 hours] or plan to go out for breakfast).

3. Please bring all materials (including this book) and diabetes supplies that you have been given with you when returning to the clinic.

Not drawn to size.

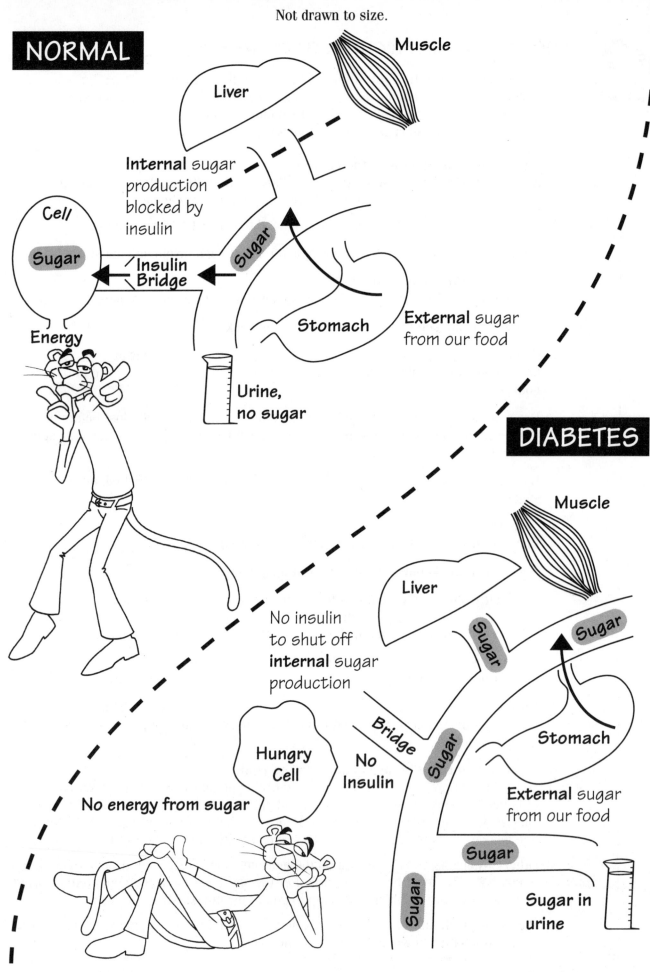

NORMAL

Liver

Muscle

Internal sugar production blocked by insulin

Cell

Sugar

Insulin Bridge

Sugar

Energy

Stomach

External sugar from our food

Urine, no sugar

DIABETES

No insulin to shut off **internal** sugar production

Muscle

Liver

Sugar

Sugar

Bridge

No Insulin

Sugar

Hungry Cell

Stomach

External sugar from our food

No energy from sugar

Sugar

Sugar

Sugar in urine

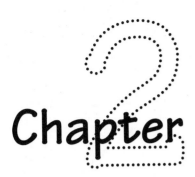

Chapter 2

WHAT IS DIABETES?

Key ideas of this chapter:

❧ Know the two main functions of insulin.

❧ Know that there are two types of diabetes that are completely different from each other.

❧ Be aware of the "honeymoon" or "grace" period.

TYPE 1 (Insulin-Dependent) Diabetes

Type 1 (insulin-dependent diabetes mellitus [IDDM] or "juvenile" or "childhood") diabetes is the usual type found in children and young adults. **It is caused when the pancreas doesn't make enough insulin. Insulin allows sugar to pass into our cells so that it can be "burned" for our energy.** Sugar comes from two places (see drawing on opposite page). "Internal" sugar comes from our body's own production in the liver or from the release of stored sugar from the liver and muscle. This sugar is released into the blood stream. "External" sugar comes from the food we eat and is absorbed from the stomach (intestine) into our blood stream. When people **do not** have diabetes, the pancreas makes insulin. People need insulin to help the "internal" and "external" sugars pass into the body's cells, where the sugar is "burned" for energy. The cells are like a furnace, which burns fuel to make energy. Our bodies constantly need energy for all of our body functions, such as allowing our heart to beat and our lungs to breathe. When people have type 1 diabetes, the pancreas does not make enough insulin. The blood sugar can't pass into the body's cells to be burned. Instead, the blood sugar rises to a high level and overflows through the kidneys into the urine. When sugar enters the urine, water must go out with the sugar. The results are the usual **SYMPTOMS** of diabetes:

❧ **Frequent passing of urine.**

❧ **Frequent drinking of liquids:** to make up for water lost in the urine.

❧ **Frequent eating of food:** because the body is hungry for the energy it isn't getting. This hunger is not always present in children. In addition, sometimes the appetite may even

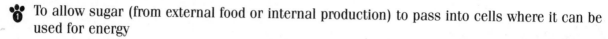

FUNCTIONS OF INSULIN

1. To allow sugar (from external food or internal production) to pass into cells where it can be used for energy

2. To shut off excess internal sugar production in liver and muscle

decrease. Ketones (see Chapter 4) can cause an upset stomach and possible vomiting.

Weight loss: when the body can't get sugar into the cells, it burns its own fat and protein for energy. This causes weight loss.

Changes in behavior: if the person is getting up frequently at night to pass urine, sound sleep will not occur. This can result in behavioral changes.

Insulin also shuts off the body's internal production of sugar. This "internal" sugar mostly comes from the liver and muscles. When the insulin level is too low, too much "internal" sugar is made. Thus, when there is not enough insulin, the blood sugar level can be high for two reasons:

1. Too much "internal" sugar being made

2. The sugar (from internal production or from external food) not being able to pass into the cells

TYPE 2 DIABETES

There is another kind of diabetes that is sometimes found in overweight teenagers, and is also the most common type of diabetes in adults over age 40 years. It is called type 2 diabetes, or sometimes "adult-onset" or "non-insulin-dependent diabetes mellitus" (NIDDM). In type 2 diabetes, **insulin is still made** in normal or increased amounts (at least initially), but it doesn't work very well in helping the body use sugar. Unlike type 1 diabetes, where insulin shots are required, diet and weight loss may be the only treatment necessary in type 2 diabetes. Adults with this disease may be treated with pills, **which are not insulin**. The pills help the pancreas to make more insulin or help the person's cells to be more sensitive to insulin. These pills cannot help people with type 1 diabetes to make more insulin because their pancreas is unable to make insulin. Insulin cannot be taken in pill form because it would be broken down by the acid in the stomach.

People who develop childhood (type 1) diabetes will always have this type of diabetes and will not convert to adult (type 2) diabetes as they grow older. The two conditions are inherited differently, have different reasons for high blood sugar and, as far as we know, are unrelated to each other. It is now possible to separate the two by doing blood antibody levels (see Chapter 3), which are only positive with type 1 diabetes. Type 2 diabetes has become more common in overweight teenagers in recent years. It is most commonly found in African-American and Hispanic youth. Ketones (Chapter 4) may still be present at diagnosis, as well as high blood sugars (Chapter 6) and an elevated HbA$_{1c}$ test (Chapter 13). If ketones are present, insulin shots are usually begun. At a later time, if the antibody tests (Chapter 3) are negative and the blood sugars and HbA$_{1c}$ test have decreased to near-normal, the oral tablets may be tried.

HONEYMOON (GRACE) PERIOD

As stated previously, type 1 (insulin-dependent) diabetes does not turn into type 2 (adult) diabetes as children become adults. According to what we now know, patients with type 1 diabetes will need insulin injections for the rest of their lives. Often, there is a "honeymoon" or "grace" period that may occur a short time after the onset of the diabetes. It commonly starts within two to eight weeks, although not all people have this honeymoon period. During the honeymoon, sugar production is turned off in the liver and a fair bit of insulin is still being made in the islet cells in the pancreas. This is a time when people often think they don't have diabetes. They may be attracted to "miracle cures." The honeymoon period may last a few weeks to a few years. During this time, the body may not need much extra insulin. After this period, the body will again need more insulin, although small amounts of insulin may still be made by some. We advise our patients to continue their insulin during the grace period, even though they may not always need it. We know from experience that the body will again need more insulin. It is usually hard to begin insulin shots again after having stopped.

The **MOST IMPORTANT RULE** for the new patient with diabetes to remember is: **I MUST TAKE MY INSULIN EVERY DAY FROM NOW ON. IF I FORGET MY INSULIN, MY DIABETES WILL GET OUT OF CONTROL. THERE IS ABSOLUTELY NO WAY I WILL NOT NEED INSULIN EVERY DAY FROM NOW ON.** Even if I get sick, I still need insulin. I may need more or less insulin, but I must have it every day. **IMPORTANT**: The only known difference about people who develop type 1 diabetes is that their bodies don't make enough insulin. THE PERSON AND EVERY OTHER PART OF THE BODY ARE OTHERWISE COMPLETELY NORMAL.

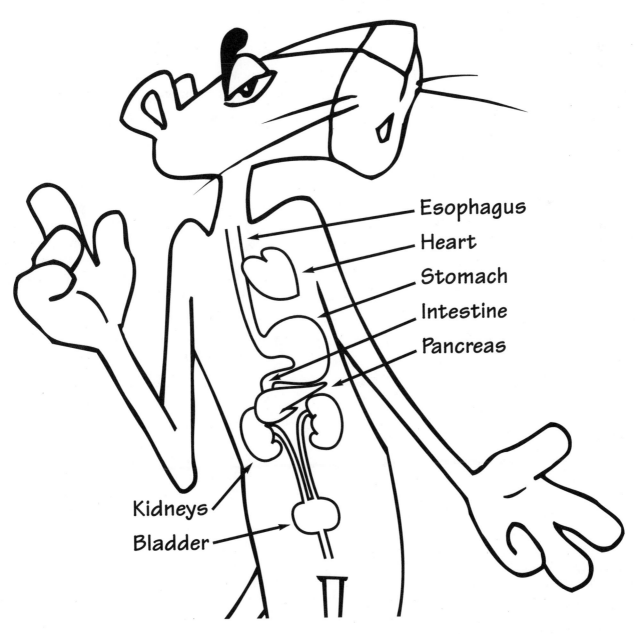

Esophagus
Heart
Stomach
Intestine
Pancreas

Kidneys
Bladder

DEFINITIONS

Bladder: The organ (sac) that collects the water from the kidneys and holds it until it is passed as urine (see the drawing).

Bloodstream: The flow of blood within the blood vessels to and from the different parts of the body.

Cells: The very smallest units of the body. You can only see them with a microscope.

Enzymes: Proteins in liver, muscle, and intestine that help make sugar. (There are many enzymes that have other functions.)

Esophagus: The swallowing tube (see the drawing).

External sugar: The sugar taken in from food. Insulin allows the external sugar to pass into the body's cells to be used for energy.

Insulin: The substance (hormone) made by the pancreas that allows sugar to pass into cells.

Internal sugar: The sugar made by the body (or sugar released from stored sugar, mainly in the liver and muscle). Insulin shuts off the excess production of internal sugar.

Intestine: The part of the GI tract (gut) below the stomach where most sugar (and other foods) are actually absorbed into our blood stream (see the drawing).

Islet cells (pronounced "eye-let"): The groups of cells within the pancreas that make insulin.

Kidneys: The two organs in the body that remove waste products and water from the bloodstream and make urine (see the drawing).

Pancreas: The organ where insulin is normally made (see the drawing). People who have type 1 diabetes cannot make enough insulin and are thus "insulin-dependent."

Stomach: Where the food is collected and made smaller after it is swallowed (see the drawing).

Type 1 diabetes: (Also called "juvenile diabetes" or "childhood diabetes" or "insulin-dependent diabetes mellitus" [IDDM].) The condition that results when the body cannot make enough insulin. The most common type of diabetes in persons under age 40 years. Insulin must be taken by shots; pills do not help. Islet cell antibodies are usually present in the blood.

Type 2 diabetes: (Also called "adult-onset diabetes" or "non-insulin-dependent diabetes mellitus" [NIDDM].) The condition in which the body still makes insulin but is unable to use it. This is the most common type in adults over age 40 years. It also occurs in overweight teenagers. Pills may be able to stimulate the pancreas to make more insulin or make the person more sensitive to insulin. The pills are not insulin. People with type 2 diabetes do not have islet cell antibodies.

Urine: Water with wastes passed from the body by the kidneys.

QUESTIONS (Q) AND ANSWERS (A) FROM NEWSNOTES

Q. When our son was diagnosed with diabetes, he had been vomiting and had kept no food down for over 24 hours. Yet his blood sugar was over 1,000 mg/dl (55 mmol/L). How could that be when he had not eaten any sugar?

A. Insulin has several actions in the body. One is to allow all (or any) sugar to pass from the blood stream into cells where it can be burned for energy. A second function, which is emphasized in this Pink Panther book, is to shut off the body's own production of sugar (primarily in the liver and muscle). When insulin is not available, as in your son at the time of diagnosis, the muscle and liver production of sugar can be enormous. This likely accounted for the high blood sugar even though no sugar had been eaten.

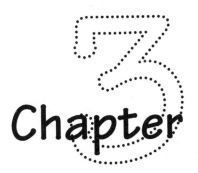

Chapter 3

WHAT CAUSES TYPE 1 DIABETES?

Key ideas of this chapter:

* Recognize the three probable reasons why type 1 diabetes develops.

* Explain the differences between type 1 and type 2 (adult-onset) diabetes.

FREQUENCY

Type 1 diabetes is one of the most common chronic disorders of childhood. It is also the most common form of diabetes to occur in people under age 40 years. The adult type of diabetes (type 2) is the most common form of diabetes after age 40 years. The list of famous people: sport stars, politicians, movie stars, and artists, who have type 1 diabetes is long. Following diagnosis, children frequently discover classmates who also have diabetes. Their looks, personalities, and activities are no different from those of anyone else.

CAUSES

We know that diabetes is not "catching" like a cold. We also know that it isn't caused from eating too much sugar. Three reasons seem to be important in determining why one person develops type 1 diabetes and another one does not. These are: 1) inherited (or genetic) factors; 2) self-allergy (autoimmunity); and 3) environmental damage (e.g., from a virus or chemical).

Inheritance (genetic)

The first important reason seems to be an "inherited" or genetic factor. This is similar to the way a person inherits the color of the eyes from a mother, father, or other relative. People with insulin-dependent diabetes are more likely to have inherited certain cell types (called HLA types). Those who don't have diabetes are less likely to have these HLA types. The HLA types are the blood types determined using white blood cells for typing. (The A, B, and O blood types are determined using red blood cells for typing.) Nearly all people with type 1 diabetes have an HLA type DR3 or DR4. Fifty-three percent of people with type 1 diabetes have one DR3 and one DR4, with one of these

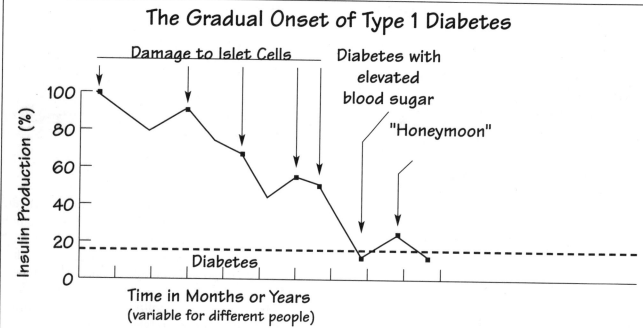

The Gradual Onset of Type 1 Diabetes

Damage to Islet Cells

Diabetes with elevated blood sugar

"Honeymoon"

Insulin Production (%)

100
80
60
40
20
0

Diabetes

Time in Months or Years
(variable for different people)

It is now believed that diabetes develops gradually, over many months or many years. It does not just come on suddenly in the week or two before the elevated blood sugars. Many insults (represented by the arrows in this figure) likely result in further damage until the diagnosis of diabetes is made. The insults may include viral infections, stress, chemicals in the diet, or other agents. These agents may work by "activating" white blood cells in the islets to make toxic chemicals that cause injury to the insulin-producing cells (beta cells). However, a "genetic-predisposition" (inherited factors) must be present for the process to start.

coming from each parent. Only 3% of people without diabetes have this DR3/DR4 combination. Thus, this particular combination makes a person more likely to develop diabetes.

Over half of the families (up to 90% in one study) have no close relative with type 1 diabetes. It may be that a family has a DR3 or a DR4 gene in their genetic makeup, but no family member previously married another person from a family with the other DR gene. When a family member with a DR3 gene marries into another family carrying the DR4 gene, the child may end up with the DR3/DR4 combination (one from each parent) and a high likelihood for diabetes. It is now known that there are also different genes that help to protect a person from developing diabetes.

Children from a family that has a child with diabetes have a greater chance of developing it than the rest of the population. A brother or sister of a child with diabetes has approximately a 1 in 20 (5%) chance of developing diabetes. However, the cause is not completely due to heredity. We know this from studies of identical twins. When one identical twin gets diabetes, only in half of the cases does the other twin also develop the disease. If it were entirely due to heredity, both twins would always develop it, as they have the same genes. Although we don't completely understand the inheritance factors, we believe that both mother and father transmit the tendency to develop diabetes to their child.

Self-allergy (autoimmunity)

The second cause that seems to be important in type 1 diabetes may be self-allergy (or autoimmunity). Normally, our immune systems protect our bodies, but in the case of type 1 diabetes and other autoimmune diseases such as lupus, arthritis and multiple sclerosis, the immune system turns against a body part. We have learned that most Anglo and about half of Hispanic and African-American children show an allergy against the cells in their pancreas (islet cells) that make the insulin when they develop diabetes. They have evidence in their blood of an allergic reaction against their islet cells. The evidence in the blood is called an antibody or, more specifically, an **"islet cell antibody (ICA)."** We now know that some people have this antibody present in their blood for many years before needing to start insulin shots. Other antibodies ("GAD" antibodies, insulin autoantibodies [IAA], and ICA 512 antibodies) have also been found in the blood of people who are in the process of developing diabetes. It is the presence of these antibodies in the blood that has made it possible to screen people who are likely to develop diabetes and to start research trials (see Chapter 26) to try to prevent diabetes. We believe it is important for brothers, sisters and other relatives to have this screening. The antibodies gradually disappear from the blood after the onset of type 1 diabetes. Thus, within one year many people no longer have them. People who develop adult-onset (type 2) diabetes do not have these antibodies.

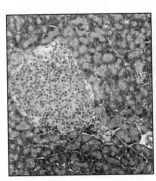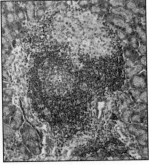

MICROSCOPIC PHOTOGRAPH OF PANCREATIC ISLET:

The photo on the left shows a normal islet (center) surrounded by other pancreatic tissue that is responsible for making digestive enzymes. The photo on the right is from a diabetic animal with white blood cells that have invaded and destroyed the islet.

Environmental (virus or chemical)

A third factor may also be important. This environmental factor may either be a virus or something in the food we eat. This factor may link the genetic (inherited) part with the allergic reaction. For example, a person may inherit a defect that allows a virus or a part of a protein (peptide) to injure the islet cells. Part of the damaged islet cell may then be released into the blood, causing the body to make islet cell antibodies (an allergic or autoimmune reaction). The damage can attract white blood cells to the area of the islet. When the white blood cells are activated, they produce chemicals that further injure the islet cells. Anything that activates the white blood cells in the following years (viral infections, certain foods, stress, etc.) may result in more islet cells being destroyed.

We now know that most people who get diabetes don't just suddenly develop it. They have been in the process of developing it gradually for many years, sometimes even from birth. It is probable that many viral infections and other factors result in damage and destroy a few more islet cells. As more and more islet cells are destroyed the person moves closer to having diabetes (see Figure on page 12).

ADULT-ONSET (TYPE 2) DIABETES

Obesity, or being overweight, is an important cause of adult-onset diabetes. It is **not** a cause of insulin-dependent diabetes. People with adult-onset diabetes (type 2) do not have a similar association with the HLA genes as do people with type 1 diabetes. They do not make islet cell antibodies. The causes of the two types of diabetes seem to be completely different. Insulin does not seem to work normally in the person with adult-onset (type 2) diabetes. However, it can still be made in normal or above-normal amounts (in contrast to insulin-dependent [type 1] diabetes, where insulin is either not made at all or is made in reduced amounts).

About half of the Hispanic and African-American children who develop diabetes do not have the antibodies. Many of these antibody-negative children initially present with very high blood sugars, ketones in their urine and, sometimes, acidosis (see Chapter 14). If this is the case, initial insulin treatment and all of the other parts of this manual are important to learn. At a later time, if the blood sugars and HbA$_{1c}$ test (see Chapter 13) have returned to normal or near-normal, it may be possible to try oral agents rather than insulin shots. The shots may still be needed during times of illness, stress, pregnancy, or further weight gain.

DEFINITIONS

Allergy: A special reaction of the body to some material. This is similar to what happens if you are allergic to something that makes you sneeze.

Antibody: The material we measure in the blood if someone has an allergy (example: milk antibodies might be present if someone has a milk allergy).

Autoimmunity (self-allergy): The process of forming an allergic reaction against one's own tissues. This happens in diseases such as lupus and arthritis. People with type 1 diabetes make an antibody against their islet cells (where the insulin is made).

Genetic (inherited): Features, such as eye color, that are passed from both parents to children.

HLA type: The way to group cell types—just as red blood cells are grouped into A, B, and O blood types. HLA stands for Human Leukocyte Antigen. A leukocyte is another name for a white blood cell, which is the type of cell used in HLA typing.

Identical twins: Twins that come from the same egg. All their features (genetics) are exactly alike.

Islet cell (pronounced "eye-let"): The groups of cells within the pancreas that make insulin.

Islet cell antibody: The material we measure in the person's blood to show that they have had an allergy against the cells in the pancreas (the islet cells) that make insulin.

QUESTIONS (Q) AND ANSWERS (A) FROM NEWSNOTES

Q. My daughter was in a car accident the week before the onset of her diabetes. Could that have caused the diabetes?

A. It is now accepted that diabetes comes on gradually over many months or many years, and is not just brought about by one event. After initial damage occurs to the islets in the pancreas (where insulin is made), the person may have positive islet cell antibodies indicating that some damage has occurred. We have followed some people with positive islet cell antibodies who have not needed to start insulin treatment for as long as ten years.

After the initial damage, many factors may cause activation of white blood cells (WBCs) in the islets. These factors may include some viral infections, dietary components or even stress. When the WBCs in the islets are "activated" by these factors, they produce toxic chemicals that destroy a few more islets each time. Gradually, a person gets closer to having full-blown diabetes. Thus, the stress of the automobile accident may have been the final precipitating event, but it was most likely only one of several insults over many years.

Chapter 4 URINE KETONE TESTING

Key ideas of this chapter:

- Know why it is important to measure urine ketones.

- Know when it is important to measure urine ketones.

- Know how to measure urine ketones.

- Recognize when to call the diabetes care provider in relation to results of urine ketone testing.

Urine ketone testing is **VERY** important. A method of testing for ketones must be kept in the home (and taken on trips) at all times. Urine ketones (sometimes called "acetone") are chemicals which appear in the urine when body fat is being broken down for energy. Fat is burned by the body when there is not enough insulin to allow sugar to be burned for the energy needed by the body. Ketones also are formed when not enough food has been eaten to provide the energy the body needs.

We usually teach families how to do the urine ketone test on the first day of diagnosis of diabetes. Frequent urine ketone tests are important in the first few days after diagnosis to determine if enough insulin is being given to turn off ketone production. **Turning off ketone production is the first goal in the treatment of newly diagnosed diabetes** managed in the outpatient setting. The second goal is to lower blood sugar levels (done primarily by turning off internal sugar production in the liver). As giving insulin helps to accomplish both goals, they usually take place, at least in part, at the same time.

Checking for urine ketones and learning about ketoacidosis (discussed in Chapter 14) might be taught together, as they are closely related. However, we have found that the concept of ketoacidosis is too difficult to understand at the time of diagnosis. Thus, we usually wait until the one-week follow-up visit to teach this (see Table 1 in Chapter 1). Urine ketone testing must be learned early.

REASONS FOR TESTING FOR URINE KETONES

It is important to test for urine ketones because they can build up in the body and result in one of the two emergencies of diabetes, acidosis, or ketoacidosis (see Chapter 14). If the urine test shows medium or large ketones to be present, the diabetes care provider should be contacted and usually extra insulin is taken to help make the ketones disappear. If the urine ketones are not detected early, particularly during illnesses, they will build up in the body and ketoacidosis will result. It is the early detection of urine ketones and the treatment with extra Humalog or Regular insulin that prevent hospitalizations for ketoacidosis (see Chapter 14 on Ketoacidosis). Hospitalizations for ketoacidosis are still listed as the number one reason for hospitalizing children in the U.S. with known diabetes. **It is our belief that if the urine ketone test is done, the diabetes care provider is called when indicated, and extra shots of insulin are given, then these hospitalizations for ketoacidosis are completely preventable.**

WHEN TO TEST URINE FOR KETONES

Urine ketones must always be checked if the blood sugar is high (above 240 mg/dl or 13.3 mmol/L), OR ANYTIME THE PERSON FEELS SICK OR NAUSEATED (especially if he/she vomits, even once). **If the person is sick, ketones can be present even when the sugar is not high.**

CALL YOUR DIABETES CARE PROVIDER IF MODERATE OR LARGE URINE KETONES ARE PRESENT, NIGHT OR DAY. TELL THE PERSON ANSWERING THE PHONE THAT THE CALL IS URGENT.

People who have been recently diagnosed with diabetes usually need to check urine ketones twice daily (or more often if they are positive). After the first week, if all urine ketone checks have been negative, daily testing of urine ketones is not needed.

People who take only one insulin injection per day should do routine morning urine ketone tests to see if their insulin is lasting a full 24 hours. Morning ketones will usually be present if an insulin injection is needed in the evening.

If the morning blood sugars vary between very high and very low values, check morning ketones. This will be discussed in more detail in Chapter 5, Low Blood Sugar. Morning ketones can be a sign of a low blood sugar during the night followed by "rebounding" or "bouncing."

WHAT TEST MATERIALS ARE AVAILABLE?

Testing for Urine Ketones

The two strips that are most frequently used in checking for urine ketones are the Ketostix® and the Chemstrip K®.

If the child is not yet toilet trained, it is usually best to press a test strip (see section on Ketostix) firmly against the wet diaper. It is also possible to place a cotton ball in the diaper near the urinary opening. Drops of urine can then be squeezed from the cotton ball.

Ketostix

The Ketostix (or Ketodiastix® with the sugar check) is reliable for urine testing IF THEY ARE CAREFULLY TIMED WITH A CLOCK WITH A SECOND HAND. The Ketostix are cheaper than the Ketodiastix and it is not necessary to do the urine sugar, as a blood sugar is now generally done. There is a place on the side of the bottle to write the date the bottle is opened. The strips are then good for six months. Individually foil-wrapped Ketostix are now available and will not expire for two or three years. This gets around the problem of having to throw unused Ketostix away once the bottle has been open for six months. Ask your pharmacist to order them if he/she does not have them. A computer scan of the box (with the Bayer order number - 2640) is shown in the figure.

The following procedure must be followed exactly:

i. Completely cover the colored square on the end of the strip by dipping into FRESH urine. Then immediately remove the strip from the

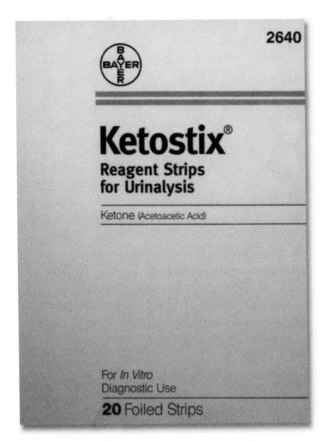

Ketostix®
Reagent Strips
for Urinalysis

Ketone (Acetoacetic Acid)

For *In Vitro*
Diagnostic Use

20 Foiled Strips

2640

urine. We prefer that the urine be collected in a cup and that the strip then be timed and read by two people. This prevents errors due to color blindness or psychological factors. A supply of small paper cups might be kept in the bathroom medicine cabinet for this purpose.

ii. Gently tap the edge of the strip against the side of the urine container to remove excess urine.

iii. Compare the test area closely with the corresponding color chart. The timing is **very** important. READ KETONES AT **EXACTLY** 15 SECONDS AFTER DIPPING THE STRIP. HOLD THE STRIP CLOSE TO THE COLOR BLOCK AND MATCH THE COLORS CAREFULLY. These tests must **always** be timed with the second hand of a clock. Counting is NOT accurate enough.

iv. Immediately record the result of the ketone test as negative, small (15), moderate (40), large (80), or large-large (160) in the notebook so that it is not forgotten.

Chemstrip K

The Chemstrip K (or Chemstrip uGK® with the urine glucose check) is the second method that can be used to check for urine ketones. The only difference from the instructions for the Ketodiastix is in the timing. Chemstrip K must be timed for one minute. Read as negative, small, moderate, or large at exactly one minute.

Acetest Tablets

Urine ketones also can be measured using Acetest tablets (these are now rarely used since the strips are easier to use). The measurement is done as follows:

Place one drop of urine on top of the Acetest tablet. Take the reading after 30 seconds. Compare to the color on the chart.

A. Light purple means "small" acetone

B. Medium purple means "moderate" acetone

C. Dark purple means "large" acetone

If the color does not reach the color of the "small" acetone on the chart at exactly 30 seconds, the test is negative. Do not record color changes that develop after 30 seconds.

DEFINITIONS

Acetest tablets: Tablets that are available for checking urine ketones (acetone). These are rarely used.

Chemstrip K: Strips for measuring urine ketones (acetone). They are also available as Chemstrip uGK (for urine ketones and sugar).

Ketoacidosis (Acidosis): What happens in the body when not enough insulin is available. Blood sugar is usually high at this time. Moderate or large ketones are present in the urine, as well as in the body. This is the subject of Chapter 14.

Ketostix: Strips for measuring urine ketones (acetone). They are also available as Ketodiastix (for urine ketones and sugar).

Ketones (Acetone): The chemicals that appear in the urine when not enough insulin is present and fat is broken down. Acetest tablets, Ketostix, or Chemstrip K measure urine ketones (acetone).

mg/dl: Milligrams of material in a measured amount (100cc). Blood sugar levels are expressed in these terms in the U.S., but are usually expressed as mmol/L in Europe. It is possible to convert mg/dl to mmol/L by dividing by 18 (or multiplying by 0.0555). The opposite is done to go from mmol/L to mg/dl.

mmol/L: Method of measuring the amount of a material (sugar) in the blood, usually used in Europe. See mg/dl for conversion factors.

Void: Passage of urine.

QUESTIONS (Q) AND ANSWERS (A) FROM NEWSNOTES

Q. Why are you now advising that we buy the foil-wrapped rather than the bottles of Ketostix for measuring urine ketones?

A. You will note that on the side of a bottle of Ketostix, you are asked to write in the date the bottle is opened and to dispose of the bottle six months later. Sometimes people forget to do this. Once the bottle is open, moisture and other factors result in a gradual loss of sensitivity. Often, a flu episode will start in the middle of the night. As one looks at the date on the side of the bottle, one finds that the strips have been open longer than six months and are unreliable. Then one has to go looking for an open pharmacy in the middle of the night. The foil-wrapped Ketostix avoids this problem. It may have an expiration date two years away.

Urine ketone measurements are **VERY** important. A method for urine ketone testing **MUST** be in the home at all times. It is **ONLY** by measuring the urine ketones that one can know if moderate or large urine ketones are present. If present, the physician must be called immediately. This may prevent a life-threatening episode of ketoacidosis (Chapter 14).

Chapter 5

LOW BLOOD SUGAR (HYPOGLYCEMIA or INSULIN REACTION)

Key ideas of this chapter:

- Recognize the common signs of low blood sugar (hypoglycemia).

- Know how to treat low blood sugar (hypoglycemia).

There are two "emergency" problems in blood sugar control for people with diabetes. The first, discussed in this chapter, is low blood sugar or hypoglycemia. (The second, discussed in Chapter 14, is acidosis or ketoacidosis.) Low blood sugar comes on quickly and must be treated by the person, family, or friends. Early treatment helps prevent a more severe reaction and possible hospitalization.

Any time a person has received a shot of insulin, there is a chance of a low blood sugar reaction. Thus, the family of a non-hospitalized person with newly diagnosed diabetes must know the signs and symptoms of hypoglycemia before going home the first night.

CAUSES OF LOW BLOOD SUGAR

Hypoglycemia (low blood sugar) occurs because the body doesn't have enough sugar to burn for energy and the level of sugar in the blood falls too low. Sometimes it is called an **"insulin reaction"** or just a **"reaction."** Frequent causes are listed below:

1. Meals and snacks that are late or missed

2. Extra exercise that burns more sugar than usual

3. An insulin dose that is too high

4. Giving a shot into muscle which results in rapid absorption of insulin

5. Making a mistake in the drawing up of an insulin dose

6. Taking a bath or shower (or hot tub) soon after taking a shot of insulin

Prevention of low blood sugars ("lows") is much wiser than having to treat the lows. When too many lows occur, the stored adrenaline (epinephrine) is depleted and then the usual symptoms of a low may not occur. In addition, the treatment (eating too much) often causes a high blood sugar and can increase the HbA_{1c} value (Chapter 13). Paying attention to the six causes of lows listed will help to decrease the number of low blood sugars. The reason for low blood sugars from taking a shot just before a hot shower or bath (or a hot tub) is that the blood vessels in the skin dilate from the hot water and cause insulin to be rapidly absorbed. It is always wise to wait to take an insulin shot until **after** a shower or bath.

SYMPTOMS OF LOW BLOOD SUGAR

The body gives a warning when low blood sugar or an insulin reaction is developing. DIFFERENT PEOPLE GET DIFFERENT WARNINGS. These signs are common warnings of an insulin reaction:

1. **Hunger:** the person may either feel hungry or have an upset stomach (nausea)

2. **Shakiness:** the person's hands or body may feel shaky

3. **Sweatiness:** the person may sweat more than usual (often a "cold" sweat)

4. **Color:** the face may become pale or red

5. **Weak,** anxious feeling

6. **Headache**

7. **Confusion:** the person may feel or look "spacy," or may appear "dazed"

8. **Drowsiness:** the person may yawn, feel sleepy, or may have trouble thinking clearly; preschoolers frequently get sleepy

9. **Behavioral changes:** changes in behavior are quite common; often the person may cry, act intoxicated, or act angry

10. **Double vision:** the person may "see double" or the pupils of the eyes may get bigger; the eyes may appear glassy

11. **Loss of consciousness**

12. **Seizure or convulsion:** both loss of consciousness and convulsion occur late in the reaction; they are usually the result of not treating a reaction quickly enough

With an insulin reaction, you may experience hunger, shakiness, and sweating.

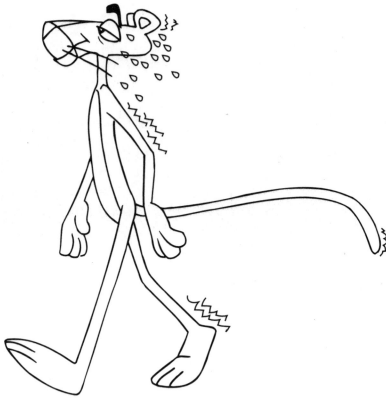

Initial symptoms (one through four) are due to the output of the excitatory hormone, adrenaline (epinephrine is another name). Later symptoms (5 through 12) are more related to the lack of sugar to the brain. Sugar is the main source of fuel for the brain. If the low sugar continues too long, the brain can be harmed. As the brain grows very rapidly in the first four years of life, it is particularly important to prevent severe low blood sugar in young children.

NIGHTTIME LOWS

People usually wake up with symptoms (infants may just cry) when lows occur during the night. The symptoms may be the same as during the daytime, although there are sometimes special "clues":

1. **Inability to sleep or waking up "alert"**

2. **Waking up sweating**

3. **Waking up with a fast heart rate**

4 Waking up with a headache

5 Waking up feeling "foggy-headed" or with memory loss

6 Unusually high blood sugar or positive urine ketones (possible rebounding)

IF ANY OF THESE DO OCCUR, TEST YOUR BLOOD SUGAR IMMEDIATELY. If low, treat appropriately and call the doctor or nurse the next day. Also think about what was different the previous day (extra exercise, extra insulin, less food, etc.). This will allow planning ahead to prevent a low with a similar occurrence in the future.

RECOGNIZING LOW BLOOD SUGAR

It is important to recognize low blood sugar (also called hypoglycemia, reaction, or insulin reaction) at the earliest possible time so that it does not progress to a severe reaction. The common symptoms are listed, but will vary from person to person. The early warning signs of a reaction are due to the release of a hormone called adrenaline. It is also called the excitatory hormone or epinephrine. Most people make it when they are excited or scared. It causes shakiness, sweating, dilated pupils, a rapid heart rate, and other symptoms. Some people tend to have only mild reactions and can easily detect symptoms. This seems to be more common in the first few years after diagnosis. Others may have more difficulty detecting symptoms. This seems to happen to people who have had diabetes longer or whose blood sugars tend to run at more normal levels. A term, **"hypoglycemic unawareness"** is sometimes applied to this condition, and is discussed in this chapter. Sometimes this is due to less adrenaline being available. In some cases, the lack of symptoms may be due to less dramatic falls in blood sugar levels, such as from 70 to 50 mg/dl (3.9 to 2.7 mmol/L) rather than from 170 to 50 mg/dl (9.5 to 2.7 mmol/L). The greater fall is more likely to cause adrenaline release and symptoms. Some people are less likely to detect low blood sugar in the morning because the sugar has fallen gradually during the night. Thus, adrenaline release and its symptoms did not occur.

Different children learn to tell if they have low blood sugar at different ages (see Chapter 17). It may be possible to train young children (or older people who have difficulty detecting low blood sugars) to recognize certain signs. Parents may frequently need to remind a young child, "Remember how you felt shaky (or whatever the feeling was) and you came and told me? You did a good job! Remember to tell a grown up if you feel that way again." For very young children, the parent can often tell when the child has low blood sugar by the type of cry or fussiness he/she presents.

False Reaction

A rapid fall in blood sugar can also cause adrenaline release and symptoms even if a low blood sugar does **NOT** occur. We call this a **"false reaction,"** as the symptoms of low blood sugar occur, but the blood sugar is not low. A common example is when children eat lunch at school and their blood sugar rises to a value of perhaps 250 mg/dl (13.9 mmol/L) after eating. They then go outside to play and the sugar might fall to 150 mg/dl (8.3 mmol/L) fairly rapidly. Adrenaline is released and the symptoms of having a reaction occur. Yet, their blood sugar is 150 mg/dl (8.3 mmol/L) and they DO NOT HAVE LOW BLOOD SUGAR. **(A TRUE LOW BLOOD SUGAR IS DEFINED AS A BLOOD SUGAR LEVEL BELOW 60 mg/dl or 3.2 mmol/L.)** It was just the rapid fall in blood sugar that caused adrenaline release and made them feel like they were having a reaction. Since the sugar is not truly low, they do NOT need to drink sugar pop or juice, which will raise their blood sugar back to 250 mg/dl (13.9 mmol/L). They might feel better if they ate some solid food, such as crackers or fresh fruit. It is important to remember that THE ONLY WAY TO TELL IF SOMEONE HAD A RAPID FALL IN BLOOD SUGAR OR A TRULY LOW BLOOD SUGAR IS BY DOING A BLOOD SUGAR TEST. Thus, whenever possible, a blood sugar test should be done when the symptoms of low blood sugar occur.

TREATMENT FOR LOW BLOOD SUGAR
(Insulin Reaction)

The general rule is to GIVE SUGAR IN SOME FORM AS FAST AS POSSIBLE. If the reaction is not severe, do a blood sugar test first. If you are not able to do a blood sugar, then just give milk, juice, or sugar pop. A person with diabetes won't get sick from excess sugar. It will just cause high blood sugar and then be passed in the urine. Insulin reactions come quickly and should be treated at once by the person, parent, friend, or teacher.

Different forms of sugar can be carried to treat low blood sugar. PEOPLE WITH DIABETES SHOULD CARRY SUGAR PACKETS OR TABLETS IN THEIR POCKETS AT ALL TIMES FOR EMERGENCIES. Candy is too tempting. It also may be taken by other children. A special pocket for sugar packets can be sewn inside of gym shorts. Some people carry them in a "jogger wallet" attached to a shoe. Others slip packets in high stockings. It is often best to wrap the packet in foil or a plastic bag in case of leaks. Insta-Glucose® comes in a tube and looks like toothpaste. It is available in most pharmacies. A tube of cake gel from the grocery store will also work. After taking in some sugar and liquids, the person should wait 10 minutes and then eat a sandwich or other longer-lasting solid food. The liquid sugar will be absorbed more quickly if the person waits to eat the solid food. Gradually, each person will become familiar with the type of reactions that occur. The person will learn how severe the reactions tend to be, when they are most likely to occur, and how best to treat them.

Eventually, as a person becomes more familiar with the diabetes, it may be possible to treat different reactions differently. Remember that, when it is possible, it is always wise to do a blood sugar if the reaction is not severe. If the level is above 60 mg/dl (3.2 mmol/L), it may be possible to treat the reaction with fresh fruit and solid food, rather than milk, juice, or sugar pop. ALSO, REMEMBER THAT IT TAKES TEN MINUTES FOR THE BLOOD SUGAR LEVEL TO RISE, AND IT IS WISE TO WAIT FOR AT LEAST TEN MINUTES TO RETURN TO NORMAL

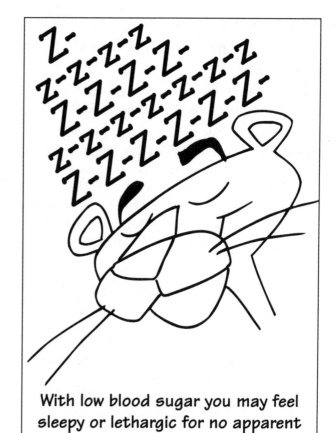

With low blood sugar you may feel sleepy or lethargic for no apparent reason.

ACTIVITY. Some sources of quick-acting sugar for people of different ages are given in Table 1. Possible variations on the usual treatment for reactions are defined below:

❶ **MILD REACTION** (such as hunger at an unusual time, shakiness, or irritability): If possible, do a blood sugar level. If below 60 mg/dl (3.2 mmol/L), give a glass of milk or a small glass of juice (4 oz). If the blood sugar is above 60 mg/dl (3.2 mmol/L), give just solid food. If below 60 mg/dl (3.2 mmol/L), wait 10 minutes for absorption of the liquid sugar and then give solid food (crackers, sandwich, fresh fruit, etc.).

❷ **MODERATE REACTION** (very confused or spacy, very pale or very shaky): Give Insta-Glucose, Reactose®, or any source of simple sugar, such as sugar pop or juice. One-half tube of the Insta-Glucose can be placed between the cheeks and gums, and the person told to swallow. Do a blood sugar level as soon as it is possible. Wait to give solid food until the blood sugar is shown to have risen above 60 mg/dl (3.2 mmol/L).

SOURCES OF QUICK-ACTING SUGAR (GLUCOSE) FOR HYPOGLYCEMIA

	AGE		
	5 years or less (10 gms)	**6-10 years (10-15 gms)**	**over 10 years (15-20 gms)**
FOOD			
Glucose Tabs (4 gms each - check label; some = 5 gms)	2	3-4	4-5
Instant Glucose (31 gm tube)	1/3 tube	1/3-1/2 tube	1/2-2/3 tube
Cake Gel (1 small tube = 12 gms)	1 tube	1 tube	1-2 tubes
Apple Juice (1/2 cup = 15 gms)	1/3 cup	1/3-1/2 cup	1/2-2/3 cup
Orange Juice (1/2 cup = 15 gms)	1/4-1/2 cup	1/2-3/4 cup	3/4-1 cup
Sugar (1 tsp = 4 gms)	2 tsp	3-4 tsp	4-5 tsp
Honey (1 tsp = 5 gms; do not use if child is less than two years old)	2 tsp	2-3 tsp	3-4 tsp
Regular Pop (1 oz = 3 gms)	3 oz	4-5 oz	5-6 oz
Milk (12 gms/cup)	3/4 cup	1 cup	1 1/2 cup
LIFE SAVERS® (2.5 gms each)	4	4-6	6-8
Skittles® (1 gm each)	10 pieces	10-15 pieces	15-20 pieces
Sweet Tarts® (1.7 gms each)	6 pieces	6-8 pieces	8-12 pieces
Raisins (1 Tbsp = 7 1/2 gms)	1-2 Tbsp	2 Tbsp	2 1/2 Tbsp

SEVERE REACTION (loss of consciousness, seizure, or convulsion): Some doctors believe that Insta-Glucose or Reactose should be placed between the gums and cheeks, with the throat stroked to encourage swallowing. Glucagon can then be given. Other doctors may prefer to use glucagon only. They may be concerned that the Insta-Glucose might get into the airway in a person who cannot swallow. Remember to do the blood sugar level as soon as possible. If the person does not improve after 10-20 minutes, it may be necessary to call 911 to get extra help. A second dose (same amount) of glucagon (from the same vial) can also be given. In the preliminary part of the Diabetes Control and Complications Trial (DCCT), one of every 10 people (10%) receiving standard treatment had a severe reaction each year. One of four people (25%) on intensive treatment (including insulin pumps) had a severe insulin reaction each year. Thus, every family must have glucagon available and know how to use it (the use of glucagon is explained below). It is wise to call the diabetes care provider prior to the next insulin injection for possible dose reductions.

We are concerned about any blood sugars below 60 mg/dl (3.2 mmol/L). When these are obtained in routine testing, the insulin dose or snacks should be changed so that further low values do not occur. In a child under five years old, we are concerned about values below 70 mg/dl (3.9 mmol/L). When values are below these levels at the time of an insulin injection, we usually recommend not giving the usual amount of Regular insulin in that injection and not giving any Humalog (at least until after eating). If two or three values below 60 mg/dl (3.2 mmol/L) are present at the same time of day in the same week, a decrease in insulin dose is probably needed. CALL THE DIABETES CARE PROVIDER IF HELP IS NEEDED.

Sometimes low blood sugars will be found on routine testing and the person will not have had symptoms. This may be due to a very gradual fall in the blood sugar or, in young children, because they have not learned to recognize the symptoms. Some adults with very strict sugar control do not release adrenaline and may have the problem medically referred to as **"HYPOGLYCEMIC UNAWARENESS."** In this case, they must not

aim for such strict blood sugar control. Sometimes the insulin dose can be lowered, and after blood sugars have been higher for two or three weeks, it will be possible to again recognize low blood sugars.

PREVENTION OF SEVERE REACTIONS

It may be possible to help prevent severe insulin reactions using the GlucoWatch® or a subcutaneous glucose sensor (see Chapters 6 and 26). An alarm can be set on the GlucoWatch to sound if the glucose value is below a certain level. The GlucoWatch may be most helpful to wear at night—particularly if the person has had previous severe lows during the night. As the new subcutaneous sensors are expensive, it is unlikely that many insurance companies will initially be willing to fund them. They may be more willing when a person has had repeated severe reactions, particularly if costly hospitalizations were required.

GLUCAGON

Glucagon is a hormone made in the pancreas, like insulin. However, it has the opposite effect of insulin and raises the blood sugar level. It is rarely needed, but we ask families to keep it handy. The expiration date on the box should be checked regularly and, if outdated, a new bottle obtained. If a very severe reaction occurs and the person loses consciousness, glucagon should be given promptly. It can be stored at room temperature or in the refrigerator at home. It should not reach temperatures above 90° or freezing. It can be taken, with the insulin and blood sugar strips, in a cooler for trips away from home.

Use of Glucagon

Glucagon comes in a bottle containing 1 mg as a tablet or powder. There is a syringe containing diluting solution in the emergency kit. The method for giving glucagon is as follows **(also see Table 4):**

Remove the flip-off cover from the glucagon vial.

It is sterile if the cap is in place. If not, wipe it off with an alcohol swab (if readily available).

3. Inject all of the diluting solution in the syringe (or from the vial) into the glucagon vial.

4. Remove the syringe and shake the vial gently until it is clear. Using a syringe with a longer needle (if available), withdraw either 0.3cc (children five and under) or 0.5cc (children 6-18 years) of the diluted glucagon. Adults can usually tolerate the full 1.0cc (1 mg). An excess of glucagon may cause vomiting. Inject the glucagon either into the front thigh or arm muscle, or into the subcutaneous fat layer (where the insulin is injected) of the abdomen, arm, leg, or buttocks (seat). **It works just as fast when given into muscle or fat.** If another syringe is not available, just use the syringe provided in the Glucagon Emergency Kit (if you have that) or an insulin syringe and inject the glucagon into the fat as instructed in the kit.

5. If the person doesn't start to come out of the reaction within 10 minutes and the blood sugar is still below 60 mg/dl (3.2 mmol/L), inject a second dose of the glucagon (same amount). Call the doctor or emergency number if help is needed. If a doctor cannot be reached, or there is any difficulty breathing, call the paramedics or 911 (if available in your area) or take the person to a hospital emergency room.

6. Call the diabetes team prior to the next regularly scheduled insulin shot. They may wish to reduce the insulin dose.

Sometimes vomiting will occur after a severe reaction. This may be from the person's own glucagon output, or from the glucagon that was injected. It usually does not last very long and, if the blood sugar is above 150 mg/dl (8.3 mmol/L), it is not a big problem. Urine ketones should be checked (see Chapter 14) as they sometimes also form. If the family is concerned about the ketones, if the blood sugar did not rise, or if the vomiting continues, the diabetes care provider should be called.

DELAYED HYPOGLYCEMIA

Delayed hypoglycemia is also discussed in Chapter 12 on exercise, as it usually occurs four to 10 hours after exercise. For some people, blood sugars tend to be high after exercise. This is because of the normal response of releasing adrenaline during exercise. Adrenaline causes sugar to come out of muscle and liver and raises the blood sugar. At some point after the exercise, the adrenaline levels go back down (sometimes not until the time of sleep) and the sugar moves back into the muscle and liver. The result is low blood sugar or **"delayed hypoglycemia."**

Prevention involves lowering the insulin dose, especially the long-acting insulin, after heavy exercise even though the blood sugar may be high. Taking extra carbohydrate at bedtime (even with high blood sugar) may also be helpful. As the exercise is essential for the heart and cardiovascular system, it is important to always be thinking about how to best prevent exercise and post-exercise lows.

REBOUNDING (reactive hypoglycemia or Somogyi reaction)

Occasionally the blood sugar will become low during the night and the person will put out hormones (epinephrine and glucagon) to raise the blood sugar. These hormones may also result in ketone output in the urine. The person may not have any symptoms during the night, or may complain of night sweats or a morning headache. Rebounding should be considered if the morning blood sugar varies frequently from being very low to being very high (and possibly even having intermittent morning ketones). Rebounding should also be considered if a person is on a very large insulin dose (above 1.5 units/kg or 0.75 units/lb body weight). Table 2 summarizes when to consider rebounding. A person may experience only one or two of the five factors listed in the table.

WHEN TO CONSIDER REBOUNDING

Table 2

1. Variable (very low to very high) morning blood sugars
2. Intermittent morning urine ketones
3. Night sweats
4. Morning headaches
5. Large insulin dosage (above 1.5 units/kg or 0.75 units/lb body weight)

If rebounding is suspected, it is important to check the blood sugar level during the night (usually between midnight and 4 a.m.) for several nights to make sure the values are not low. Table 2 in Chapter 6, Blood Sugar Testing, gives blood sugar levels to aim for at bedtime (before the bedtime snack) and in the morning. If bedtime blood sugar values are below the desired ranges, extra food should be eaten at bedtime to prevent low blood sugars during the night. If the values are **VERY** low at bedtime (e.g., below 60 mg/dl or 3.2 mmol/L), the value should be rechecked during the night. If bedtime or morning values are below the desired ranges two or more days in a week, the insulin dose working at that time should be reduced (see Chapter 20, Adjusting the Insulin Dose). The diabetes care provider should be called during office hours if there are further questions.

RECORD ALL INSULIN REACTIONS

Record insulin reactions in your record book. If occasional mild reactions occur, discuss them with your doctor or nurse at clinic visits. If more than two mild insulin reactions occur in a short time period, call the diabetes care provider to adjust the amount of insulin. It is usually possible to call during office hours, but if severe reactions occur, call the care provider prior to giving the next regularly scheduled insulin shot.

PREVENTING INSULIN REACTIONS (THINKING AHEAD)

Snacks before heavy physical exercise and at the time of day when there have been previous reactions may help prevent insulin reactions. When you are going to do an all-day exercise such as hiking or skiing, you can reduce the insulin dose, do extra blood sugar tests, and take extra snacks (see Chapter 12 on Exercise and Diabetes). If there are questions about how much to reduce the dose, look at your records to see what was done previously or call your diabetes care provider. Be careful to take shots of insulin after the shower or bath **AND NOT BEFORE.** Often the blood sugar rises to a high level due to eating high sugar foods after an insulin reaction. Sometimes reducing the number of reactions can be an effective way to improve overall sugar control (see Chapter 13). Some factors that change blood sugar levels are listed in Table 3.

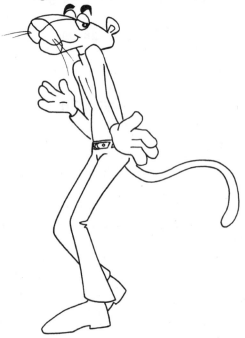

Table 3 SOME FACTORS THAT CHANGE THE BLOOD SUGAR

- 1   Sugar intake raises blood sugar

- 2   Exercise usually lowers blood sugar, although, for some people, the values may be higher immediately following exercise

- 3   Insulin lowers blood sugar

- 4   Glucagon raises blood sugar

- 5   Illness usually raises blood sugar and may cause ketones

- 6   Emotions such as anger, excitement, etc., generally raise blood sugar; some younger children have lower blood sugars with extra excitement

- 7   Rapid growth raises blood sugar; teenagers usually require more insulin with increased growth

- 8   Hormones such as glucagon, adrenaline, growth hormone, and cortisol all raise the blood sugar; their action is opposite to that of insulin

- 9   Menstrual periods may raise blood sugar or cause ketones

- 10   Hot baths or showers may increase insulin absorption and cause a low blood sugar

MEDICAL IDENTIFICATION

In case of a severe insulin reaction, EVERYONE needs to know about the diabetes. This includes teachers, strangers, police, co-workers, friends, and medical personnel. The person with diabetes should wear a bracelet or necklace with this information. A card in the wallet is not good enough; this may not be found by paramedics. A diabetes ID card can also be stapled to the registration of the car in the glove compartment. Bracelets or necklaces can be found at most pharmacies or medical supply houses. The MedicAlert Foundation, P.O. Box 1009, Turlock, California 95381 provides MedicAlert tags. The MedicAlert tag includes a number that can be called 24 hours a day for information concerning both the person and the doctor. The minimum charge for the bracelet or necklace and keeping the information readily available 24 hours per day is $35, then the annual membership renewal after the first year is $15.

There is a second company called Medi-Check that provides stainless steel bracelets or necklaces for a donation of $25 or more. The person's name, address, phone number, condition (Diabetes) and the doctor's name and phone number can all be put on the neck tag or bracelet for this price. In this case, the doctor is called and not Medi-Check. The address is: Medi-Check International, Inc. Foundation, 800 Lee Street, Des Plaines, Illinois 60016. An application is in Appendix 2 in the back of this book. Dog tags (similar to the ones soldiers wear) have gained in popularity and instructions for ordering them are in Appendix 2 in the back of the book. A bracelet, necklace or medallion with your personal medical information (name, condition, and medications) can be engraved and ordered through the American Medical Identifications, Inc. The prices for an identification tag starts at $18.95. The address is: American Medical Identifications, Inc., P.O. Box 925512, Houston, Texas 77292. An application is in Appendix 2. Colorful "sports bracelets" are sometimes preferred and can be ordered from FIFTY 50 PHARMACY. The cost per bracelet is $16.95 plus $3.50 for shipping. Mail your order with payment to FIFTY 50; 1740 South IH35, Suite 112, Carrollton, Texas 75006, or call 800-746-7505.

GLUCAGON INJECTIONS-When To and How To

1. Use only when child is unconscious or having a seizure.

2. Keep in a convenient, known place. Store in refrigerator during hot weather. Protect from freezing.

3. Keep a 3cc syringe available or use the fluid-filled syringe in the Lilly Emergency Kit®. An insulin syringe and needle can also be used (preferably a 1.0cc syringe).

4. If you have the emergency kit, the fluid does not need to be withdrawn from bottle 1 (diagram below) as it is already in the syringe.

5. Withdraw:
   0.3cc for a child less than six years old
   0.5cc for a child 6-18 years of age
   1.0cc for an adult over 18 years of age
   from the mixed glucagon bottle
   (Estimate if using the emergency kit syringe.)

6. Inject either deep into muscle (in front of leg or upper, outer arm) or into the subcutaneous fat (just as you would an insulin shot). If a blood sugar has not yet been done, it can be done now.

7. Wait 10 minutes. Check blood sugar. If still unconscious and blood sugar is still below 60 mg/dl (3.2 mmol/L), inject second dose of glucagon (same amount as first dose).

8. If no response to glucagon, or any difficulty breathing, call paramedics (or 911).

9. Give sips of juice, sugar pop, or sugar in water initially as soon as he/she awakens. Honey may help to raise the blood sugar. After 10 minutes, encourage solid food (crackers and peanut butter or cheese, sandwich, etc.).

10. Notify diabetes care team of severe reaction prior to next insulin injection (so dose can be changed if needed). Complete recovery may take 1-2 hours.

You may copy this page as often as you wish.

Tape a copy to the box of glucagon.

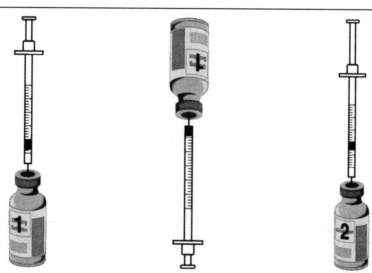

Insert 1/2cc of air into fluid bottle (1cc won't fit).

Draw out 1cc of fluid from bottle.

Inject the 1cc of fluid into bottle with tablet. Mix.

DEFINITIONS

Adrenaline (epinephrine): The excitatory hormone. This is released with a low blood sugar or a rapid fall in blood sugar, which then causes the symptoms of low blood sugar (shaking, sweating, pounding heart).

Glucagon: A hormone also made in the pancreas (like insulin) that causes the blood sugar to rise. It is available to inject into people when they have severe (unconscious) insulin reactions.

Hypoglycemia: The term used for a low blood sugar (insulin reaction).

Hypoglycemic Unawareness: The term used to describe low blood sugars without the person having any warning signs or symptoms.

Insta-Glucose, Monojel®, or Reactose: Source of concentrated sugar that can be purchased. It can be given to a person in case of low blood sugar.

Ketoacidosis (Acidosis): What happens in the body when not enough insulin is available. Blood sugar is usually high at this time. Moderate or large ketones (acetone) are present in the urine. See Chapter 14.

Rebounding ("Somogyi" reaction or "bouncing"): The process of blood sugars falling to low levels and then rebounding to high levels. Ketones may sometimes be present when this occurs.

Seizure (convulsion): Loss of consciousness with jerking of muscles. This can occur with a very severe low blood sugar (insulin reaction).

QUESTIONS (Q) AND ANSWERS (A) FROM NEWSNOTES

Q. Do we still need to keep glucagon?

A. YES. The current statistic (from three studies) is that 4% to 13% of standard insulin-treated patients have one or more severe episodes of hypoglycemia each year. With intensive insulin therapy in the DCCT, 25% (one in four) of subjects had a severe reaction each year. Glucagon should be given anytime there is loss of consciousness without being able to arouse the person. If paramedics are to be called, it is still wise to give the glucagon before they arrive.

The biggest change in giving glucagon is that two studies have shown it will work just as fast when given subcutaneously (the same place as insulin) as when given into muscle. People used to think it always had to be given into muscle.

The Eli Lilly Company Glucagon Emergency Kit comes with the diluting solution already in the syringe—ready to be injected into the bottle with the powdered glucagon for mixing. The syringe and needle they provide can then also be used for the subcutaneous or intra-muscular injection (either is fine).

Some people have rebounding, a high blood sugar, and even ketones after glucagon. Vomiting can also occur, but these side effects can be handled.

Q. Since I have changed to three injections of insulin per day, and my Hemoglobin A_{1c} has come down, I don't seem to feel low blood sugar reactions. Is this common?

A. Unfortunately, this is not unusual. It is called "hypoglycemic unawareness." People on intensive insulin therapy often do not make the "counter-regulatory" hormones as effectively as they previously did. Adrenaline (epinephrine) output is sometimes reduced in people with very tight sugar control. This is probably the most important hormone, which normally increases with low blood sugar and then causes the symptoms (shakiness, sweatiness, rapid heart beat, etc.). Sometimes it is possible to reduce the insulin dose to let the blood sugars run a bit higher for two or three weeks in order to regain the ability to feel low blood sugars.

Other hormones that normally help to raise the blood sugar may also have reduced output following intensive insulin therapy. Production of the hormone glucagon, made in the pancreas like insulin (normally), is reduced in most people who have had diabetes for longer than one year, so it also may not be available to help raise the blood sugar.

It is important to let your diabetes care provider know if you are having low blood sugars without symptoms.

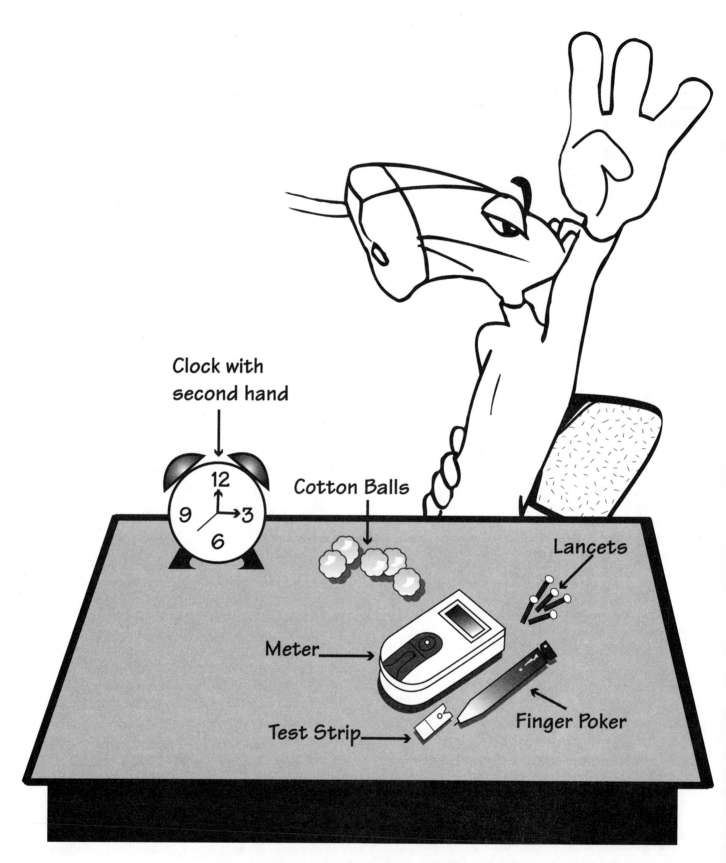

Clock with second hand

Cotton Balls

Lancets

Meter

Test Strip

Finger Poker

Blood sugar testing should be done at least three or four times a day.

Chapter 6

BLOOD SUGAR (GLUCOSE) TESTING

Key ideas of this chapter:

- 🐾 Show awareness of the importance of measuring blood sugar levels.

- 🐾 Perform accurate blood sugar tests.

SELF BLOOD-GLUCOSE (SUGAR) MONITORING (SBGM)

The ability of people (or families) with diabetes to check blood sugar levels quickly and accurately has changed diabetes management more than anything else in the past 20 years. Prior to this, diabetes was primarily managed by measuring urine sugars, which were very unreliable. The people in the intensive treatment group of the Diabetes Control and Complications Trial (DCCT) did at least four blood sugars every day. They were able to achieve excellent diabetes control as a result of frequent blood sugar testing, more frequent dosages of insulin, and following a dietary plan. The improved glucose control was shown to reduce the risk for the eye, kidney, and nerve complications of diabetes. Clearly, for people who are able to check blood sugars more frequently and practice good follow-through, improved sugar control (Table 1) is now possible. The Standards of Diabetes Care (see Chapter 19) recommends "frequent blood-glucose monitoring" (at least 3-4 times per day). This is a reasonable goal for all people with diabetes.

Figure 1: Blood Sugars

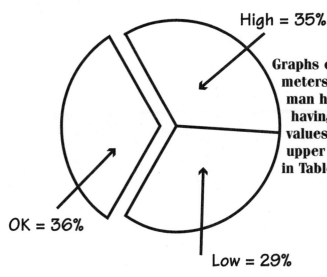

High = 35%

OK = 36%

Low = 29%

Graphs can be obtained from some of the blood sugar meters when they are brought to the clinic. This young man had a HbA_{1c} (see Chapter 13) of 7.1%, but was having too many lows. We like no more than 14% of values to be low and for less than 50% to be above the upper range (see suggested ranges for different ages in Table 2).

REASONS FOR BLOOD SUGAR (GLUCOSE) TESTING

Table 1

1. Safety
2. Improve sugar control
3. Adjust the insulin dosage
4. Manage illnesses
5. Understand the effects of various foods, exercise, or stress
6. Determine a rapid fall in blood sugar from a truly low blood sugar value
7. Know the blood sugar level immediately
8. Sense of control
9. Indicate a need to test for urine ketones

WHY DO SELF BLOOD-GLUCOSE MONITORING (SBGM)?

There are many reasons why measuring blood sugars at home has become a "cornerstone" of diabetes care. A few of these will be discussed here (and are listed in Table 1):

1. **Safety:** A big reason for the use of blood sugar testing relates to safety. Almost no one feels all the low blood sugars that occur (and very young children may not report feeling any lows). Checking the blood sugar before the bedtime snack may help in choosing ways to prevent low blood sugars during the night.

2. **Improving sugar control:** Studies have clearly shown that testing a minimum of four blood sugars daily and using the results wisely can result in improved sugar control. This results in a lesser risk for diabetic eye, kidney, and nerve complications.

3. **Adjusting the insulin dosage:** If regular blood sugars are checked, and the results recorded to look for patterns of lows or highs, the insulin dosage can be intelligently adjusted as needed. Similarly, people who take Humalog or Regular insulin before meals should use the blood sugar level (along with the amount of food and planned exercise) to decide how much insulin to take.

4. **Managing illness:** Being able to check blood sugars at home when a person is sick (or before or after surgery) allows for safe management at home. In the past, people with diabetes were sometimes kept in the hospital because accurate blood sugars could not be done at home.

Figure 2:

Blood Sugar Levels in mg/dl (mmol/L)

400-800 (22.2-44.4)	Very High
200-400 (11.1-22.2)	High
GOAL	
80-200 (4.4-11.1)	Under 5 years
70-180 (3.9-10)	5-11 years
70-150 (3.9-8.3)	12 years and up
70-120 (3.9-6.6)	Normal
below 60 (below 3.2)	Low

To understand the effects of various foods, exercise, or stress: By checking a blood sugar two hours after eating a certain food or doing a certain amount of exercise, one can better plan the insulin dose the next time. Pizza, for example, tends to raise blood sugars more than other foods for some people. If this is found to be true, extra Humalog or Regular insulin can be considered for the next time it is to be eaten. Similarly, some people raise their blood sugar with a certain exercise, whereas others do not. Knowing the blood sugar value after doing the exercise a few times will help in future planning.

To separate a rapid fall in blood sugar from a truly low blood sugar value: Some people report frequent symptoms of, or insulin reaction (see Chapter 5). This occurs when the blood sugar falls rapidly (for example from 300 to 150 mg/dl [16.6 to 8.3 mmol/L]) or when a low blood sugar truly

occurs. A blood sugar test at the time of a reaction will help determine whether the symptoms are due to a rapid fall **(false reaction)** or a seriously low blood sugar. We consider a truly low blood sugar to be **below 60 mg/dl (3.2 mmol/L)** or, in a preschooler, **below 70 mg/dl (3.9 mmol/L)**. Sugar can be given if the level is low, but is not needed if the symptoms are just due to a rapid fall in sugar. If the level is between 60 and 100 mg/dl (3.2 and 5.5 mmol/L), it is often helpful to eat food that is not high in sugar. These differences will not be known unless a blood sugar level is tested at the time of insulin reactions.

To know the blood sugar level immediately: A blood sugar test will give immediate results when the value is important to know. For example, a child may be irritable and the cause may be unknown. A blood sugar test will quickly help the parent decide if the irritability is due to a low blood sugar level or another cause. Another person may have an important event and just want to know the blood sugar prior to the event.

Blood sugar testing gives people a "sense of control" over their diabetes: Many people feel better knowing how their blood sugars are running. However, it is important to remember that there may not always be an exact relationship between the blood sugar level and what one expects it to be. There are always unknown factors that result in occasional high or low levels. This can be very upsetting for the person who expects blood sugars to always be in the target range. It is important not to become discouraged when blood sugars do not always match the expected results. Questions or concerns about the blood sugar tests should be discussed with the diabetes team.

As an indicator to do a urine ketone test: A fasting blood sugar above 240 mg/dl (13.3 mmol/L) or a value above 300 mg/dl (16.6 mmol/L) during the rest of the day should indicate a need for a urine ketone test. (Some meters now even flash this advice.) Testing for urine ketones when the blood sugar is high may help to prevent an episode of ketoacidosis (see Chapter 14).

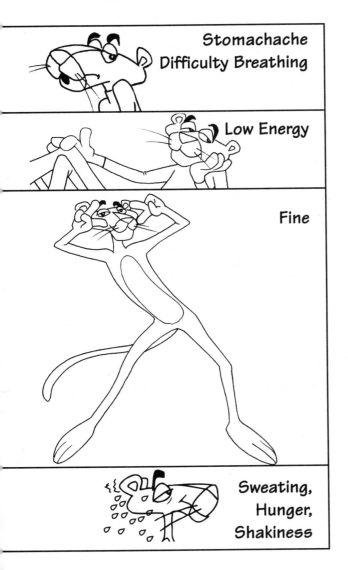

Stomachache
Difficulty Breathing

Low Energy

Fine

Sweating,
Hunger,
Shakiness

SUGGESTED BLOOD SUGAR LEVELS

	Fasting (a.m.) or no food for 2 hours		Bedtime (before bedtime snack)	
Age (years)	mg/dl	mmol/L	mg/dl	mmol/L
Below 5	80-200	4.5-11.1	Above 150*[80**]	8.3*[4.4**]
5-11	70-180	3.9-10.0	Above 120*[70**]	6.6*[3.9**]
12 and above	70-150	3.9-8.3	Above 100*[60**]	5.5*[3.2**]

*If values are below these levels, milk or other food might be added to the solid protein and carbohydrate bedtime snack.

**If values are below these levels, the test should be rechecked between midnight and 2 a.m. If this happens more than once within a week, either reduce the dinner Humalog or Regular insulin or call the diabetes care provider for advice.

Note: A normal fasting blood sugar (or when no food has been eaten for two hours) for people without diabetes is between 70 mg/dl (3.9 mmol/L) and 120 mg/dl (6.6 mmol/L).

WHEN TO DO BLOOD SUGAR TESTS

We now encourage people to do three to four blood sugar tests every day, with occasional "off-days" for a rest.

If four blood sugar tests are done each day, they are often scheduled before breakfast, before lunch, before the afternoon snack or before dinner, and before the bedtime snack. The morning blood sugar test reflects the values during the night and is probably the most important blood sugar related to diabetes control. The short-acting insulin dosages at breakfast and dinner are sometimes based, at least in part, on blood sugar results at these two times. A blood sugar test before lunch helps to decide if the morning Humalog and/or Regular insulin dosage is correct. The blood sugar test prior to the bedtime snack is important for people who tend to have reactions during the night, children who play outside after dinner, and anyone who did not eat well at dinner. It also gives information about the short-acting insulin dosage given at dinner. The more often you measure your blood sugar level, the more information you and your diabetes care provider will have for making the right decisions regarding your diabetes management.

A test should not be done unless it has been at least two hours since food was eaten. Otherwise, the result will be high from the food eaten in the previous two hours. If it is time for dinner and the person had an afternoon snack one hour earlier, it is best to just wait and do the test prior to the bedtime snack. If this is a common occurrence, change to doing the blood sugar tests before the afternoon snack. Some physicians routinely request that a test be done prior to eating lunch. For some children (and schools), this is not a problem and can be done without interfering with the child's normal school life. Our major aim at school is to have the child be as normal as possible. If reactions do occur at school, it is helpful to do a blood sugar level at the time of the reaction (see Chapter 22 on The School and Diabetes). It may be necessary to occasionally do blood sugar tests in the middle of the night (see Chapter 5 on Low Blood Sugar) to make sure the value is not getting too low. The diabetes care provider may suggest this if very erratic results are noted for the morning blood sugars.

The bedtime blood sugar is particularly important for people who tend to have reactions (low blood sugars) during the night. Higher values are usually aimed for at bedtime (Table 2) than during the rest of the day. If the bedtime values are low (e.g., below the values in Table 2), an additional snack should be given in addition to the usual solid protein and carbohydrate. If the values are below the levels shown in the brackets in Table 2, it is wise to recheck the blood sugar between midnight and 2 a.m.

HOW TO DO SELF BLOOD SUGAR TESTS

Finger-poking

A finger-poking (lancing) device is used to get the drop of blood. There are many good devices on the market, and these can now often be set at different depths for different people. The ultraTLC® adjustable lancing device by MediSense has an adjustable cap and can be used with the B-D ULTRA-FINE® II lancets. The Softclix® by Accu-Chek also has an adjustable cap (but must use their lancets). The adjustable pokers are particularly good for young children who have tender skin and may not need much lancing depth. Lancets that people in our clinic currently prefer are the B-D ULTRA-FINE II lancet, the Monolet® Original or Thin Lancet, and the E-Z JECT® color lancet.

The hands should be washed with warm water (to increase blood flow and to make sure they are clean). Any trace of sugar on the finger may give a false elevated reading. We do not recommend routinely wiping with alcohol, as any trace of alcohol left on the skin will interfere with the chemical reaction for the blood sugar test (Table 3). Occasionally, when away from home (e.g., camping, picnics), it is necessary to use alcohol to cleanse the finger. In that situation, dry the finger and, when possible, discard the first drop of blood.

It is often helpful to place the finger to be used on a table top (to prevent the natural reflex of withdrawing the finger and not getting an adequate poke). The side of the finger should be used rather than the fleshy pad on the fingertip, which is more painful. The first drop of blood should be wiped away, as it may be diluted with water (or alcohol). If the drop is not coming easily, hold the hand down to the side of the body to increase the blood in the finger. OBTAINING TOO SMALL A DROP OF BLOOD THAT FAILS TO COMPLETELY COVER THE PAD IS ONE OF THE MOST COMMON ERRORS AND CAUSES INACCURATE RESULTS. If the fingers become sore, the toes may be used.

Blood Sugar (Glucose) Meters

Most people in the U.S. now have blood glucose meters to test their blood sugars. In some countries where meters are not as readily available, blood sugar strips are used alone and are compared to a color chart. The method for Chemstrip bG® strips is included in the Appendix at the end of this chapter. We do not recommend one meter over another. Most meters read within 10% of a hospital laboratory determined value. Some meters read the sugar in the plasma (the clear part of the blood), whereas others read whole blood sugar (including the red cells which have a lower sugar level). As a result, meters reading plasma glucose usually give values that are 15% higher than for meters reading whole blood glucose. Thus, results from different

COMMON PROBLEMS CAUSING INACCURATE BLOOD SUGAR TEST RESULTS

METER READING

- Finger is not clean and dry (sugar on finger will raise result; alcohol will interfere)
- Adding more blood after the first drop has been put on pad (now ok for some meters)
- Meter parts are dirty (e.g., with dried blood)
- Codes on strips and meters are not matched (some meters now read the codes automatically)
- Too small a drop of blood on pad

meters are often not comparable. It does not matter which type of meter, plasma or whole blood, is chosen for use.

We do request that families choose a meter with a memory for at least the last 100

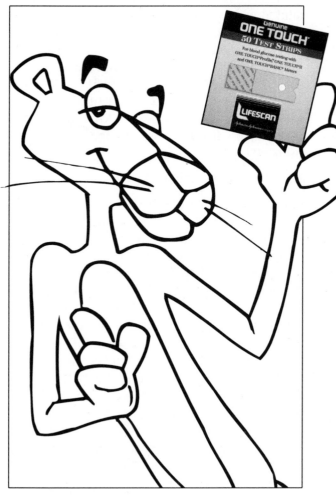

Blood glucose testing strips

glucose values. **The meter must always be brought to the clinic visit** so that it can be downloaded and graphs, such as the pie-chart (Figure 1), can be printed. Research from our Center showed that if at least half of blood sugar values are below the upper limit of the goal for age (see Figure 2 and Table 2), the HbA_{1c} values will usually be in the desired range for age (see Chapter 13). The HbA_{1c} test does not reflect the average blood sugar, but only how often the blood sugar has been high over the past 90 days. During the "honeymoon" phase (Chapter 2), or when one still makes much of their own insulin, most of the blood sugars will be in the desired range for age. For other people with diabetes, it is a reasonable goal to try to get half of the blood sugar values at any time of day within range for that person's age.

Some of the desirable features in selecting a meter are listed in Table 4. Families tend to prefer small meters that are easy to slip into a pocket. They also prefer meters that take a short time for the glucose determination. Particularly for younger children, the need for only a small amount of blood is helpful. Some of the strips now have a capillary action to pull the blood into the strip. This may be helpful for a small child who has difficulty holding still. This type of strip may also result in less of a need for cleaning the meter at regular intervals. For some people, accuracy in cold, heat, high humidity or high altitude is important. If a strip has been in a cooler or refrigerator (most strips spoil at above 90° or

DESIRED FEATURES OF BLOOD GLUCOSE METERS

1. Accurate (in environment where it is to be used)
2. Storage of at least the last 100 values
3. Able to be downloaded at clinic and/or at home
4. Small in size
5. Short determination time
6. Small drop of blood (± capillary action of strip)
7. Cleaning is easy or not necessary
8. A control solution or strip can be used to check for accuracy
9. Strips are paid for by the family's insurance

if they freeze), they should always be brought to room temperature before using.

Some families like to download their blood glucose results in their homes. Current programs and meters that are able to do this are listed in Table 5.

Unfortunately, often the main reason one meter is selected over another in the U.S. is that the family's health insurance will pay for that meter and its strips. The glucose strips usually add up to a cost of $2-3 (U.S.) per day, so insurance coverage is important. The cost of strips is usually a more important factor than the cost of the meter.

It is important with most meters to test a control strip or solution at regular intervals to make sure reliable results are being obtained. Some clinics with a more accurate meter may wish to intermittently check the family's meter with the clinic's. Some common problems causing inaccurate blood sugar test results are shown in Table 3.

RECORD KEEPING

Examples of daily record sheets are included in this chapter. The pages record either the last one week or the last two weeks of blood sugars. Many families will now fax the page to their diabetes care provider at regular intervals. If this is done, make sure the insulin dosages and instructions for return fax or phone contact are included. These sheets may be copied and stored in a notebook to bring along to clinic visits. Keeping good records to look for patterns in blood sugars is essential. It is wise to keep written records even if your meter is able to store results (these may be lost if the meter malfunctions). **Patterns of high or low blood sugars will be missed if results are not recorded.** It is important to note all reactions and possible causes. Some people also circle all values below 60 mg/dl (3.25 mmol/L) or put a star on days of reactions so that these can be easily noted by the diabetes care providers. If times of heavy exercise are recorded, it may be possible to see the effects of exercise on blood sugars. Illnesses, stress, and menstrual periods may increase the blood sugar and should be noted. It may be helpful to record what was eaten for

the bedtime snack or any evening exercise to see if these are related to morning blood sugars. Hopefully, occasional tests will also be done at the time(s) when routine tests are not usually done. Also included is a way to record urine ketone checks, as newly diagnosed people must check their ketones frequently. Ketone checks are essential with any illness **or** anytime the blood sugar level is above 240 mg/dl (13.3 mmol/L). We realize, however, that most people will not need to routinely check urine ketones after the period of new diagnosis.

The insulin dose can be recorded with the units of short-lasting insulin on top (e.g., 5H or 5R) and the units of longer lasting insulin on the bottom (e.g., 15N or 15L).

Good record keeping and bringing the results to clinic visits allow the family and diabetes team to work together most effectively to achieve good diabetes management.

Non or Minimally Invasive Glucose Monitoring

As discussed in Chapter 26, two minimally invasive meters are now close to becoming available. Both are accurate and read subcutaneous (not blood) glucose levels, which take about 10 minutes longer than blood glucose levels. This is generally not a problem.

The Continuous Glucose Monitoring System® (CGMS) by MiniMed was approved by the FDA in 1999. This system involves the insertion of a small plastic tube with a needle that is then removed. It can stay in place for three days (like the insulin pump cannula). It is usually put under the abdominal skin. Readings are done every 10 seconds and are summarized every five minutes. Unfortunately, as discussed in Chapter 26, the initial model will not allow reading the glucose levels at home. The pager-sized monitor will instead need to be taken into the doctor's office to be downloaded. It also does not have an alarm to warn of highs or lows. The company hopes to return to the FDA in a year or two to seek approval for a device that corrects these two deficiencies. Probably its main initial use will be for:

i. Helping to monitor people who have had severe hypoglycemia (blood sugar testing will still be necessary, but this will allow values between the blood sugar tests to be evaluated).

ii. Changing people from two shots per day to intensive therapy, multiple shots of insulin or an insulin pump.

iii. Monitoring glucose levels when a medicine, such as prednisone (steroids), is needed (which greatly increases blood sugars).

iv. Attempting to improve glucose control in people whose HbA_{1c} level (Chapter 13) is too high.

v. Checking to make sure sugar levels during the night are not too high or too low.

vi. Monitoring sugar levels during illness or after surgery.

vii. Monitoring sugar levels after periods of strenuous exercise.

The GlucoWatch®, by Cygnus, pulls extra-cellular fluid from under the skin by a small current from a battery within the watch. As discussed in Chapter 26, it is completely non-invasive in that a needle is not put through the skin. However, many people have temporary areas of irritation, either from the pad under the watch (where the fluid is drawn) or, more commonly, from the adhesive material around the outer edges of the watch. After a three-hour equilibration period and one blood sugar determination, the watch can check three glucose readings per hour for 12 hours. Any reading is cancelled if there is excessive sweating. The company has submitted the GlucoWatch to the FDA, with the ability to read the glucose levels as they are determined and an alarm that can be set for a desired level of high or low glucose values. Probably the main initial uses will be similar to those outlined above for the CGM system.

Even with the limitations of the CGM system and the GlucoWatch, as discussed above and in Chapter 26, they represent important advances.

SUMMARY

Whichever method of blood sugar testing you use, WRITE DOWN THE TIME OF THE TEST, THE DATE, HOW YOU FEEL, AND THE BLOOD SUGAR VALUE. BRING THESE RESULTS TO CLINIC APPOINTMENTS. Samples of daily record sheets are found in this chapter. If the results are consistently outside of the desired range, change your insulin dose, call, mail, or fax your test results to your diabetes care provider to obtain help. **Don't wait for your next scheduled appointment.** Try to do the tests at the same time each day, preferably before breakfast, before lunch, before supper, and before the bedtime snack. Do the test when no food has been eaten for at least two hours.

The use of blood sugar testing adds an extra expense to diabetes management. In most cases, insurance companies will help to cover this expense. Most knowledgeable doctors and nurses believe that diabetes control can be improved through the use of blood sugar testing. It is necessary for the whole family to be supportive in this effort. Family members must never show displeasure when a reading is high, or testing will become a negative experience. The only response is, **"THANK YOU FOR DOING THE TEST."**

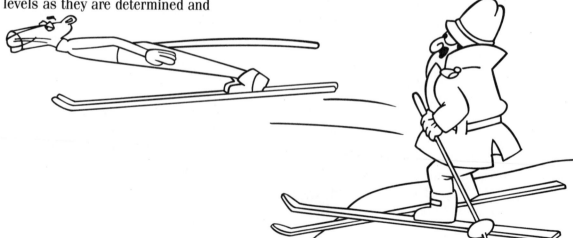

SOME METERS WITH PROGRAMS TO ALLOW DOWNLOADING AT HOME*

PROGRAM AND COST	VENDER/ADDRESS/ PHONE/WEB SITE	METER SUPPORT
In Touch Diabetes Management 1.2.3.0., $89.99 (including cable)	**LifeScan, Inc.,** 1000 Gibraltar Drive, Milpitas, CA 95035, 800-382-7226, http://www.lifescan.com/lsprods/intouch.html	LifeScan Profile® and One Touch II®
Precision Link 1.3, $139-$149 (as sold through pharmacies; including cable)	**MediSense, Inc.,** 4A Crosby Drive, Bedford, MA 01730, 800-527-3339, http://www.abbottdiagnostics.com	MediSense Q.I.D.®, MediSense 2®
WinGlucofacts 1.01, $49.95 (including cable)	**Bayer Corp.,** 511 Benedict Avenue, Tarrytown, NY 10591, 800-348-8100, http://www.glucometerdex.com/Sftwre.html	Bayer Glucometer Dex®
Accutility 1.01C, $34.95 (including cable)	**Roche Diagnostics,** 9115 Hague Road P.O. Box 50457, Indianapolis, IN 46250-0457, 800-858-8072, http://www.accu-chek.com	Accu-Chek Complete®
Camit for Windows 1.1, $59.95 (including cable)	**Roche Diagnostics,** Same as above	Accu-Chek Advantage®, and Accu-Chek III®
Acculink™ Modem (for faxing to MD) $95.00 (including cable)	**Roche Diagnostics,** Same as above	Accu-Chek Advantage or Accu-Chek Complete

*Adapted in part from an article by Rick Mendosa in the *Diabetes Wellness Letter*, Vol. 5, April, 1999.

Daily Record Sheet

Name _____

Fax To _____ At _____

Bring these results to your clinic visit

		Breakfast		Lunch		Dinner		Bedtime		Comments: Reactions, exercise, illness, bedtime snack
		Results	Insulin Dose	Results	Insulin Dose	Results	Insulin Dose	Results	Insulin Dose	
Sun	Time									
	BG/Ket									
Mon	Time									
	BG/Ket									
Tues	Time									
	BG/Ket									
Wed	Time									
	BG/Ket									
Thurs	Time									
	BG/Ket									
Fri	Time									
	BG/Ket									
Sat	Time									
	BG/Ket									
Sun	Time									
	BG/Ket									
Mon	Time									
	BG/Ket									
Tues	Time									
	BG/Ket									
Wed	Time									
	BG/Ket									
Thurs	Time									
	BG/Ket									
Fri	Time									
	BG/Ket									
Sat	Time									
	BG/Ket									

Reminder: 1. Make sure insulin doses are included under the Insulin Dose Heading.

2. How to reach you: FAX _____ or Phone _____

if by phone, best time to reach you: _____ (between 8 a.m.- 5 p.m.)

3. Person to be reached: _____

Daily Record Sheet

Name _____

Fax To _____ At _____

Bring these results to your clinic visit

		Breakfast		Lunch		Dinner		Bedtime		Comments: Reactions, exercise, illness, bedtime snack
		Results	Insulin Dose	Results	Insulin Dose	Results	Insulin Dose	Results	Insulin Dose	
Sun	Time									
	BG/Ket									
Mon	Time									
	BG/Ket									
Tues	Time									
	BG/Ket									
Wed	Time									
	BG/Ket									
Thurs	Time									
	BG/Ket									
Fri	Time									
	BG/Ket									
Sat	Time									
	BG/Ket									

Reminder: 1. Make sure insulin doses are included under the Insulin Dose Heading.

      2. How to reach you: FAX _____ or Phone _____

         if by phone, best time to reach you: _____ (between 8 a.m.- 5 p.m.)

      3. Person to be reached: _____

Concerns:

_____

_____

_____

_____

_____

_____

_____

_____

_____

_____

The Daily Record Sheets may be photocopied as often as desired.

DEFINITIONS

DCCT: Diabetes Control and Complications Trial. This trial was completed in June 1993 and clearly showed that eye, kidney, and nerve complications of diabetes were related to glucose control.

Glucose: The scientific name for the sugar in the blood or urine.

Insulin reaction (hypoglycemia): Another term for a blood sugar level that is too low. See Chapter 5.

Monitoring: Keeping track of and following blood sugar levels at home and writing them down in a record book.

SBGM: Self blood-glucose monitoring. Checking one's own blood sugar tests rather than going into a clinic or hospital to have the tests done.

Subcutaneous: Under the skin (but not in a blood vessel).

ultraTLC or Softclix: Instruments that prick the finger to get a blood sample.

QUESTIONS (Q) AND ANSWERS (A) FROM NEWSNOTES

Q. What range should my blood sugars be within?

A. This is not an easy question to answer. It depends on the individual person and family, as well as the age of the person with diabetes. Most textbooks list a normal fasting level (or when no food is taken for two or more hours) as 70-120 mg/dl (3.9-6.6 mmol/L). It is unrealistic for most people with diabetes to aim for normal non-diabetic sugar levels. *Understanding Insulin-Dependent Diabetes* (the Pink Panther book) suggests ranges by ages:

Under five years old: 80-200 mg/dl (4.5-11.1 mmol/L)

5-11 years old: 70-180 mg/dl (3.9-10.0 mmol/L)

12 years old and above: 70-150 mg/dl (3.9-8.3 mmol/L)

However, these are "generally suggested ranges" for fasting or if there is no food intake for at least two hours, and they do not take individuals or families into account. For example, a 10 to 11-year-old who does blood sugar testing regularly so that the chances of unrecognized low blood sugars occurring are unlikely, and who does not have severe insulin reactions (e.g., unconscious episodes), can probably safely aim for a level of 70-150 mg/dl (3.9-8.3 mmol/L). The reason for aiming for the lower level would be so that the glycohemoglobin (HbA_{1c}) levels may be lower with a reduced long-term likelihood of complications.

On the other hand, an adult who has severe episodes of unrecognized hypoglycemia might be wiser to try to achieve the middle range of 70-180 mg/dl (3.9-10.0 mmol/L). This might help to reduce the severe insulin reactions.

It is generally wise to discuss the level of blood sugar to aim for with your physician at each clinic visit.

Q. Should bedtime blood sugar values be in the same range as morning blood sugars?

A. No! Table 2 in Chapter 6, Blood Glucose Testing, lists suggested blood sugar levels for the morning and bedtime. We ask that values be 50-70 mg/dl (2.7-3.9 mmol/L) higher at bedtime for the three age groups in comparison to the morning values.

This is particularly important for the spring and early summer. As the good weather comes and children play outside in the evening, it is important to reduce the pre-dinner Humalog or Regular insulin and to check the blood sugar before the bedtime snack. If the blood sugar value is below the suggested lower limit for age, an additional snack should be given (and the insulin dose further reduced the next afternoon). Levels are also suggested in Table 2 for when it would be wise to check another blood sugar during the night. It is only by constant monitoring that some families are able to prevent severe insulin reactions in their children.

Q. With the data from the DCCT being in everything we read about diabetes, what can we do to improve glucose control for our 17-year-old son? His morning blood sugars are fine, but he is extremely variable (60-340 mg/dl or 3.2-18.9 mmol/L) before dinner.

A. Blood sugars before dinner are influenced by lots of factors. For example:

• The size and sugar content of the afternoon snack

• If it has been two hours without food intake when the blood sugar is done

• Exercise, which makes some people's blood sugar higher due to adrenaline (epinephrine) output while causing other people's to become lower

One helpful practice is to do a blood sugar before the afternoon snack. If the value is high, the snack can be limited to low calorie foods such as diet pop, popcorn, carrots, celery, etc. Then see if the value is down by dinner. Obviously, if the value is low, calories are needed. Each family has to decide (on the basis of exercise, school lunch, stress, etc.) what a low value is at that time of day for their child.

Another alternative might also be considered. I know a 17-year-old (whose father asked this question) whom I would guess is going to eat regardless of the blood sugar level! He might take some Humalog or Regular insulin if the value is above a certain level to hold him until dinner. In this boy's case, I suggested he take four units of short-acting insulin if the blood sugar is 150-200 mg/dl (8.3-11.1 mmol/L) and six units if greater than 200 mg/dl (11.1 mmol/L). The dose would vary for different sized people and different sized appetites.

A third alternative which works for many people is to exercise for 30 or more minutes (shooting baskets, riding an exercise bike, or doing other activities). This brings the sugar down for many people, and the exercise is obviously important for many other reasons.

I should also stress that with the DCCT data and the push for better control, more frequent blood sugar monitoring and extra insulin when the value is high may be the key for many patients. Sometimes this may be in the afternoon or at lunch. This adds extra pressure to families who have children 13 years old or above (as studied in the DCCT), but the results will be rewarding in the long run.

Q. Do I need to test my child's blood sugar every morning at 2:00 a.m.?

A. For most children, this is NOT necessary. Occasional checks during the night (e.g., once every one or two weeks) are helpful. Special circumstances that make nighttime checks important are:

❶ An illness. A sick child who may not have eaten well during the day, or who had urine ketones and/or extra (or less) insulin secondary to the illness.

❷ A low pre-bedtime snack blood sugar. If values are below 80 mg/dl (4.4 mmol/L) in a preschooler, below 70 mg/dl (3.9 mmol/L) in a 5 to12-year-old, or below 60 mg/dl (3.2 mmol/L) in a person age 12 or above, the blood sugar should be checked later—when the parents go to bed or during the night—to make sure the value has risen. This is recommended in Table 2 in Chapter 6. It might also be good to give an extra snack (or a larger amount) at bedtime.

❸ Variable morning blood sugar levels. When some morning blood sugar values are low (e.g., below 60 mg/dl [3.2 mmol/L]) and other values are high (e.g., above 200 mg/dl [11.1 mmol/L]), many care providers suggest doing a value during the night to make sure "rebounding" from low values is not causing the high values. Other care providers believe that rebounding is very unlikely and that the difference in morning values is due to other factors, such as variability in insulin absorption.

❹ Frequent low blood sugars during the night. If a child is awakening two or more times per night during the week with symptoms of low blood sugar, it may be wise to routinely do some middle-of-the-night blood sugars to make sure this is not happening more frequently. The physician caring for the child should also be called.

If blood sugars are fluctuating without explanation. A more intensive testing schedule for a week or more, including early a.m., can often determine where the insulin dosage needs to be adjusted.

Q. **With all of the good glucose meters having memories of blood sugar values which can be printed out in clinic, do I still need to write down every blood sugar value?**

A. Unfortunately, the answer is **YES**. It is just as important to write values down now as it was when meters did not have memories. It is important to look for "trends" in blood sugar levels in order to know when to make changes in insulin dosages. If a person or family does not do this, they are not doing a good job of home diabetes management. One of my top "pet peeves" in diabetes care is to have a patient (or family) who does blood sugars and constantly have values that are too high or too low, but doesn't make changes between clinic visits or fax the values to a diabetes care provider who can make suggestions.

Our general rule of thumb is that if more than half of the values at any time of day are above the upper level (usually 180 for 5-11 years old, or above 150 if 12 years or older), an increase in the insulin dose is needed. For example, if a 11-year-old has all morning values above 180 mg/dl (10 mmol/L) for a week, the evening long-lasting insulin should be increased by one

unit. Similarly, if the pre-dinner values are all above 180 mg/dl (10 mmol/L) for a week, the morning long-lasting insulin dose should be increased by one or two units. If the values are not being recorded in such a way that values done at the same time of day can be easily compared, it is possible that these trends will be missed. The opposite is also true; if there are more than one or two values in a week below 60 mg/dl (3.24 mmol/L) at any time of the day, the insulin dose working at that time can be reduced. If there is a question whether doses should be changed, the fax page in this chapter can be faxed to the health care provider (most schools and work places now have fax machines). The faxing of the blood sugars saves valuable doctor/nurse time in having to sit at a phone and write down results. Our Center now averages over twenty patient faxes per day, and it is considered part of the service of the clinic visits every three months.

For the young child or teen who does not want to write values down, it is often acceptable for the parent to push the "M" (memory) button at the end of the day and record the values. This is a way for the parents to stay involved and most teenagers agree to accept this help. The parent is often the family member who does the faxing to the health care team as well.

Blood Sugar Goals

Under 5 years old:	5-11 years old:	12 years old and older:
80-200 mg/dl	70-180 mg/dl	70-150 mg/dl
(5.5-11.1 mmol/L)	(3.9-10 mmol/L)	(3.9-8.3 mmol/L)

APPENDIX TO CHAPTER 6

VISUAL METHOD TO DO BLOOD SUGARS USING CHEMSTRIP bG Strips

The nurse educator will explain how to use the strip. There are several products available for doing blood sugar tests. The Chemstrip bG strips can be used without a meter by comparing the color change of the strip to a color chart. They also may be used with several blood sugar meters (see below). Chemstrips can be cut in half (lengthwise) for visual reading (not meter reading) to save some money.

The directions for using the Chemstrip bG strips are on the side of every can, but will be summarized here:

1. Place a large drop of blood on the white-yellow pad at the end of the strip, covering the entire pad (essential if the strip is to be meter-read). Do not add a second drop of blood if the first drop was not large enough. The strip can still be visually read.

2. Note the time on the second hand of a clock as the drop is put on the strip. If using a meter, push the timer button. A clock with a second hand or a digital timer must always be used for visual reading.

3. After EXACTLY 60 seconds, wipe off all visible blood with a dry cotton (or rayon) ball. Wait another 60 seconds and then compare the colors to those on the side of the can. If a meter is being used, place the strip in the slot at 100-110 seconds. This allows drying time before inserting the strip into the meter.

4. In contrast to the directions on the can, we suggest using only the green block at the top of the strip if this block turns color. If it doesn't, only the blue (lower) block is used when comparing to the colors on the side of the can. We do not recommend trying to average the results of the two blocks.

5. When the green color is darker than the 240 mg/dl (13.3 mmol/L) comparison block, it is

necessary to wait another minute before comparing the color on the strip with the three blocks in the second row on the can. Some meters also have a way to do a later reading.

6. Values can be estimated when colors of the strip are between those of the blocks on the can.

7. The Chemstrip bG strips hold their color for two hours after the test, so others can check to see if they agree with the reading. The strips can also be dated and put back in the can if it is desired to keep them longer than two hours.

8. If the meter will not read the strip (the Accu-Chek II gives an "S -" reading), it can still be read visually. Reasons for a meter not giving a reading are outlined in Table 3 in this chapter.

9. Remember to always record the results of the test in your book and to bring your record book with you to clinic visits.

Note: *Problems with visual readings can result from improper timing, wiping too hard or too lightly, and not using the correct material (dry cotton or rayon) for doing the wiping.*

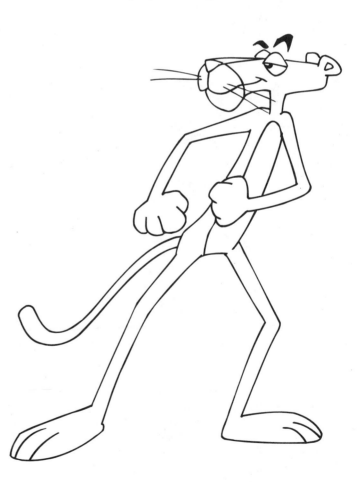

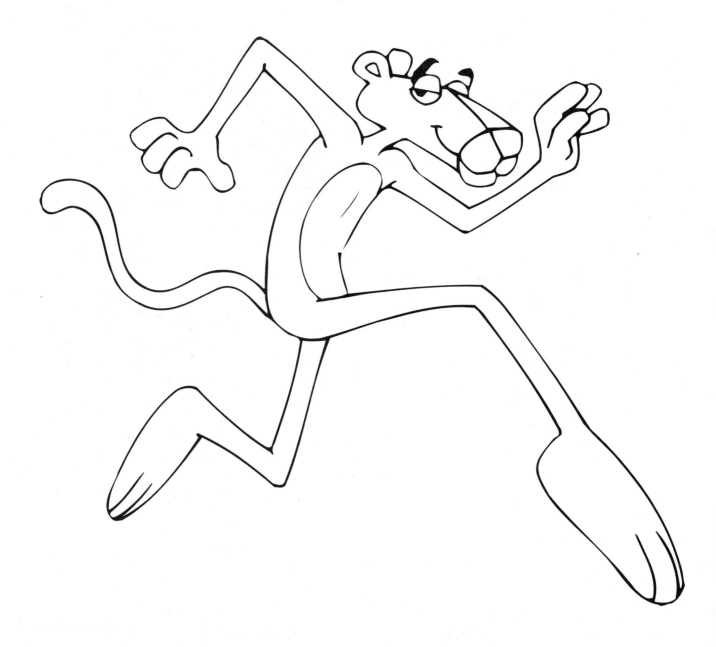

Chapter 7: Insulin Types and Activity

Chapter 7 INSULIN: TYPES AND ACTIVITY

Key ideas of this chapter:

* Recognize the different types of insulin.

* Be aware of when different insulins have their activity.

WHAT IT IS

Before insulin was discovered in 1921, there was little help for people who had type 1 diabetes. Since then, millions of people all over the world have been helped by insulin.

Insulin is a hormone made in the pancreas, an organ inside the abdomen (see picture in Chapter 2). Special cells called "beta cells," located in a part of the pancreas called the "islets" (pronounced eye-lets), make the insulin. When a person has type 1 diabetes, these cells stop making insulin. Other cells in the pancreas and throughout the body continue to work normally.

Most people with diabetes now use human insulin. The human insulin does not come from humans, but has the same "make-up" as human insulin. It is produced by bacteria (Lilly) or by yeast (Novo-Nordisk) using complicated "genetic engineering." There are no known advantages of one brand of insulin over another brand.

WHAT IT DOES

Food (carbohydrate) is converted to sugar for the body's energy needs. The insulin allows the sugar to pass from the bloodstream into the cells where it is burned for energy. The body cannot turn sugar into energy without insulin (see diagram in Chapter 2). Insulin has a second function—to turn off the production of sugar in the liver and muscle (see Chapter 2). If insulin is not available, the sugar builds up in the blood until it spills into the urine.

People who have type 1 diabetes don't make enough insulin and have to take injections of insulin. People who have adult-onset (type 2) diabetes still make insulin and can take pills to help them make even more insulin. However, the pills are not insulin. There are no known vitamins, herbs, or other medications which can take the place of insulin injections.

TYPES OF INSULIN

Several companies make many different types of insulins. The two broad classes of insulin are "short-acting" (such as Regular and Humalog) and "longer-acting" (such as NPH, Lente and Ultralente). Insulins are grouped by how long they last in the body. Insulin action (when it begins working, when it peaks in activity and how long it lasts) may vary from person to person. There is also some variability from one day to the next in the same person. The site of the shot and exercise may influence the insulin action as well.

🐾① Short-Acting Insulins

Regular insulin begins to act approximately 30-60 minutes after being injected. It has its peak effect 2-4 hours after the injection and lasts 6-9 hours. There is again, considerable variability in these times from person to person.

Humalog insulin is more rapid in onset of activity (10-15 minutes), has peak activity in 30-90 minutes and lasts four hours. The figures show the activities of Regular and Humalog insulins.

Humalog insulin has several advantages over Regular insulin. Because it starts to work in 10 minutes rather than in 30-60 minutes, it can be taken just prior to eating rather than 30 minutes before meals. The blood sugar levels two hours after meals are lower when Humalog, rather than Regular insulin, is taken prior to meals. Because it does not last as long, there is less danger of lows during the night when Humalog insulin is used at dinner rather than Regular insulin. Finally, as discussed in Chapter 17, use of Humalog **after meals** in toddlers who eat varying amounts can help to prevent hypoglycemia, as well as food struggles.

The main disadvantage of the Humalog insulin is its shorter time of action. Regular insulin can be mixed with the Humalog insulin (with either one going into the syringe first) to extend the period of action. The long-acting insulin can then also be added to the syringe.

We have used the term "insulin cocktails" to refer to the mixing of three or more insulins in the same syringe. This is discussed in more detail in Chapter 20.

It is fine to use Humalog just before a meal on one day when one plans to eat right away and to use Regular insulin (same dosage) on another day because the meal will not be eaten right away.

When Humalog and Regular insulins are combined in the same syringe, it does not matter which of the two insulins goes into the syringe first. However, they should both be drawn up before the long-acting insulin (see Chapter 8). This allows for an immediate effect on the blood sugar and on food about to be eaten (the Humalog insulin), as well as for coverage of a later snack or meal (the Regular insulin). Examples of mixtures of Humalog and Regular insulin are given in Chapter 20.

🐾② Longer-Acting Insulins

NPH insulin is made with a protein that allows it to be absorbed in the body more slowly. The letters NPH stand for **N**eutral **P**rotamine **H**agedorn. Protamine is the protein added to the insulin to make it long-acting. Hagedorn is the name of the man who developed it. Human NPH has its peak activity 6-8 hours after the injection in most people. If it is taken in the morning, the peak action comes before supper. Human NPH insulin lasts an average of 13 hours. The peak in NPH insulin activity and the duration of activity may vary for some people. NPH insulin can be premixed with Regular insulin without changing the activities of either insulin.

Ultralente insulin is also a long-lasting insulin. Human Ultralente insulin lasts 15-18 hours and, for some people, up to 24 hours. It is primarily a flat-acting insulin with almost no peak in activity. It is now frequently taken at dinner as the long-acting insulin to turn off sugar production in one's own body ("internal" sugar production by the liver—see Chapter 2) during the night. This is shown in the figures that follow. The methods to adjust all insulin dosages are discussed in Chapter 20.

Ultralente and Humalog insulins can be mixed in the same syringe without delaying the onset of the activity of the Humalog insulin. In contrast, Ultralente insulin does slightly delay the onset of activity of Regular insulin. Two shots per day (breakfast and dinner) of Humalog and Ultralente insulin, with Humalog insulin by pen at noon, has now become a popular insulin therapy (see Figures under Three Injections Per Day).

LANTUS® (Insulin Glargine) is a new, clear, long-acting insulin analog made by Hoechst that may soon become available. Genetic engineering has been used to change the amino acids in the insulin. The result is an insulin that lasts 24 hours and has almost no

🐾 Pre-Mixed Insulins

Lente insulin is a pre-mixed combination of seven parts of Ultralente (long-acting) insulin and three parts of Semilente (short-acting) insulin (see Table 1). Similarly, different combinations of premixed **NPH** and **Regular** insulin are available. The most frequently used are 70/30® and Mixtard®, both of which have 70% NPH and 30% Regular insulins. The usual times of activity are shown in Table 1. Whereas NPH and Regular insulins can be pre-mixed without the NPH insulin binding the Regular insulin, this is **NOT** true for the Lente insulins and Regular insulin. The Lente insulins will bind Regular insulin and make the Regular insulin slightly longer acting.

Figure 1: Longer-acting Insulins

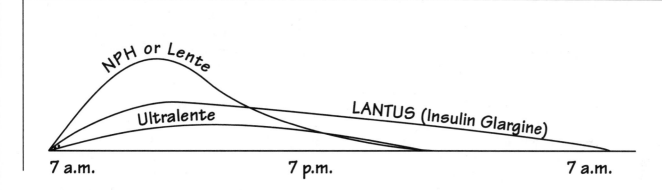

NPH or Lente

Ultralente

LANTUS (Insulin Glargine)

7 a.m.   7 p.m.   7 a.m.

peak in activity (very flat). It will be a more reliable basal insulin, without the occasional build up of insulin or the plugged needles (see Chapter 8) that can occur with Ultralente insulin. However, the pH of the insulin is different than for other insulins, and it must be given in a syringe without other insulins. It will generally be taken (alone) at bedtime with use of Humalog (by pen) before meals. Care will need to be taken not to accidentally draw up one of the other clear insulins (Regular or Humalog), which would obviously act much differently.

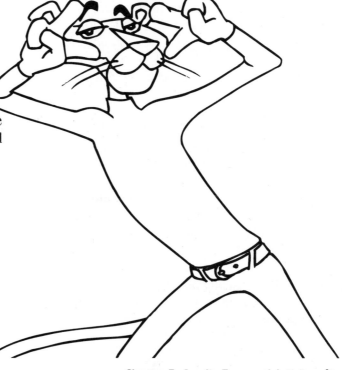

Table 1 INSULIN ACTIVITIES

Type of Insulin	Begins Working	Main Effect	All Gone
SHORT-ACTING			
Regular	30-60 minutes	2-4 hours	6-9 hours
Humalog	10-15 minutes	30-90 minutes	4 hours
LONGER-ACTING			
NPH	2-4 hours	6-8 hours	12-15 hours
Ultralente	4-6 hours	6-12 hours	15-18 hours
LANTUS (Isulin Glargine)	2-4 hours	4-24 hours	24 hours
PRE-MIXED INSULINS			
Lente (3 parts Semilente and 7 parts Ultralente)	1-2 hours	6-12 hours	15-24 hours
70/30 NPH/Regular	30-60 minutes	2-4 and 6-8 hours	12-15 hours

HOW OFTEN IS INSULIN GIVEN?

 One Injection Per Day

A few people have good blood sugar control by taking insulin once a day. This is particularly true during the "honeymoon" period that occurs shortly after diagnosis, or for some people with type 2 (adult-onset) diabetes who need insulin. The combination of insulins usually used are a long-lasting insulin (Lente, Ultralente or NPH) and a short-lasting insulin (Humalog or Regular). The two insulins are combined in one syringe for a single injection to provide insulin activity over several time periods. The morning shot of NPH, Lente and Ultralente insulins have their main activities in the afternoon and evening. They must last through the night. This is often not possible and thus, two injections per day are usually necessary. People who take one insulin injection per day may do better on two injections per day if they do not have a good level of sugar control, have frequent insulin reactions, or have many changes in their daily lives. Ultralente is sometimes more likely to last through the night than NPH insulin. Animal insulins (such as pork insulins from pigs' pancreases) usually last longer than human insulin and are sometimes used if only one injection per day is taken.

Two Injections Per Day

Most people obtain better sugar control using two or more injections of insulin per day. We recommend that very young children, under four years old, routinely receive two injections per day to lessen the likelihood of low blood sugars from one or two large peaks of insulin. The exception may be during the honeymoon period. We also recommend that most teenagers receive at least two injections per day. Most doctors now believe it is best to treat all patients with type 1 diabetes with two or more injections per day. When a person receives two injections per day, there are four (or more) small peaks of insulin activity (see drawing for two shots each day). Each of the small peaks in insulin activity can be adjusted to fit the person's schedule.

During adolescence, individuals usually need more insulin because the sex and growth hormones make it more difficult for insulin to work and diabetes control may become more difficult. These hormones also seem to increase the likelihood of blood vessel changes in people with diabetes. Better sugar control at this time is a goal that can often be achieved more easily with two or more injections of insulin per day.

Either NPH, Lente or Ultralente insulins can be used as the long-acting insulin when two or three injections of insulin are taken each day. We will sometimes even mix NPH and Ultralente in the same syringe (see Chapter 20, Insulin Cocktails). If Humalog and Regular insulins are also being used, there could be four insulins in the same syringe. NPH insulin is often used in the morning, with the peak in activity helping to allow the food eaten during

Most people over age 12 years now receive three (or more) shots of insulin each day (see Figure 3). When this is combined with checking blood sugar levels four or more times per day, paying attention to diet and frequently communicating with the health care provider, it's called **intensive diabetes management**.

Three (or more) shots of insulin per day can be done with Humalog (H) and/or Regular (R) and Ultralente in the morning, Humalog (and/or Regular) at noon, and Humalog (and/or

Figure 2: Two Injections Per Day

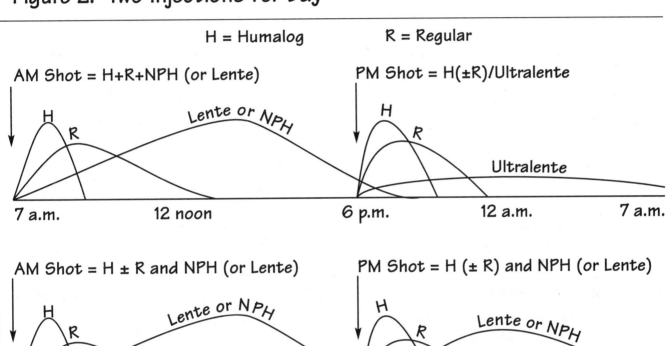

H = Humalog   R = Regular

AM Shot = H+R+NPH (or Lente)   PM Shot = H(±R)/Ultralente

Lente or NPH   Ultralente

7 a.m.   12 noon   6 p.m.   12 a.m.   7 a.m.

AM Shot = H ± R and NPH (or Lente)   PM Shot = H (± R) and NPH (or Lente)

Lente or NPH   Lente or NPH

7 a.m.   12 noon   6 p.m.   12 a.m.   7 a.m.

Many people still receive two injections per day of NPH or Lente as their long-acting insulin. They can then take Humalog or Regular or both with the NPH or Lente (see figure above).

the day to be utilized for energy. Ultralente is often used at dinner, as less of a peak of activity is needed during the night. Also, the Ultralente insulin usually lasts a few hours longer than NPH insulin, so that it may be more apt to last during the night. When only Humalog (not Regular) insulin is used in the dinner shot with the Ultralente, there is a lesser risk for low blood sugars between 10 p.m. and 2 a.m.

Regular) and Ultralente again at dinner. Using only Humalog with the evening shot and no Regular insulin reduces the likelihood of low blood sugars in the 10 p.m. to 2 a.m. period. When the HOE 901 (Insulin Glargine) which is clear and lasts 24 hours becomes available, it will have a flat line curve similar to these two shots of Ultralente insulin. It cannot be given with other insulins and will probably be best given at bedtime. The Humalog pen can then be used prior to (or after) each meal to cover the food eaten.

Figure 3: Three Injections Per Day

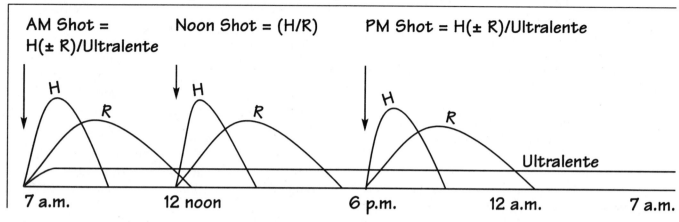

The above diagram shows Humalog (± Regular) and Ultralente in the morning and at dinner, with Humalog (± Regular) at lunch. Other people prefer Humalog (and/or Regular mixtures) with NPH or Lente insulins in the morning, Humalog (and/or Regular) at dinner, and NPH (or Lente) at bedtime (see diagram below).

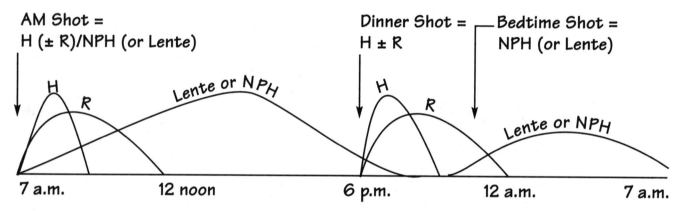

A third regimen for people taking three shots per day is to use Humalog/Regular with NPH or Lente in the morning, a shot of Humalog at 3:30 p.m. to cover "grazing" in the afternoons and Humalog and Ultralente at dinner (see below). A modification of this third regimen is to take a mixture of Humalog and Regular at 3:30 p.m. to cover the afternoon snack and dinner and then to take the longer-acting insulin—NPH, Lente or Ultralente at bedtime.

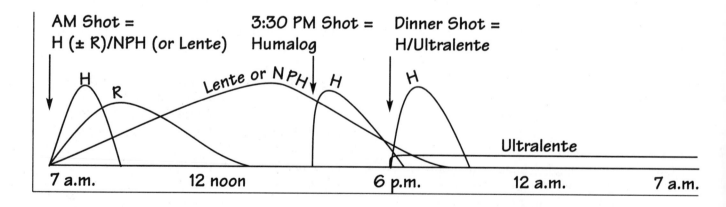

INSULINS WE FREQUENTLY USE

Table 2

Type	Name	Color of Box or Cap	Manufacturer
Humalog	Humalog	Purple Cap	Lilly
Regular	Humulin-R	White Box With Black Print	Lilly
NPH	Humulin-N	" "	Lilly
Lente	Humulin-L	" "	Lilly
Ultralente	Humulin-U	" "	Lilly
Regular	Novolin-R Human	White Box With Blue Markings	Novo Nordisk
NPH	Novolin-N Human	" "	Novo Nordisk
Lente	Novolin-L Human	" "	Novo Nordisk
Regular	Novolin R PenFill Human	" "	Novo Nordisk
NPH	Novolin N PenFill Human	" "	Novo Nordisk
NPH	Purified Pork N	" "	Novo Nordisk
Regular	Purified Pork R	" "	Novo Nordisk

AMOUNT OF INSULIN

Insulin is measured in "units" per cc. All U.S. insulin now contains 100 units per cc (ml). It is called U-100 insulin. Standard insulin syringes hold either 3/10cc (30 units), 1/2cc (50 units) or 1cc (100 units). The 3/10cc syringes have larger distances between the unit lines and are easier to use if it is necessary to measure small doses.

Insulin dosage is based on body weight and blood sugar test results. After the initial diagnosis and treatment, people are usually started on approximately 1/4 unit of insulin per pound (1/2 unit per kilogram [kg]) of body weight per day. The dose is then gradually increased as needed up to 1/2 unit per pound body weight (1 unit per kg body weight). After a few weeks to months, many children go into a "honeymoon" or "grace" period, when very little insulin is required (see Chapter 2). This usually lasts 1-3 months. Frequent telephone contact with the diabetes team is important when the honeymoon starts, as indicated by dramatic reductions in blood sugar levels. The insulin dosage must then be reduced to prevent low blood sugars. We generally recommend continuing the injections during this period. After the honeymoon, most people gradually increase to an **average** insulin dosage of 1/2 unit per pound body weight (1.1 units per kg

body weight). During the teenage growth spurt, the growth hormone level is high and blocks insulin activity. The insulin dosage may increase to 1.5 units per kg body weight (0.7 units/pound). The dosage then goes back down after the period of growth is over.

Insulin dosages can be adjusted to fit the person's lifestyle and needs. For example, seasonal changes are common. In the winter, when it is cold outside, children do not go out to play after dinner. They may need more Humalog or Regular insulin before the evening meal. In the summer, when they go outside to play after dinner, the evening Humalog or Regular insulin dose often can be decreased. Chapter 20 deals with how to adjust insulin dosages.

INTENSIVE DIABETES MANAGEMENT

Intensive diabetes management refers to the routine use of more than two shots of insulin per day (or insulin pump therapy) combined with very frequent blood glucose monitoring (four or more times per day), careful adjustment of food intake and frequent communication with the health care provider. Now that the Diabetes Control and Complications Trial (DCCT) research has proven that sugar control "closer to normal" helps prevent the complications of diabetes

(Chapter 13), more individuals are selecting intensive diabetes management. The purpose of intensive insulin therapy is to try to keep the blood sugars closer to normal than can be done with one or two injections per day. For intensive therapy to be safe, frequent blood sugar tests are needed. When people tell us they are ready for intensive insulin therapy, we often test their commitment by first asking them to do four blood sugar tests per day for one month. It is pointless to recommend intensive insulin therapy until people decide that they are ready and willing. Insulin pumps have become safer and more popular in recent years and Chapter 25 now discusses insulin pump use.

DEFINITIONS

Analog: A new form of insulin with a slightly different make-up that results in different times of onset and duration of activity. (Humalog is an example of an insulin analog modified to have rapid onset of activity. LANTUS (Insulin Glargine), recently submitted to the FDA for routine use, is an example of an analog modified to have a long duration of activity.)

Antibodies: A reaction in the blood against materials to which a person is allergic.

Beta cells: The cells in the islets of the pancreas that actually produce insulin.

cc (cubic centimeter; same as ml or milliliter): A unit of measurement. Five cubic centimeters (cc) equals one teaspoon; 15cc equals one tablespoon; 30cc equals one ounce; 240cc equals one cup.

DCCT: The Diabetes Control and Complications Trial. A very large research trial that showed that better sugar control reduced the likelihood of the eye, kidney, and nerve complications in people over age 13 years with type 1 diabetes.

Hormone: A chemical found in the blood and made in certain glands. An example is insulin that is produced by the pancreas.

Humalog insulin (insulin Lispro): This is a synthetically made insulin with two amino acids in the insulin molecule, lysine and proline, reversed in order. As a result, the insulin molecules do not bind as tightly to each other and the insulin has a more rapid onset of action (10-15 minutes) and a shorter duration

of meaningful activity (about four hours).

Islet (eye-let): The part of the pancreas where the beta cells (which make insulin) are located.

Insulin pump: A machine designed to give a preset steady (basal) injection of insulin throughout the day, as well as before-meal supplements (boluses) that are regulated by the user. Current pumps do not stop injecting insulin when blood sugars are low.

QUESTIONS (Q) AND ANSWERS (A) FROM NEWSNOTES

Q. I know I'm supposed to take my insulin and then wait to eat, but there's no way. My life just isn't that structured. I inject right before I eat. Would Humalog insulin work better for me than Regular insulin?

A. You're in good company. Most people don't wait the recommended 30-60 minutes between injecting Regular insulin and eating. In one survey, 90% of the respondents didn't wait.

Humalog is the no-wait insulin. It starts acting much more quickly than Regular, so you take it right before you eat. It starts working about the time the glucose from your meal hits your bloodstream. In contrast, if you inject Regular right before you eat, the glucose from your meal will hit your bloodstream way before the Regular does, and your glucose level will be high after the meal. So if you prefer to inject right before you eat, you're going to get better blood glucose control with Humalog than with Regular.

Q. I sometimes have low sugars in the middle of the night. Do you have any suggestions to prevent this?

A. People who use Regular at dinner time and who tend to have hypoglycemic episodes between 10 p.m. and 2 a.m. will likely have fewer lows when they change to Humalog. This is because Humalog lasts only about four hours. A shot of Humalog taken at 6 p.m. won't be active in the middle of the night. In contrast, Regular insulin may still be lowering the blood sugar 6-10 hours later, and sometimes even 14 hours later. Our research shows that the total number of hypoglycemic events is reduced by half in people taking Humalog compared with Regular insulin users. The frequency of nighttime lows, in particular, is reduced. A consistent bedtime snack is also helpful.

Q. My Ultralente insulin at dinner seems to be keeping my sugars down much better than the NPH insulin that I take in the morning. Would I be wise to use Ultralente insulin in the morning too?

A. Two shots a day of Ultralente insulin provide essentially a "flat" line of insulin activity (good for suppression of liver glucose production). It is then essential to take injections of Humalog (or Regular) insulin prior to meals to cover the second source of blood sugar—the food we eat. The Humalog (or Regular) insulin can be taken in the same syringe as the Ultralente insulin before breakfast and dinner, and can be taken by insulin pen before lunch. For someone planning to remain on two shots per day, Ultralente insulin in the morning does not peak adequately to cover daytime meals, and morning NPH insulin usually works better.

Q. What are the main advantages of the new insulin analog, Humalog? Should everyone just switch to it?

A. First, the advantages: Humalog is quick-acting and starts working in 10 minutes. With the human Regular insulin, we ask people to wait 30-60 minutes to eat after taking their shot. This would allow insulin to work as the food was absorbed, rather than first sending the blood sugar to 300-500 mg/dl (16.6-27.7 mmol/L). Unfortunately, this was inconvenient and most people (90% in one survey) just took their shots and ate. The high blood sugars in the hour or two after eating added to higher HbA_{1c} values at clinic visits. Now, with Humalog, the waiting is not necessary. People can take their shots and immediately eat their meals. This will result in lower blood sugars in the two hours after meals, as well as less guilt from not following rigid instructions.

A second major advantage of Humalog is that it only lasts four hours. When people take human Regular insulin before supper, it is not unusual to get late peaks of activity (and hypoglycemia) between midnight and 2:00 a.m. This will not happen with Humalog, as activity is gone in four

hours. Our research at the Barbara Davis Center over three years showed the total number of low blood sugars to be reduced in half in people using Humalog. The lows from midnight to 6:00 a.m. were particularly reduced.

Should everyone switch to Humalog? The answer is definitely NO. It is a prescription medication and the switch should be made with the help of health care providers at the time of clinic visits. A recent example of a person who should not switch was that of a college student who wanted to take his insulin shots in the dorm room and then walk across the street to stand in line to eat at the cafeteria. It would be likely that this person would be experiencing low blood sugars before the first bite was ever eaten if he was using Humalog. Another example of someone who should not switch is a teenager who receives two shots of insulin daily but who does not eat breakfast!

It is fine to use Humalog at one meal and human Regular at another meal on the same day. As people learn more about how Humalog works in their body, they will likely use "THINKING SCALES" (see Chapter 20) more and more. For example, they may use Humalog on Saturday morning when getting up a bit late with a high blood sugar (and planning to eat right away). Or, they may use human Regular insulin on another morning when the blood sugar is low and there will be six hours between breakfast and lunch. Or, they may use a mixture of the two insulins in the same situation when the morning blood sugar is high! All kinds of alternatives will now be possible!

Q. How do you decide when someone is ready for intensive diabetes management?

A. This is a decision that is made by the person with diabetes and the diabetes care provider. Intensive management takes extra time and effort; the patient has to be ready to make this commitment (not the parents). It involves taking insulin shots before meals, adjusting for carbohydrate intake, and doing frequent blood sugar monitoring to determine if insulin dosages are correct. We often start by asking the person to do a minimum of four blood sugar values per day and ask them to bring the values to the clinic in one month. Motivation to proceed can then be discussed.

Injection Rotation Chart

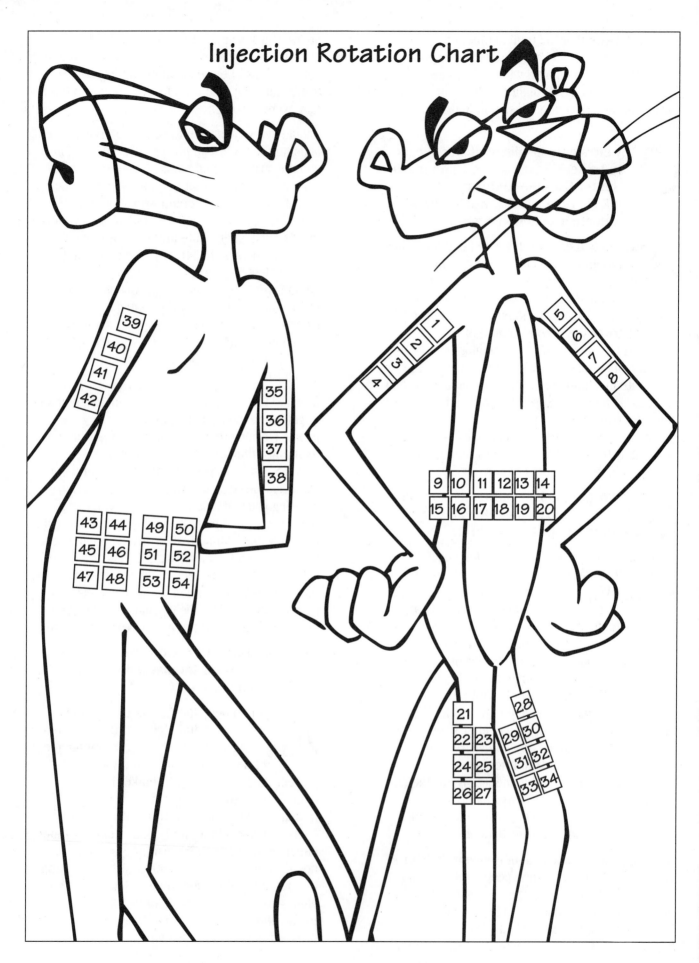

Chapter 8

DRAWING UP INSULIN AND INSULIN INJECTIONS

Key ideas of this chapter:

🐾 Demonstrate drawing up and injecting insulin.

🐾 Appreciate when and where the shot should be given.

🐾 Understand why "leak-back" of a drop of insulin on the skin occurs, and how to prevent it.

🐾 Know what happens when insulin is injected into muscle.

WHERE TO INJECT THE INSULIN

Insulin is injected into the fat layer beneath the skin. Proper techniques must be learned so that the insulin is not injected too close to the outer skin (which may cause a lump, pain, or a red spot) or too deep into the muscle (which may cause pain and insulin to be absorbed too quickly). If the injections are given in the recommended areas (see diagram of the Pink Panther), it is very unlikely that a large artery or vein will be entered. The only problem if this were ever to happen would be that the insulin would last only a matter of minutes rather than hours. Also, it is not true that injecting a bubble of air into someone (even into an artery or vein) would harm them. These are common, but unnecessary worries.

INJECTION SITES

The best places to give insulin are the abdomen, arms, thighs, and buttocks. Rotation of injection sites used to be a frequent area of conflict between parents and children. It is now possible to select two or three of the usual four areas for injections (arms, thighs, abdomen, buttocks) and to skip areas that are not well tolerated. Injections should be moved around within the sites that are used (example: six to nine areas in each thigh site). If there are swollen (hypertrophied) areas, injections should not be given into these sites, as the insulin may be absorbed at a different rate.

Insulin is absorbed more rapidly from the abdomen than from the arm, and more rapidly from the arm than from the thigh or buttock. However, the differences are not great for most people. Some people who do notice a difference will use one site for morning shots and another site for dinner shots. For example, the abdomen or arm might be used in the morning when more rapid insulin uptake is desired. The thigh or buttock might be used in the evening when less rapid insulin uptake is desired so that the insulin will last through the night.

There is some increase in uptake of insulin when the shot is given in an area that is then exercised. Injecting into an arm or leg which will be used in an activity may result in low blood sugars during exercise. Therefore, if you are to play tennis, don't inject into the arm that will be used to swing the racquet. More blood will go to this arm during the exercise and more insulin will be absorbed into the blood. A low blood sugar could occur.

Insulin should also not be injected just prior to a bath, shower or hot tub. The warm water will draw more blood to the skin, causing a rapid absorption and resulting in a serious low blood sugar.

INSULIN SYRINGES

(See picture diagram below and Table 1)

There are now several brands of disposable insulin syringes with varying needle widths (measured in gauges with a larger number for a thinner needle) and varying lengths. The needles are thin and are sharp for easy insertion. If money is short, the syringes can be reused. The amount of insulin the syringe will hold varies. There are 3/10cc and 1/2cc syringes for people using less than 30 or 50 units of insulin per injection, or 1cc syringes for those using more than 50 units per injection (see drawings). The B-D Ultra-Fine II short needles are just 5/16 inch in length (compared to the usual 8/16 inch length) and at 30 gauge are very thin. They are available in 3/10cc, 1/2cc or 1cc syringes.

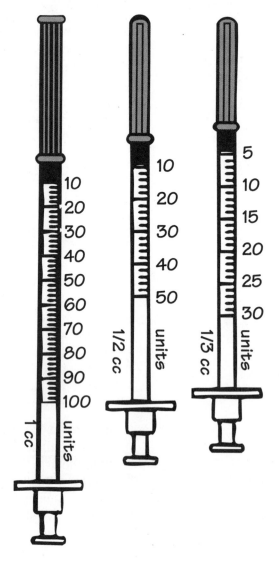

DRAWING UP THE INSULIN

The nurse will show you how to draw the insulin into the syringe. YOU SHOULD LEARN BY PRACTICE AND FORM GOOD HABITS FROM THE START. When possible, wash your hands first. The picture diagrams show how to give an injection. In addition, Table 1 gives you a checklist to follow. The nurse will go over the checklist with you at regular intervals. These are the steps:

1. Get everything together: alcohol, cotton, insulin, and a syringe.

2. Wash your hands.

3. Push the plunger of the disposable syringe up and down before drawing in the insulin. This will help soften the rubber at the end of the plunger and smooth the plunger action.

4. Wipe the top of the insulin bottle(s) with alcohol.

5. Before you insert the needle into the bottle, draw back the plunger to the number of units of long-acting (cloudy) insulin to be used.

6. Insert the needle through the rubber top of the bottle of long-acting insulin with the bottle right-side-up on a counter. Inject the same number of units of air as the number of units of insulin to be drawn out. It can remain sitting upright on the counter while the air is injected. Do not bubble air through the insulin. If you are using more than one type of insulin, always remember to inject air into the bottle of cloudy/long-acting insulin first. Then, remove the needle from the bottle.

7. Next, draw back the same number of units of air as the amount of Regular and/or Humalog insulin to be drawn from the bottle. Insert the needle and inject the air into the bottle of short-acting insulin. Leave the needle in the bottle. An alternative to adding air is just to "vent" the bottles once weekly by putting a sterile needle (or syringe without the barrel) into each bottle of insulin (with the bottles sitting upright on the table).

8. If both Humalog and Regular insulins are to be drawn up, either can go into the syringe first (but both should go in prior to the long-acting insulin).

9. Turn the bottle upside down and withdraw the amount of clear/short-acting insulin needed. You may have to push the insulin back into the bottle several times to remove air bubbles. (If you are using more than one type of insulin, do this only with the first insulin.) To get the correct dose, align the top edge (the very end) of the rubber plunger tip with the desired dosage mark on the syringe. Air bubbles can change the insulin dose but will not harm your body. By drawing the short-acting insulin into the syringe first, you will prevent a drop of the cloudy/long-acting insulin from getting into the bottle of short-acting insulin. If the bottle of short-acting insulin does become cloudy, throw it out.

10. Turn the bottle of cloudy/long-acting insulin gently up and down with 10-12 twists of the wrist to thoroughly mix. This must be done even if the cloudy insulin was mixed at the beginning. Some settling of the insulin occurs in this short time. This could result in some difference in concentration of the insulin.

11. Insert the needle into the long-acting insulin bottle, turn the bottle upside down, and carefully withdraw the amount desired, again aligning the top edge (the very end) of the plunger with the desired dosage mark on the syringe. Know the total amount of the two or more insulins so that you will know the right point to stop on the syringe. Many people make mistakes in adding, so you should double check this total.

Blood sugars should be watched carefully when the insulin bottle is almost empty. If the blood sugars start to be unusually high or low, the last bit of insulin should be discarded. Some people prefer to just routinely discard the last bit of insulin in a bottle. The expiration date on the bottle should always be checked and the insulin discarded if that date is reached.

In summary, BE PRECISE ABOUT THE DOSAGE. An overdose can cause an insulin reaction or low blood sugar. If you ever take an incorrect dose, be sure to notify your diabetes care provider. It is wise to have the morning and afternoon dosages posted on the refrigerator or some obvious place to prevent confusion. Children below age 10 years do not usually have the fine motor abilities and concern for accuracy to draw up insulin by themselves (see Chapter 17).

DRAWING UP INSULIN

A. <u>Gather supplies:</u> Insulin, syringe, alcohol wipe for tops of bottles, log book with current tests and insulin dosage (please record each blood sugar result in log book after each test).

B. <u>Technique:</u>

1. Know correct insulin dosage (based on "thinking" scales if appropriate)

2. Wipe tops of insulin bottles with alcohol swab

3. Put air into the long-acting (cloudy) insulin with the bottle upright and remove the needle*

4. Put air in the clear insulin and leave the needle in*

5. Draw up clear (short-acting) insulin, get rid of air bubbles, and remove the needle

6. Mix cloudy (long-acting) insulin vial by gently turning the bottle up and down 10-12 times; this ensures that the insulin gets well mixed

7. Draw up cloudy insulin into syringe making sure not to push any insulin already in the syringe back into the vial

8. If insulin vials have been in the refrigerator, you can warm up the insulin once it is mixed in the syringe by holding the syringe in the closed palm of your hand for a minute; it will be less apt to sting if brought to room temperature

9. Give insulin injection

*An option now used by some people is to not put air into the bottles, but to just "vent" the bottles to remove any vacuum once weekly (see text).

HOW TO INJECT THE INSULIN

(See Table 2 and picture diagrams)

1. Many people clean the site of injection with soap and water or an alcohol swab (particularly if camping or in a hospital). Most of our patients do not use alcohol or wash the skin (assuming the skin is relatively clean) prior to giving their shots at home, and infections almost never occur. Store cotton balls and rubbing alcohol in a container with a lid. Others use disposable alcohol swabs. If alcohol is to be used, let it dry on the skin before injecting or it may cause stinging. Bacteria (germs) will be killed as the alcohol dries. Seventy percent alcohol is a better germ killer than 90% alcohol. If you don't use alcohol and the area is not clean, use soap and water. If skin irritation occurs from alcohol, it may be better to just use soap and water.

2. Pinch the skin and fat tissue between the thumb and the first finger. Touch the needle to the skin, holding the syringe at a 45° angle (or less) for the 5/8 inch needles. **If you are using the B-D ULTRA-FINE II (0.3, 0.5 or 1.0cc) syringe with short needles (5/16 inch) and the fat in the area of injection is adequate, the needle can be inserted at a 90° angle to the skin without pinching**. It is generally best to push the needle all the way into the skin. If the needle is not in far enough, the insulin may not be injected into the fatty layer. If it goes into the layer directly under the skin rather than into the fatty layer, it will sting and may cause a bump or redness and itching. **Let go of the pinched tissue before injecting the insulin**, or you will be squeezing the insulin out at the same time you are trying to inject it. This is one of the most common reasons for a drop of insulin leaking from the injection site (leak-back). After you let go of the pinch, check again to make sure the needle is still all the way in.

3. Inject the insulin by pushing the plunger down with a SLOW and steady push as far as it will go. Some people like to wait a few seconds to let the insulin "spread out" after each five units of insulin is injected. AFTER THE INSULIN IS IN, WAIT FIVE TO TEN SECONDS BEFORE REMOVING THE NEEDLE. COUNT SLOWLY TO FIVE. THIS WILL HELP PREVENT INSULIN FROM LEAKING FROM THE INJECTION SITE. A loss of one drop of insulin may be equal to two to five units. Loss of insulin is a common reason for variations in the blood sugar levels. If "leak-back" continues to be a problem, two units of air can be drawn into the syringe after removing the needle from the insulin bottle. Then flick the side of the syringe with a finger to make the air rise up under the plunger. The air will then be injected after the insulin and will help to prevent "leak-back."

4. After the injection, place a finger or dry cotton swab over the site of injection. Hold for a few seconds to prevent any bleeding. Rub the site gently to close the needle track. Some bleeding may occur after the needle is pulled out; this is not harmful, although some insulin may be carried out with the blood. Press the dry cotton firmly on the site. Some people put their finger over the site where the needle came out and rub gently. The finger should be clean.

5. The plastic syringes can be used for two to four days, although we usually don't advise this. The needle may become dull after the second or third shot. If they are to be reused, after giving the injection, push the plunger up and down to get rid of any insulin left in the needle. Wipe the needle off with an alcohol swab. Put the cap over the needle and store the syringe and needle in the refrigerator until ready for the next use.

Table 2 provides a summary for injecting the insulin.

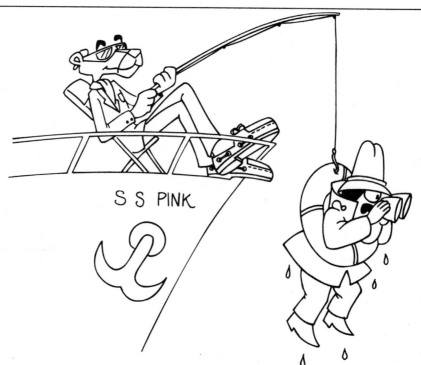

INJECTING THE INSULIN

Table 2

1. Choose injection site; use a good site rotation plan

2. Make sure the site is clean

3. Relax the chosen area

4. Pinch up the skin (not necessary for the 5/16 inch short needles)

5. Touch the needle to the skin and gently push it through the skin. Use a 45° angle for the 5/8 inch needle or **a 90° angle for the 5/16 inch (short) needle**

6. Release the pinch (unless injecting into the "tent" below)

7. Push the insulin in slowly and steadily

8. Wait five to 10 seconds to let the insulin spread out

9. Put a finger or dry cotton over the needle as it is pulled out; gently rub a few times to close the track

10. Put pressure on the site if bruising or bleeding are common

11. Observe for a drop of insulin ("leak-back"); note in record book if a drop of insulin is present

S S PINK

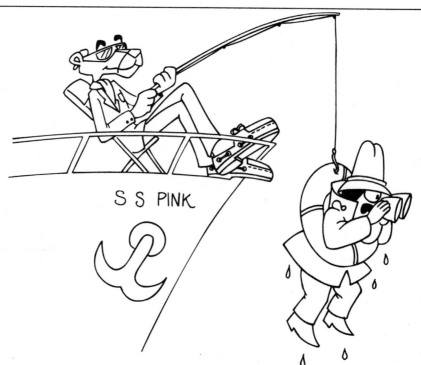

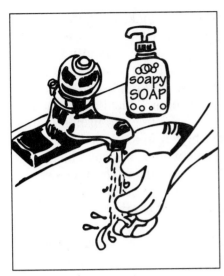

A. Wash hands

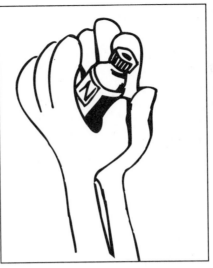

B. Warm and mix insulin

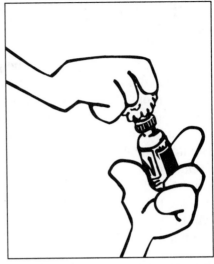

C. Wipe top of insulin bottle with alcohol

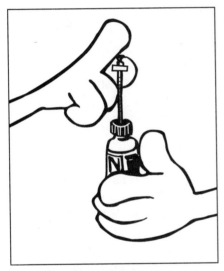

D. Air = insulin dose in units

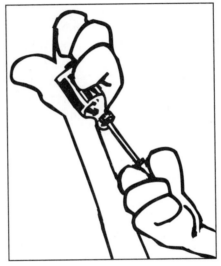

E. Pull out dose of insulin

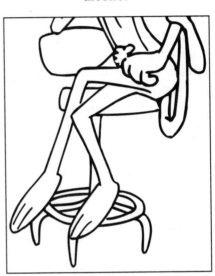

F. Make sure injection site is clean

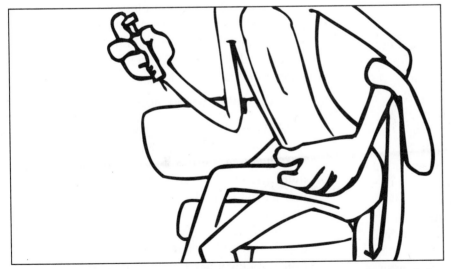

G. Pinch up skin and fat tissue if using 5/8 inch needle. **Go straight in (no pinch) if using the 5/16 inch (short) needle.**

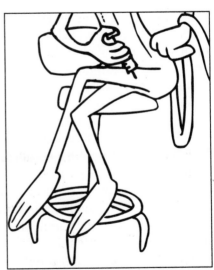

H. Inject insulin at 45° (5/8 inch) or 90° (5/16 inch needle)

WHEN TO INJECT THE INSULIN

Regular and NPH insulins can be premixed and are even sold in bottles of premixed combinations. Lente insulins bind Regular insulin and should not be mixed together until it is time to give the shot. NPH insulin binds Humalog insulin, so they should not be premixed. Humalog and Ultralente (or Lente) can be premixed. If insulin is mixed in a syringe prior to giving the shot (premixed), it will be necessary to roll the syringe between the hands to mix it thoroughly.

With Regular insulin, it is best to take the shot 30 to 60 minutes before eating. This allows the Regular insulin to start working at the time food is eaten. It will prevent the blood sugar from going very high in the half-hour or hour after eating. When the pre-meal blood sugar level is known, the time can be varied between the shot and eating the meal, as shown in Table 3. It has been our experience that using a time scale such as this can improve blood sugar control.

Other people routinely use Humalog insulin and they must eat immediately after taking their shot. An exception is with the toddler or a picky eater who has variable food intake, when it is better to wait to give the shot until after seeing how much food has been eaten (see Chapter 17).

STORAGE

Ideally, insulin should be stored in the refrigerator and warmed to room temperature prior to giving the shot. However, most people keep the bottles they are using at room temperature (except in a very hot summer). It will not be as likely to sting or to cause red spots after injection if it is kept at room temperature. After drawing up insulin that has been in the refrigerator, the filled, capped syringe can also be warmed in the closed palm of your hand to avoid stinging. A drawer in the kitchen might be identified for storage of all diabetes supplies. Research has shown that if it is stored at room temperature, it loses 1.5% of its potency per month (after one month 1cc U-100 insulin would have 98.5 units of insulin rather than 100 units). For most people, this

small change would not make a difference (9.85 units rather than 10.0 units). One of the insulin manufacturers wrote: "**Insulin vials currently in use may be kept at room temperature for 30 days, in a cool place and away from sunlight.**" Insulin will spoil if it gets above 90° or if it freezes. Insulin bottles (or pens) cannot be left in a car in the hot summer or the cold winter. If insulin has spoiled, sometimes clumps will then be seen sticking to the sides of the long-acting insulin bottle. That bottle and the accompanying bottle of short-acting insulin should not be used if this occurs. Unfortunately, the short-acting (clear) insulins do not have any tell-tale signs when they spoil. A clear insulin should be thrown away if it becomes cloudy. It may have bacteria (germs) growing in it. We have also suggested throwing away bottles of insulin that have been opened for three or more months, even if refrigerated. Families using low dosages of a particular insulin may find it more effective to draw out of 150 unit insulin cartridges (for Humalog, Regular or NPH insulins).

INSULIN PENS

Use of insulin pens has increased greatly in recent years. In the U.S., this is related to people wanting an easy method to take supplements of short-acting insulins (Regular or Humalog) with food intake during the day. In Europe, many people use pre-mixed insulins from the time of diagnosis and may not even learn to draw up mixtures of insulins. If they use pre-mixed short and long-lasting insulins (e.g., 70/30 NPH/Regular), they cannot then change the individual insulin dosages for food intake and exercise. There are now several types of pens available:

Lilly Pre-filled Disposable Pens:

Lilly disposable pens for Humalog, Humulin NPH and 70/30 NPH/Regular insulins were introduced in the U.S. in February, 1999. The pens are simple to use and will take a small B-D 31 gauge (5/16 inch) Ultra-Fine III® needle or a NovoFine® 30 gauge (1/3 inch) disposable needle (both are able to be used on all pens discussed in this chapter). The instructions are to use a new needle each time as follows:

i. Wipe the cap on the insulin chamber with an alcohol pad

ii. Remove the paper tab and screw the needle onto the pen

iii. Turn the dose knob until the larger arrow lines up below the tiny magnifying glass

iv. Pull back on the plunger and dial in a two unit priming dose

v. Push the plunger in all the way while holding the needle pointed upward (to fill the needle with insulin)

vi. Repeat steps iii and iv to dial in the desired insulin dose

vii. Assuming fat is adequate and a short needle is being used, angle at 90° to inject this dose under the skin; keep the plunger pushed down all the way for approximately five seconds after hearing a "click"

With any pre-filled insulin pen, rub the injection site with the finger as the needle is removed. This helps to close the track from the needle and reduce leak-back. If the needles are to be reused, the priming (as described in iv and v above) would be wise to do for all insulin pens. The amount of insulin wasted would be minimal, and it would help assure accuracy.

Novolin Pre-filled Disposable Pens

The **Novolin Pre-filled pens** already contain 150 units (1.5cc) of insulin, so there is no cartridge of insulin to insert. The pens are fairly simple to use and the following is a summary of the Novo Nordisk directions:

i. Pull off the cap and wipe the rubber stopper with an alcohol swab

ii. Remove the paper tab and screw the needle onto the pen

iii. If using a long-acting insulin (NPH or 70/30 NPH/Regular), turn the syringe up and down at least 10 times to thoroughly mix; (this is not necessary if only a clear insulin is being used)

iv. Remove the plastic outer cap of the syringe and the needle cap and hold the syringe with the needle pointing upward. Tap the syringe to make any bubbles rise. Turn the insulin reservoir clockwise (in the direction of the arrow) to the first notch where resistance is felt (1/5 of a full rotation). Slowly press the button to see if insulin appears at the needle tip. If not, repeat this step.

v. Replace the syringe cap, lining the "0" up with the dosage indicator knob. Turn the cap clockwise to the desired dose (do not pull cap apart from syringe while setting the dose). The maximum dose is 58 units and the insulin dose is measured in two-unit increments. Note that the push button rises as the cap is turned to set the dose. The dosage display rises 10 units with each full turn of the cap (see numbers on inner barrel). This dose <u>plus</u> the number opposite the dosage indicator represent the total dose that will be given (e.g., two complete turns of cap = 20 units [as shown] and if dosage indicator is at four units, the total would be 24 units of insulin to be given).

PRE-MEAL BLOOD SUGAR AND TIME TO WAIT BEFORE EATING

Blood Sugar Level		Time to Wait Before Eating (Minutes) Type of Insulin	
mg/dl	mmol/L	Regular	Humalog
above 200	above 11.1	60	10
151-200	8.4-11.1	45	5
80-150	4.5-8.3	30	don't wait
below 80	below 4.5	don't wait (take the shot and start eating right away)	don't wait (take the shot and start eating right away)

If a wrong dose is indicated, just turn the cap forward or backward until corrected; it is not necessary to start over. After the desired dose is dialed in, once again remove the cap (and the needle cover) to give the injection.

vi. Give the injection after inserting the needle as instructed. Just push down on the button (all the way) to push the insulin in and hold it for a few seconds.

vii. The company advises discarding the needle and using a new pen-needle with each injection. This prevents small inaccuracies in dosage due to air entering the needle. In reality, most people use the needle three or four times until it becomes dull. After giving the shot, replace the cap with the "0" opposite the dosage indicator.

🐾 Cartridge Pens

The NovoPen 1.5® is a third generation pen from Novo Nordisk and, along with the new B-D pen, offers the chance to use cartridges of Regular, NPH, 70/30 NPH/Regular or Humalog insulin (not of Lente or Ultralente insulin). The cartridges contain 1.5 ml of insulin (150 units) and are replaced into the pen when the 1.5 ml is used up. The NovoPen 1.5 delivers a maximum dose of 40 units and the B-D pen a maximum dose of 30 units, both in one-unit increments. The B-D Pen Mini® delivers in 1/2 unit doses with a maximum of 15 units at one time.

The directions for the NovoPen 1.5 are, once again, fairly simple:

i. Remove the cap (the part with the pocket clip) and unscrew the silver bottom to drop the cartridge of insulin down into the holder (metal cap first). Make sure the piston rod is flat (even) at the end of the top of the plunger. Then screw the silver bottom back on tightly.

ii. Wipe the rubber stopper with alcohol, remove the paper tab from the needle and screw the needle on the end of the pen (until tight).

iii. Turn the dial to one or two units. Pull off both needle caps and, holding the needle upward, push the button on the end to see if insulin comes out. If not, repeat the procedure until insulin appears (to get rid of all air). Do this with each usage of the pen.

iv. For giving the shot, starting at "0," turn the dial-a-dose selector to the required dose, pinch up the skin (as directed earlier) and insert the needle at a 90° angle (assuming adequate fat). Press the button on the end down firmly to deliver all insulin. Wait five seconds, pull the needle out, and rub gently. Place the small plastic cover over the needle and put the cap with the pocket clip back on the pen.

PROBLEMS THAT MAY ARISE WITH INSULIN INJECTIONS

🐾 ① Hypertrophy (swelling) of Skin

Swelling of the skin, or hypertrophy, occurs when too many injections are given in one area over a period of months to years. You can inject insulin into the body anywhere there is enough fat under the skin. Usually there isn't fat over the joints and bones, so these areas are not used. If swelling in an area does occur, you should not give further injections in that area until the swelling is gone. This may take several months and varies for different people.

The swelling will alter the uptake of insulin. Fortunately, swelling at injection sites is now less common with the use of human insulins.

🐾 ② Skin Dents (atrophy or lipoatrophy)

You may develop "dents" at the injection site. This is different from skin swelling, and is due to a loss of fat in that place. "Denting" is now very rare when human insulin is used. When dents do occur, it is possible to help them go away. If you inject human insulin into the dent four times in a row each week, the dent will gradually go away. This may take several weeks. To inject into the dented area, pick the skin up at the side of the dent and slide the needle under the center of the dent. These dents are not harmful; they just don't look very good.

🐾 ③ Plugged Needle

Occasionally, a small piece of fat or the insulin (particularly Ultralente insulin) will plug the end of the needle during the injection. Sometimes it is possible to pull out the needle a little and then push the needle back into a slightly different place. If you still cannot push down the plunger to finish the injection, you will have to pull the needle completely out of the skin. **NOTE VERY PRECISELY THE UNITS**

OF INSULIN REMAINING IN THE SYRINGE.
After you fill a new syringe with the total insulin dose as originally drawn, discard the amount of insulin you have already injected. Inject the rest into another site.

When new clear long-acting insulins become available (e.g., HOE 901), plugging of needles will be much less common.

Giving the Wrong Insulin Dose

"To err is human" is very true. If the morning insulin dose is accidentally given in the evening, usually an excess of insulin results. This results in a very long night, as the person must be awakened every two or three hours, blood sugars checked, and extra juice and food must be given. Obviously, if the blood sugar is low, more frequent checks will be needed.

Bleeding After the Injection

A small capillary blood vessel is probably hit with every injection. Sometimes a drop of blood or a bruise under the skin will be seen after the injection. This will not cause any problem except for the possible loss of some insulin with the blood. Some teenagers are upset by the bruises. As noted earlier in this chapter, place a dry piece of cotton or a clean finger over the injection site and rub gently after removing the needle. This will usually stop any bleeding. Sometimes applying pressure for 30 to 60 seconds will help to reduce bruising.

Injecting Insulin into Muscle

If a person is very thin or very muscular, there may be little fat under the skin. Injections may go into the underlying muscle, causing more rapid absorption of insulin and low blood sugar. There may then be less insulin to act later in the day, resulting in high blood sugar. Injections into the muscle are most apt to occur if the syringe is held at a 90° angle to the body (unless the short needles are used). Sometimes extra pain will occur when shots go into muscle, but this is not always the case. Thus, the pain is NOT a good indicator of shots given into muscle. If injection into muscle is a problem, it may be necessary to pull the skin away from the muscle and insert the needle into the "tent" below (while still holding the pinch of skin). Since the entire pinch is not being held, just the upper tip, the insulin should not leak-back. This technique can be taught by your diabetes nurse. Occasionally, it may be helpful to give an injection in the presence of your diabetes care provider to have your injection technique checked.

Injection Devices

Some people have difficulty pushing the needle through the skin. Others would like to inject in a difficult to reach area such as the buttocks, but can't. Placing the syringe in an injection device such as the Inject-Ease® (B-D) or the B-D Automatic Injector® may help with both of these problems. After putting the syringe in the device and pushing a button, the needle is automatically pushed through the skin very quickly. It is still necessary to push down on the plunger of the syringe to inject the insulin. If the 5/8 inch needles are being used, it may still be important to hold the device at a 45° angle with the skin pinched to prevent intramuscular shots. However, the depth can be changed, so that for some sites, this is not a worry. The Inject-Ease has a cap for 30 unit syringes with short needles. If 50 or 100 unit syringes are to be used with long needles, the extra rings can be added and the cap and the needles then resemble the short needles. Injections are then made at a 90° angle to the skin. It is still important to count before removing the needle and to briefly rub the site to close the needle track and prevent "leak-back." Other devices are available (such as the Ulster Auto Injector®) that push both the needle through the skin and push down on the plunger of the syringe to inject the insulin. Finally, there are air-pressure devices that "blow" the insulin into the body. These are expensive, but may be covered, at least in part, by insurance. They are most useful for people with needle phobia or those who cannot adjust to the insulin shots. The insulin dose may need to be changed since part of the insulin from air-pressure injections usually goes into muscle. More irregular blood sugar values may result. If you wish to see any of these devices, you should ask your diabetes nurse educator.

DEFINITIONS

Atrophy (or lipoatrophy): Areas of fat loss under the skin which appear as "dents" in the skin. Although they are believed to be due to a form of insulin allergy, they can occur in areas where insulin has never been injected.

Buttocks: The seat; the part of the body that one sits on.

Hypertrophy: Areas of swelling of the skin, which occur in places where too many shots are being given. Injecting insulin in areas of hypertrophy may cause altered insulin absorption.

Leak-back: The leaking out of a drop of insulin after the insulin injection is completed. This can be a cause of variation in day-to-day blood sugar levels.

Needle Phobia: The intense fear of needles. Working with a social worker or psychologist around "needle desensitization" may help this, as well as use of the air-pressure injector.

QUESTIONS (Q) AND ANSWERS (A) FROM NEWSNOTES

Q. **I often note that a drop of insulin comes back after I withdraw the needle when giving the morning insulin to my child. Is this of any importance and what can I do to prevent it?**

A. We are frequently asked this question. We call this "leak-back." One drop of insulin is equivalent to 1/20th of 1 ml of insulin. As 1 ml contains 100 units (U-100 Insulin), each drop would contain approximately five units of insulin. This can be a significant amount and it is therefore important to try to avoid the loss of the insulin following injections. The six main methods to prevent this loss are listed below:

1. Letting go of the pinch of skin before injecting the insulin so that pressure is not forcing the insulin out from under the skin at the same time it is being injected.

2. Making sure the needle is in the full length and that one does not start to pull the needle out until after the injection is completed.

3. Making sure there is not excessive pressure on the site of injection. For example, if the child is sitting on a chair, he/she should sit on the edge of the chair when injecting in the leg rather than on the back of the chair where the pressure beneath the leg might force the insulin out of the injection site. Having the leg straight rather than bent at the knee may also result in less pressure.

4. Injecting the insulin slowly.

5. Routinely counting for five seconds or longer (as is needed) after the insulin is injected before removing the needle.

6. Rubbing the needle track for two or three seconds as the needle is removed to "close off" the track.

If these six principles are followed, it is unusual for drops of insulin to leak-back.

Q. **My teenager read about the air-pressure device to give insulin without having to use needles. Should we be considering one of these for her?**

A. The latest models of the air-pressure injectors are greatly improved over the earlier models. The short- and long-lasting insulins do not have to be pre-mixed as they did for the earlier models. The new models are simpler and are much easier to clean.

We have had mixed reactions from the families that have tried the air-pressure injectors. One complaint has been that the insulin did not last as long. This is probably due to some of the insulin being given into muscle. Irregular blood sugars may result. A second problem has been bruising of the skin when the intensity was set high enough to make sure a drop of the insulin was not left on the skin. Expense has been another problem, with most models costing between $600-$800. Insurance will sometimes cover a part of this.

The families which have seemed to like the apparatus the most are those with very young children. When a two- or three-year-old undergoes much stress with needle injections, it may be lessened by using the air-pressure injectors. Also, when fear of needles (needle phobia) is a real problem, the air-pressure injector may help. It is not for everyone, but some people do seem to benefit.

Q. We notice that when we give the shot to our daughter in the upper outer arm, she frequently has a low blood sugar at school that morning, but is then very high before dinner. Is this possible?

A. It sounds like you are injecting the shot into muscle. This is common in the deltoid muscle (upper lateral arm) area as there is not much fat. I would guess that you are also going straight in (not at a 45° angle) with the 5/8 inch needle, which almost always results in the insulin being given into muscle. When the insulin does go into muscle, it is absorbed more rapidly so that low blood sugars are common. Then there is not enough insulin left to have its normal effect 6-10 hours later. Sometimes, use of the short needles (5/16 inch) helps to prevent injections into muscle.

Q. We just gave our son his afternoon shot and accidentally gave the morning dose rather than the afternoon dose. What should we do?

A. We hear this question almost every week. The answer is to eat more at dinner and at the bedtime snack (pizza is particularly effective). In addition, it is wise to set the alarm for every two or three hours, get up, do a blood sugar and give extra juice or food. If the value falls to very low levels (below 70 mg/dl or 3.9 mmol/L), it is necessary to stay up and keep doing the blood sugars every 20 or 30 minutes until the value is above 120 mg/dl or 6.7 mmol/L. This problem can be handled and, in our experience, has never required hospitalization or resulted in a severe insulin reaction. Some families find that having the a.m. and p.m. insulin doses taped to the front of the refrigerator can be a helpful reminder. It may also be a good way to communicate or remember recent dosage changes. It is also effective to routinely have a second person check the dose.

Q. Lately, our needle has plugged half-way through the shot several times. What causes this and what should we do?

A. The plugging may be due to a small piece of fat getting into the needle. Occasionally, the insulin can also cause the plugging, particularly Ultralente insulin (Lente insulin is 70% Ultralente). Some people have also noted a greater likelihood of plugging with one brand of syringes compared to another, so you might consider a different brand and see if it makes a difference.

As noted in bold print in the section on "Plugged Needles," if plugging does occur, note precisely the number of units of insulin remaining in the syringe. It is then necessary to start over with a new syringe. Draw up the full injection dose of insulin and discard the extra down to the number of units of insulin still needed. Then inject this as with any shot.

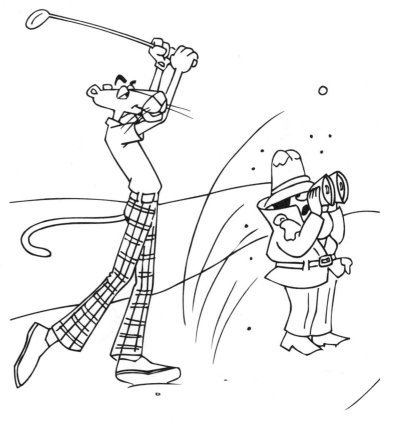

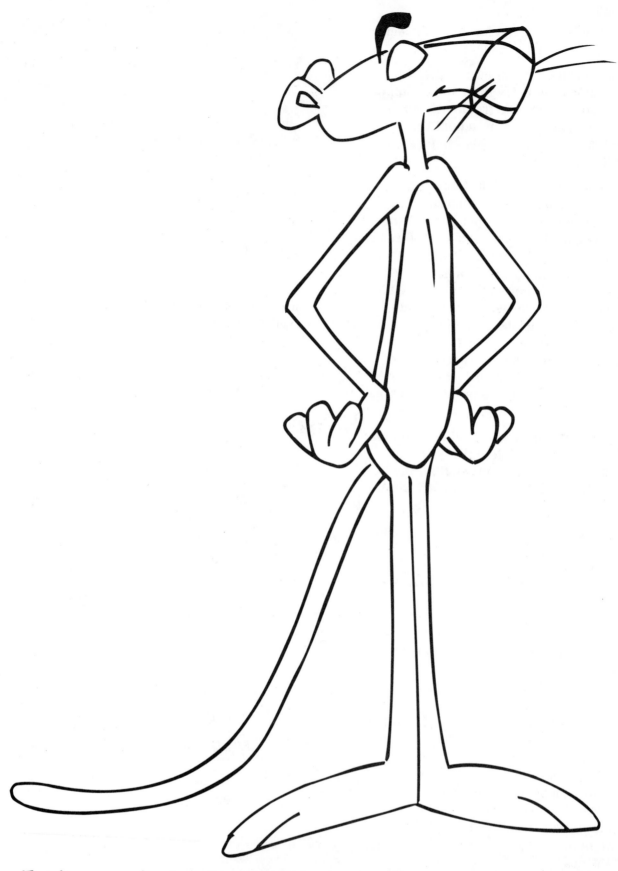

Feelings of shock, denial, and sadness are common reactions for people who learn they have diabetes.

Chapter FEELINGS AND DIABETES

Key ideas of this chapter:

🐾 Show awareness of the normal feelings that occur at the time of diagnosis of type 1 diabetes.

🐾 Realize that family members may be having different feelings, and that these are important to discuss.

🐾 Assist family members to identify and communicate their feelings.

This chapter deals with the normal feelings people have when they learn that a family member has diabetes. (Chapter 16 will cover other family concerns related to diabetes that may occur.) The emotions that one deals with at the diagnosis of diabetes are common with the onset of any serious medical condition. They are present in some form in **all** families who have a family member with diabetes. If families do not deal with the way they feel at the time of diagnosis, the feelings may linger and cause problems for many years. In our clinic, we ask **EVERY** newly diagnosed family to meet with the social worker or psychologist to discuss these feelings. Dealing with the feelings openly at the time of diagnosis will help with long-term adjustment.

CONFUSION, OR SHOCK, are common feelings for families. Some families feel like giving up when diabetes is diagnosed. They feel there is no hope and that this is the end of everything. The person that they thought was "perfect" will now be "different." The person will never be the same. This kind of sadness is similar to the process of mourning. The family mourns the loss of the person's health. These feelings are very natural. Diabetes may be the worst thing that has happened to the family. If the family learns as much as possible about the cause and the management of diabetes, and talks together about their feelings, everyone will do much better.

Because of the shock, it is often hard for families to think about what the medical team is saying in regards to diabetes. Sometimes they will ask to have things repeated. The medical team understands what the family is going through and is happy to go over the information several times. Because of the shock, and often a lack of sleep, many clinics teach only survival skills in the first day or two. They can then go into more depth at the one-week visit.

DENIAL is often expressed in comments such as, "This can't happen to us," or "This can't be happening to my child; there must be a mistake in the diagnosis." As a result, a family may want to seek second opinions from other doctors, hoping to be told that their family member doesn't have diabetes. This denial may make the person's and the family's struggle to adjust to the diagnosis much longer and more difficult. It may even interfere with medical treatment and education. Some family members may want to deny that they have any feelings at all about the diagnosis. Family members may not want to talk about the diabetes. If this happens, the person with diabetes may feel alone and the family members may not be able to help each other through a very stressful time. Sometimes people try to hide their feelings to be "strong" for a newly diagnosed person. Doing this may cause the person to feel that others don't care. IT IS IMPORTANT FOR CLOSE FRIENDS AND FAMILY TO SHARE THEIR FEELINGS ABOUT THE DIABETES.

SADNESS is a feeling that can be felt by any family member. Any member may cry, feel depressed, or feel hopeless. One teenager, shortly after she was diagnosed as having diabetes, began to cry each time she talked about living with diabetes and giving daily shots "for the rest of my life." A mother did well for three months after she learned her child had diabetes. She helped manage the diabetes and also cared for her other children. After three months, she began to cry often and had trouble caring for her family. It was important for this mother to share her feelings and to talk about her sadness. When she did, she began to feel better. A father expressed much sadness when his son was diagnosed with diabetes. Several days later, after discussing exercise and diabetes, he felt much better as he realized his son would still be able to participate in sports activities. Feeling sad is normal and brief periods of sadness can reoccur years later (see adjustment in this chapter).

ANGER is a feeling many families have. They may vent the anger toward the doctors, nurses, God, a husband or wife, the person who has diabetes, other family members, or even themselves. The person with diabetes often feels, "Why me? Why did I have to get diabetes? Did I do something wrong?" He or she may feel anger toward other healthy family members, or toward others for no apparent good reason. The anger may be expressed or it may be buried. Such anger, although it seems to have no reason, is a very normal feeling. It is important to find positive ways to let it out. This may be through talking with others or through sports or other activities. If it lasts for a long time, the person and family may have a hard time managing the diabetes. When these feelings are too strong or last a long time, family or individual counseling may be helpful.

FEAR may be felt by all the family members. The parents or spouse may fear the extra responsibilities and expenses associated with diabetes. Parents also fear not being able to manage the diabetes and doubt their abilities. Brothers and sisters may fear they might have or might get diabetes. The person with diabetes may fear such things as injections, hospitalizations, or death. He/she may fear being different from friends or family. Many of the fears may not be realistic. The family members should talk about their fears, both with each other and with the diabetes team. Then they can learn which fears are not realistic. If fears and concerns are shared with other people, they don't get "bottled-up" inside. This makes them easier to manage.

GUILT is a feeling common to many family members. Parents often feel that they "gave" their child diabetes. This idea occurs even though parents have been told that autoimmunity (self-allergy), viral infections, and other unknown factors are important in causing diabetes. We do not completely understand why someone develops diabetes. There is no proven way at this time to prevent it. Earlier diagnosis after the beginning of symptoms would not have prevented the diabetes from developing or changed the way diabetes is treated. One mother felt that because there was diabetes in her family, and not in her husband's, he must be blaming her for their child's diabetes. After months of worry and concern, she finally shared her feelings with her husband. He had not felt that way at all. Some young children feel that their diabetes is a punishment for bad behavior. Some family members may feel that "eating too much sugar" caused the child's diabetes. It didn't! These ideas can cause unnecessary guilt for everyone.

ADAPTATION OR ADJUSTMENT to the diagnosis of diabetes takes a long time. In an earlier edition of this book, the word "acceptance" was used. A knowledgeable parent related: "I won't accept the diagnosis, but I'll adapt or adjust to it." Often one parent will have stronger or more obvious feelings than the other parent. It helps to talk and share feelings within the family and with members of the diabetes team. We have every newly diagnosed family meet with a member of our psych-social staff. As the child and family live with diabetes, they become more used to it. They will feel more sure that they can manage it. Fears that have no reason will go away. Sadness and anger may still come and go at times. The parent may feel sadness when a child is hospitalized or when he or she sees pictures of the child before the diagnosis. Sometimes the parent may feel very sad for a moment, such as when kissing the child at bedtime. These feelings decrease with time. The continued love for the family member is the most important feeling and does not change.

As the family adjusts, the members begin to feel more hopeful. They may want to help in diabetes research studies or help diabetes support groups raise money. It is important not to look at diabetes as the end of the world. If all family members have a positive attitude, life with diabetes will be much easier. Fitting diabetes care into as normal a lifestyle as possible is a major goal.

DEFINITIONS

Adjustment (adaptation): Gradually learning to live with something (such as the diagnosis of diabetes).

Denial (deny): A refusal to believe something. A person may refuse to believe that he or she has diabetes.

Diagnosis: The process of finding that a person has a disease.

Guilt: A feeling that one caused something to happen.

QUESTIONS (Q) AND ANSWERS (A) FROM NEWSNOTES

Q. Why is the Pink Panther character used in the educational manual, *Understanding Insulin-Dependent Diabetes?*

A. Having a family member develop diabetes is often **the** most traumatic event that has happened to a family. If a child were pictured to demonstrate a side effect, such as hypoglycemia, it might be harder for a family member to accept than a picture of the Pink Panther having a reaction. Also, a bit of humor at this time of intense emotions can often be a big help.

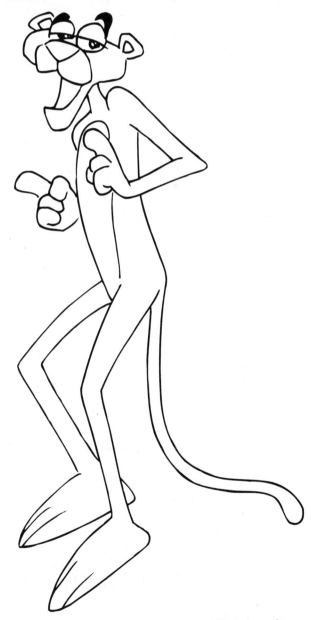

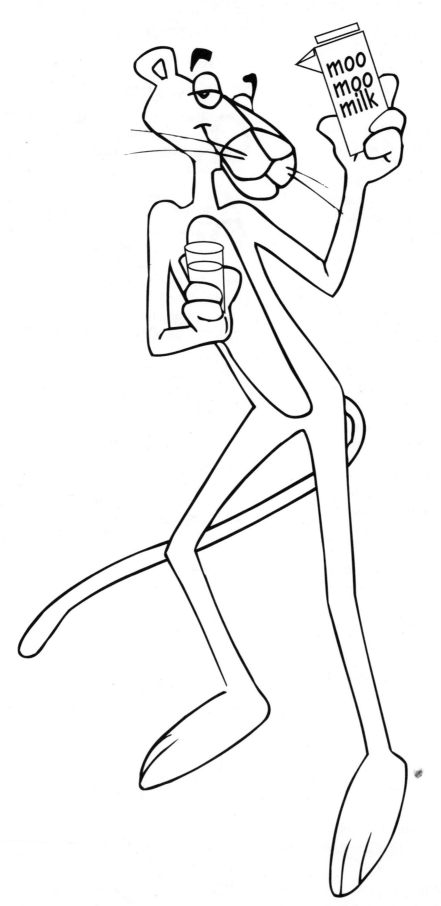

Eating nutritiously will benefit all family members.

Chapter 10 NORMAL NUTRITION

Key ideas of this chapter:

- Identify the main parts of a normal healthy diet.

- Assist family members to learn to read food labels so that they can make wise food choices.

TYPES OF NUTRIENTS

Families of a newly diagnosed person with diabetes are usually overly concerned and worried about what someone with diabetes should eat. They shouldn't be, as **the ideal diet for someone with diabetes is really just a healthy diet from which all people would benefit**. This chapter is meant to be a review of normal nutrition, which will help to improve the entire family's nutrition. It may be a good introduction to Chapter 11, Food Management and Diabetes. It may also make some of the words used by the dietitian easier to follow.

Foods provide different nutrients necessary for growth and health. If you know about these nutrients, you can help your family eat the right foods. Learn to read labels and know what you are buying at the grocery store. Types of nutrients include: 1) proteins; 2) carbohydrates; 3) fats; 4) vitamins and minerals; 5) water; and 6) fiber. Our bodies need some of all of these nutrients, but in differing amounts.

Proteins

Proteins are important for muscle and bone growth. However, eating extra protein does **not** cause increased muscle growth. Muscles only grow as a result of proper exercise. Foods high in protein include milk, meats, fish, chicken, turkey, egg whites, cheese, and cottage cheese. In addition to fish being a good source of protein, the fish oils (fats) are believed to help prevent heart disease (see "Fats" in this chapter). Protein should provide 10-20% of the total caloric intake. Proteins from animal sources are called **complete** proteins. This means they contain all of the essential building blocks of protein called amino acids.

Adults can receive adequate protein eating only a vegetarian diet, but this is more difficult for growing infants and children. Many people do not realize that protein also is available from non-meat sources. Dried beans, legumes, nuts, and seeds are fairly good sources of protein. However, most vegetable proteins are not complete proteins because they lack one or more of the essential amino acids. Vegetable proteins can be improved, however, when they are mixed with other foods. Thus, wheat (cereal, bread, tortillas) is not a complete protein by itself. However, when the cereal and milk are mixed, the cereal protein becomes a complete protein with all of the essential factors. The same happens when beans are eaten with a tortilla. Both the beans and the tortilla (wheat or corn) become complete proteins as a result of being combined.

Most people eat more protein than they need. In a review of three-day diet records from our clinic, the young men were getting approximately three times, and the young women two times the amount of protein needed. High protein intake usually results in high animal fat intake, which may be bad for the heart. It may also provide an extra stress for some people's kidneys. If only 10-20% of calories are to be from protein, the amount of meat and poultry eaten is quite often excessive (more than needed).

🐾 Carbohydrates

Carbohydrates are important mainly as an energy source for the body. It is currently recommended that carbohydrates make up 50-60% of our caloric intake. They are usually divided into two main types, starches ("complex" carbohydrates) and sugars ("simple" carbohydrates). It used to be believed that simple sugars were rapidly absorbed and complex carbohydrates were slowly absorbed. This is an easy concept to explain and to believe, but it is NOT true. Research has shown that there is no difference in absorption of a simple sugar as compared to a complex carbohydrate. This is because the intestine has such high levels of digestive enzymes that the complex carbohydrates are rapidly broken down to simple sugars. Thus, **"a carbohydrate is a carbohydrate is a carbohydrate..."** What is important is 1) **how much** carbohydrate is eaten; 2) **when** the carbohydrate is eaten; 3) **with what** the carbohydrate is eaten; and 4) **if adequate insulin activity is available** at that moment to allow the sugar to pass into the cells to be used for energy. Insulin is essential to allow sugar to pass into the cells of the body to be burned for energy. Thus, the balance between all carbohydrates eaten and the insulin dosage is one of the major keys to diabetes management. These concepts will be discussed in detail in the next chapter, Food Management and Diabetes.

More detailed knowledge about starches and simple sugars is helpful.

Starches (complex carbohydrates): Starches are substances made up of hundreds of sugar units. The sugar from starches is now known to be absorbed as quickly as from simple sugars (when each is taken alone without other foods). Sources of starch are breads, noodles, pasta, rice, cereals, potatoes, and starchy vegetables such as corn and legumes.

Simple sugars: The U.S. Dietary Guidelines recommend that all people should limit simple (refined) sugar intake to less than 10% of calories. A diet high in simple sugars contributes to dental cavities and provides few vitamins and minerals. As well as providing few vitamins and minerals, many high sugar foods also contain large amounts of fat. Thus, a nutritious diet limits the amount of high sugar foods. There are many different kinds of sugars found in foods. People with diabetes need to be aware of how much of all of these sugars they are eating (see Chapter 11). They are often added to foods as sweeteners and are not noticed unless labels are read. The names for sugars often end in "—ose." Some of the common sugars are listed below.

Glucose: Glucose is the name for the main sugar in our body. When we talk about blood and urine sugar, we really mean glucose. Table sugar is half glucose and half fructose. Another name for glucose is dextrose. Corn sugar is primarily glucose.

Fructose: Fructose is sometimes called "fruit sugar," as it is the main type of sugar found in fruits. It is sold in pure granulated form and is a part of many food products. Fructose has the same number of calories per gram as table sugar (sucrose). The liquid form is sweeter than table sugar, but the taste is the same in baked products. Generally, only one-half to one-third the amount of fructose needs to be used to have the same degree of sweetness as table sugar.

Fructose has some advantages. It is more slowly taken up from the intestine than is glucose. It does not need insulin to get into the cells to be burned for energy. However, it will raise blood sugar levels in a person who is not receiving enough insulin or in a person with poorly controlled diabetes. It may also increase one of the blood fats (triglycerides).

"High-fructose" corn syrup is different from pure fructose and contains large amounts of sucrose. People with diabetes need to be aware of how much of this is eaten.

Sucrose or table sugar: The body breaks down sucrose to glucose and fructose. Foods high in sucrose and glucose include cake, cookies, pie, candy, soft drinks, and other desserts.

Lactose or milk sugar: Lactose is found in milk and other dairy products. Children and adolescents should drink three to four 8 oz glasses of milk per day for calcium and vitamin D.

Maltose: One-hundred percent glucose. People with diabetes need to be aware of how much of this sugar they eat.

Syrups: Corn syrup, corn syrup solids, high fructose syrups, maple syrup, sorghum syrup, and sugar cane syrup are all primarily glucose and must be consumed carefully by people with diabetes.

❦ Fats

Fats are an important energy source and are needed for growth. However, fats should provide only 25-30% of total caloric intake. A major emphasis in nutrition in the past decade has been the reduction of the total daily fat intake. Higher fat intake may lead to elevated blood fat levels (see "cholesterol" in this chapter) and a higher risk for heart attacks. People may consume as much as 40-50% of calories from fat rather than the recommended 25-30%. Food eaten in fast-food restaurants is usually very high in fat. Fats have more calories (nine calories per gram) than proteins or carbohydrates (four calories per gram). Thus, they are more likely to lead to weight gain and obesity. Most effective long-term weight reduction programs emphasize the limiting of total fat intake.

The main fats in the diet are divided into three types. They are **polyunsaturated, monounsaturated** (mainly vegetable oils), and **saturated** (mainly animal fats). It is important to eat more of the polyunsaturated and monounsaturated than the saturated fats. Less than 10% of total calories eaten per day should be from saturated fat. As with reducing total fat intake, increasing this ratio of polyunsaturated to saturated fats can help to reduce blood cholesterol levels and to prevent heart attacks. Increasing the intake of monounsaturated fats (e.g., olive oil and canola oil) is also considered beneficial.

There are high amounts of polyunsaturated fats in most vegetable oils (coconut and palm are exceptions). Margarines made from vegetable oils are also polyunsaturated. In general, the softer or more liquid a fat is at room temperature, the less saturated it is. For example, liquid margarine is a better choice than stick margarine, and vegetable oil is better than vegetable shortening.

The saturated fats include most animal fats, such as the fat in meats, milk, butter, and lard. Animals are now less apt to be "fattened" (e.g., cows in a feed lot) and the fat content of some meats is decreasing. Chicken, turkey, and fish are lower in saturated fat than beef or pork, particularly when the skin is removed. Chicken, turkey, and fish also contain some polyunsaturated fat.

High levels of the two main blood fats, **cholesterol** and **triglyceride**, can lead to early aging of the large blood vessels. These vessels carry blood to the heart, legs, and other body parts. Other causes of early aging of large blood vessels are diabetes, smoking cigarettes, high blood pressure, lack of exercise, and being overweight. As people with diabetes already have one risk factor (by having diabetes), they do not need another. Research from the Barbara Davis Center has

MAKING FOOD CHOICES FOR FAT CONTENT

Table 1

Food Group (Amount)	Decrease	Instead Choose
Meat, Poultry, and Fish ≤5-6 oz per day	Beef, pork, lamb—regular ground beef, fatty cuts, spare ribs, organ meats	Lean beef, pork, lamb—lean cuts, well-trimmed before cooking
	Poultry with skin, fried chicken	Poultry without skin
	Fried fish, fried shellfish	Fish, shellfish
	Regular luncheon meat (e.g., bologna, salami, sausage, frankfurters)	Processed meat—prepared from lean meat (e.g., lean ham, lean frankfurters, lean meat with soy protein or carrageenin)
Eggs ≤2 yolks per week	Egg yolks: limit to two per week (includes eggs used in cooking and baking)	Egg whites (two whites can be substituted for one whole egg in recipes), cholesterol-free egg substitute
Dairy Products 2-3 servings per day	Whole milk (fluid, evaporated, condensed), 2% fat milk (low-fat milk), imitation milk	Milk—skim, 1/2%, or 1% fat (fluid, powdered, evaporated)
	Whole milk yogurt, whole milk yogurt beverages	Yogurt—nonfat or low-fat yogurt or yogurt beverages
	Regular cheeses (American, blue, Brie, cheddar, Colby, Edam, Monterey Jack, whole-milk mozzarella, Parmesan, Swiss), cream cheese, Neufchatel cheese	Cheese—low-fat natural or processed cheese
	Cottage cheese (4% fat)	Low-fat or nonfat varieties of cottage cheese (e.g., cottage cheese—low-fat, nonfat, or dry curd [0-2% fat])
	Ice cream	Frozen dairy dessert—ice milk, frozen yogurt (low-fat or nonfat), nonfat ice cream
	Cream, half & half, whipped cream, nondairy creamer, whipped topping, sour cream	Low-fat coffee creamer, low-fat or nonfat sour cream
Fats and Oils ≤6-8 teaspoons per day	Coconut oil, palm kernel oil, palm oils	Polyunsaturated oils—safflower, sunflower, corn, canola*, olive*, peanut
	Butter, lard, shortening, bacon fat, hard margarine	Margarine—made from unsaturated oils listed above, light or diet margarine, especially soft or liquid forms

*High in mono-saturated fats.
Adapted from Powers, MA; Handbook of Diabetes Medical Nutrition Therapy, Aspen Publishers, Inc. Gaithersburg, MD, 1996 p. 354.

shown that children with poorly controlled diabetes have higher blood cholesterol and triglyceride levels than children who have good diabetes control or who don't have diabetes. In addition to poor diabetes control, eating foods high in total fat, trans-fatty acids, animal (saturated) fat, or high in cholesterol (see Table 1) often results in higher blood cholesterol levels. The trans-fatty acids are the partially hydrogenated fats found in solid margarines, salad dressings, commercial cookies, crackers and other foods made with hydrogenated shortenings. More information is still needed about trans-fatty acids, but there seems to be an association with heart disease. **We recommend a low fat diet that allows no more than 30% of total calories from fat.** We also recommend limiting intake of foods that are high in cholesterol and animal (saturated) fat. This is discussed in more detail in the next chapter. Reduction of total fat, animal (saturated) fat, and cholesterol intake are good nutrition practices whether a person does or doesn't have diabetes. Fish and poultry (with the skin removed) should be included in the diet. Studies have shown that eating cold-water fish, which have omega-3 fatty acids, twice a week will reduce the chance of heart attacks. Milk should have no more than 1% fat. Canola, olive, corn, safflower, or soy oils should be used for salads and cooking. Suggestions for improving the fat content of food choices are shown in Table 1.

🐾 Vitamins and Minerals

These are important for growth, formation of blood cells, healthy skin, good vision, and strong teeth and bones. Fruits and vegetables are rich in vitamins. Vitamins E and C have antioxidant properties that may be important in preventing heart or blood vessel disease. Minerals are found in milk, meats, and vegetables. Calcium is a mineral that is important for the bones and teeth. People who do not drink milk may need to take a calcium supplement. The calcium content of some common foods is shown in Table 2. Children ages 1–3 years need 400 mg of calcium per day and those who are 4–10 years need 800 mg of calcium per day. Most people 10-20 years old need 1300 mg of calcium per day.

Zinc is a mineral that is lost in the urine in proportion to sugar in the urine. Zinc is important for growth. Some children with diabetes may grow better with a zinc supplement.

Sodium is also a mineral which, in some "salt-sensitive" people, may relate to higher blood pressure. It is now recommended that all people limit their sodium to no more than 3000 mg (1 1/4 tsp of table salt) per day. If the blood pressure is elevated, this amount should be even lower (2,400 mg of sodium or about 1 tsp of table salt). Salt in the food we eat (e.g., chips, hamburgers, hot dogs, and prepared foods) is often "hidden," but may be a significant source of salt.

Generally, people who eat a well-balanced diet do not need extra vitamins. If a child does not eat a balanced diet (e.g., not liking yellow or green vegetables), a vitamin supplement may be helpful. Also, vitamins and minerals often are recommended in the month following onset of diabetes as the body rebuilds. In general, "mega" doses of nutrients should be avoided, and the vitamins should not contain more than 100% of the recommended daily allowance (RDA). The fat soluble vitamins (A, D, E and K) are stored in the body and excessive doses can be harmful. If you do take vitamins, choose a multi-vitamin with trace minerals that includes zinc, iron, and calcium.

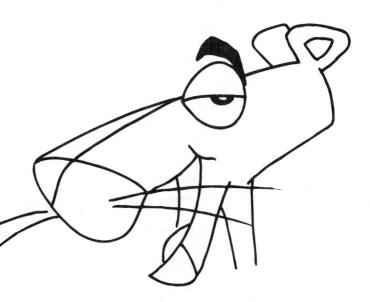

CALCIUM CONTENT OF COMMON FOODS

Food	Quantity	Calcium (mg)
Milk and Dairy Products		
American Cheese	1 oz	174
Cheddar Cheese	1 oz	204
Cottage Cheese, creamed	1 cup	126
Mozzarella Cheese, part skim	1 oz	195
Swiss Cheese	1 oz	272
Ice Cream, hard	1 cup	176
Whole Milk	1 cup	291
Low-fat Milk (2%)	1 cup	297
Skim Milk	1 cup	302
Low-fat Plain Yogurt	1 cup	415
Low-fat Plain Yogurt, with fruit	1 cup	345
Ricotta Cheese, part skim	1/2 cup	337
Green Leafy Vegetables		
Broccoli, cooked	1 cup	178
Spinach, cooked	1 cup	244
Turnip Greens, cooked	1 cup	198
Other Vegetables		
Beans, canned with pork and tomato	1/2 cup	68
Beans, green, cooked	1 cup	58
Sweet Potato, baked in skin	1 small	40
Nuts		
Almonds, roasted and salted	1/4 cup	92
Sesame Seeds, dried, hulled	1/4 cup	40
Sunflower Seeds, dry roasted	1/4 cup	22
Seafood		
*Sardines, in oil, drained	3 oz	372
Scallops, steamed	3 1/2 oz	115
Shrimp, raw	3 1/2 oz	63
*Salmon, canned	3 1/2 oz	249
Other Foods		
Bread, white or whole wheat	2 slices	46
Chili con Carne, with beans	5 oz	61
Cream of Celery Soup, made with milk	1 serving	135
Figs, dried	5 medium	126
Orange	1 medium	56
12 inch cheese pizza	1 slice	56
Raisins, seedless	5/8 cup	62
Tofu	4 oz	154
Waffles, plain, enriched	1 medium	85

Children and adults need 400-1300 mg of calcium per day (see text).

* The bones of sardines and salmon must be eaten to get the full calcium value.

Water

Water is the most important nutrient for the survival of humans. It makes up much of the blood, the body fluids and the body's transport system. It serves as a coolant, shock absorber, and waste remover. It has many other important functions. Since the body is made-up of about two-thirds water, it is important to drink a good deal of it. We recommend at least six 8 oz glasses of liquid per day, including allowed juices and milk. When a person with diabetes is spilling urine ketones, it is important to drink more water and sugar-free liquids. This helps to replace body fluid loss.

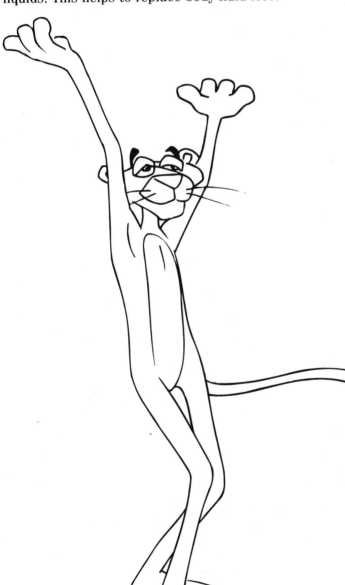

Fiber

Dietary fiber is the part of plants ("roughage" or "bulk") that is not digested and is not absorbed into the body. Foods vary in the amounts and kinds of fiber they contain (see Table 3). Fiber in the diet supplies bulk (without calories) and roughage, which helps satisfy the appetite and keep the digestive system running smoothly. In people with type 2 (adult-onset) diabetes, increased fiber intake has been helpful in slowing the absorption of sugar. Fiber has not been as helpful in lowering blood sugar levels in people with type 1 diabetes.

Fiber often is divided into two types. The first is **water-soluble fiber**, such as parts of oats and beans, seeds, citrus fruits, and apples. These may help lower the blood cholesterol levels. They also may help reduce the blood sugar levels in the period after meals in people with type 2 diabetes. The other type, **water-insoluble fiber**, such as parts of wheat bran, most grains, nuts, and vegetables, helps prevent constipation and may help other digestive disorders. Examples of the fiber content of various foods are shown in Table 3. The current recommendation is to eat between 20 grams and 35 grams of fiber in the daily diet. Note that a serving of the cereal shown in Table 3 has 2.5 grams of fiber. If eaten along with two slices of whole wheat bread and a whole banana, the fiber intake would be 8.1 grams (Table 3) for breakfast. Teenagers (and most Americans) do not eat the recommended eight exchanges of fruits and vegetables (combined) as outlined in the 2500 to 3500 calorie diets in Table 7, Chapter 11. Total fiber intake, as a result, is usually lower than recommended.

DIETARY FIBER IN FOODS*

Bread and Crackers	Amount	Weight (gm)	Fiber (gm)
Graham cracker	2 squares	14	1.4
Pumpernickel bread	1 slice	24	1.4
Rye bread	1 slice	25	0.8
Whole wheat bread	1 slice	25	1.3
Whole wheat cracker	6 crackers	19	2.2
Whole wheat roll	3/4 roll	21	1.2
Cereal			
All Bran, 100%	1/3 cup	28	8.4
Bran Chex®	1/2 cup	21	4.1
Corn Bran	1/2 cup	21	4.4
Corn Flakes	3/4 cup	21	2.6
Grapenuts Flakes®	2/3 cup	21	2.5
Grapenuts®	3 Tbsp	21	2.7
Oatmeal	3/4 package	21	2.5
Shredded Wheat®	1 biscuit	21	2.8
Wheaties®	3/4 cup	21	2.6
Fruits			
Apple	1/2 large	83	2.0
Apricot	2	72	1.4
Banana	1/2 medium	54	1.5
Blackberries	3/4 cup	108	6.7
Cantaloupe	1 cup	160	1.6
Cherries	10 large	68	1.1
Dates, dried	2	18	1.6
Figs, dried	1 medium	20	3.7
Grapes, white	10	50	0.5
Grapefruit	1/2	87	0.8
Honeydew melon	1 cup	170	1.5
Orange	1 small	78	1.6
Peach	1 medium	100	2.3
Pear	1/2 medium	82	2.0
Pineapple	1/2 cup	78	0.8
Plum	3 small	85	1.8
Prunes, drained	2	15	2.4
Raisins	1 1/2 Tbsp	14	1.0
Strawberries	1 cup	143	3.1
Tangerine	1 large	101	2.0
Watermelon	1 cup	160	1.4
Rice			
Rice, brown (cooked)	1/3 cup	65	1.6
Rice, white (cooked)	1/3 cup	68	0.5
Leaf Vegetables			
Broccoli	1/2 cup	93	3.5
Brussel sprouts	1/2 cup	78	2.3
Cabbage	1/2 cup	85	2.1
Cauliflower	1/2 cup	90	1.6
Celery	1/2 cup	60	1.1
Lettuce	1 cup	55	0.8
Spinach, raw	1 cup	55	0.2

DIETARY FIBER IN FOODS*

Root Vegetables	Amount	Weight (gm)	Fiber (gm)
Beets	1/2 cup	85	2.1
Carrots	1/2 cup	78	2.4
Potatoes, baked	1/2 medium	75	1.9
Radishes	1/2 cup	58	1.3
Sweet potatoes, baked	1/2 medium	75	2.1
Other Vegetables			
Beans, green	1/2 cup	64	2.1
Beans, string	1/2 cup	55	1.9
Cucumber	1/2 cup	70	1.0
Eggplant	1/2 cup	100	2.5
Lentils, cooked	1/2 cup	100	3.7
Mushrooms	1/2 cup	35	0.9
Onions	1/2 cup	58	1.2
Tomatoes	1 small	100	1.5
Winter squash	1/2 cup	120	3.5
Zucchini squash	1/2 cup	65	2.0

Adapted from: Anderson, J.W.: Plant Fiber in Foods, University of Kentucky Medical Center, 1980.

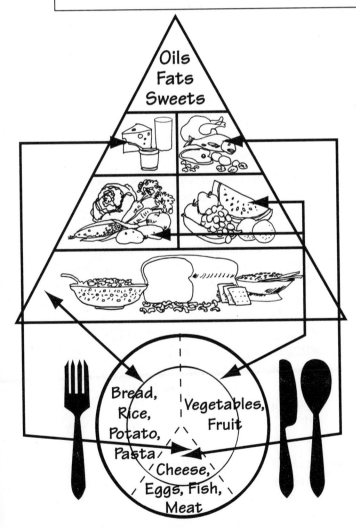

The Daily Plate of Food.

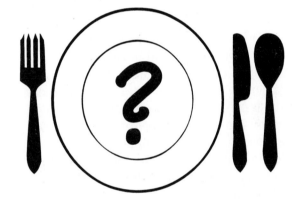

What does your plate for a day look like?

You probably need to:

1. Eat more starchy foods (e.g., bread, rice, potato, and pasta);

2. Eat more fruits and vegetables;

3. Eat less protein and fat (particularly red meat).

Others

Foods such as tea with no sugar, diet pops, clear broth, fat-free bouillon, unsweetened gelatin, mustard, unsweetened pickles, and spices have few or no calories and little sugar. As long as you don't eat too much of these foods, you will not need to count them in your diet.

Food Groups

Foods are often divided into groups or exchanges (see Chapter 11). The common divisions include the milk, meat, bread, fruit, vegetable, and fat groups. The milk and the meat groups are important sources of protein, and the milk group is a major source of calcium and vitamin D. Some of the minerals such as iron and zinc are high in the meat groups. Vitamins are generally highest in the fruit and vegetable groups. Just be aware that some foods from each of the food groups should be eaten daily to have a well-balanced diet.

Three-day Food Record

It is good to keep a three-day food record once a year. This will show you if you are eating the right foods. Write down all foods and the amounts you eat for three days, as shown in the Appendix in this Chapter. The dietitian can use the record to suggest changes in your diet. While you are doing the recording, eat as you usually do; this way you will get the right information. If you would like to do this and feel you need more help with instructions, ask your dietitian for help.

SWEETENERS (Sugar-substitutes)

Thousands of foods are now available which contain sweeteners that either do not raise the blood sugar, or which may cause less of an increase than would a similar amount of table sugar. They are divided into the **nutritive sweeteners** (including table sugar), which do provide calories and carbohydrate, and the **non-nutritive sweeteners,** which essentially provide no calories or carbohydrate.

🐾 Nutritive Sweeteners

These include all sugars and all sugar-alcohols. They contain four grams of carbohydrate and 16 calories per level teaspoon. The two main sugars used as sweeteners are sucrose (table sugar) and fructose. Both are discussed earlier in this chapter under Carbohydrates, and both cause an increase in blood sugar levels. High-fructose corn syrup is a combination of both sugars and raises the blood sugar more than pure fructose. Foods sweetened with fruit juices, dates or raisins may have the label "no added sugar." This is misleading as there is sugar in these food-additives.

The sugar alcohols include sorbitol, xylitol, mannitol, and others (often ending in—ol). They provide about two grams of carbohydrate and eight calories per teaspoon. They are more slowly absorbed than sugar, and eating an excessive amount can cause diarrhea. They are often found in "sugar-free" candies.

🐾 Non-nutritive Sweeteners

The non-nutritive (or "artificial") sweeteners do not provide any calories or carbohydrate. The five currently on the market are:

Saccharin: Saccharin is 200-700 times sweeter than table sugar. Saccharin can cause bladder tumors in mice (but this has not been found in humans). It is found in Sweet'N Low®, other table top sweeteners and in some diet pops.

Aspartame: Aspartame is 200 times sweeter than table sugar. It is broken down into aspartic acid, methanol and phenylalanine. (Rare patients with a condition called phenylketonuria cannot metabolize phenylalanine and cannot eat foods with this sweetener.) People have suggested that the methanol (or its breakdown product, formaldehyde), could be bad for one's health, but there is **NO SCIENTIFIC DATA TO SUPPORT THIS IN HUMANS**. The products that contain aspartame include: Equal®, NutraSweet®, diet pop, sugar-free JELL-O®, Kool-Aid®, ice cream, Crystal Light® and many others. Use in moderation is generally advised (no more than two diet pops per day!)

Acesulfame-K (Ace-K): Ace-K is 200 times sweeter than table sugar. It is approved for use as a table-top sweetener (Sweet-One® or

Sunnette®) and for use in chewing gum, desserts, beverages and other products. It is used in PEPSI-ONE®, along with aspartame.

Sucralose: Sucralose was approved for use in 1998 and is 600 times sweeter than sugar. It is used as a table-top sweetener (Splenda®) and is found in RC Cola® and in Ocean Spray Lightstyle Juices®.

Stevia: Stevia is a natural alternative sweetener from the herb, Stevia Rebaudiana. It is 300 times sweeter than sugar.

LABEL READING

Label reading has become easier for people in the U.S., as labeling the nutrient content of products is now required by law. Thus, smart buyers can learn a lot about the foods they are considering to buy by learning to read labels. The information that can be gained from reading a label is discussed in Table 4.

If you are interested in the carbohydrate content for carbohydrate (or "carb") counting (see Chapter 11), it is listed under "total carbohydrate" on most labels. In the U.S., one carbohydrate count is considered to be 15 grams of carbohydrate. The counts are approximate so that a food having 12 grams may be rounded off to one exchange. Grams of fiber (which are not absorbed) can be subtracted from the grams of total carbohydrate. Carbohydrate counting is discussed in detail in the next chapter.

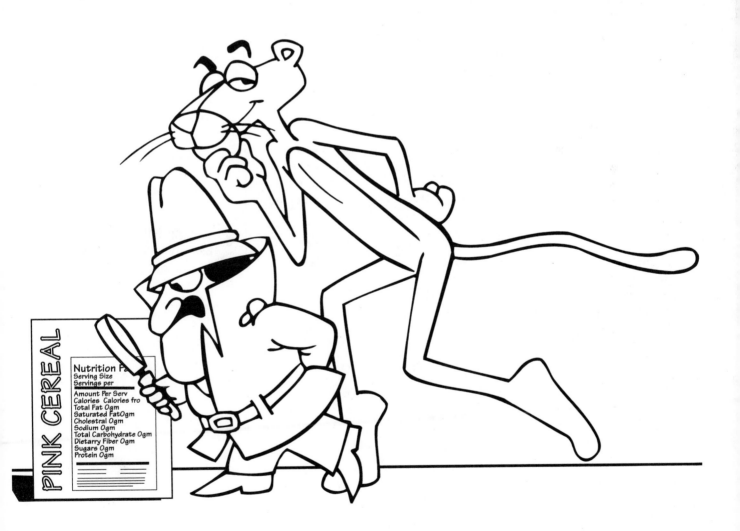

Table 4

READING A NUTRITION LABEL

- The serving size is shown at the top. It is important to observe the serving size. (This is often less than the amount people eat. If you eat two cups rather than one, you would need to double all of the daily values eaten.)

- The total calories and the calories from fat per serving are routinely given and are important.

- The total fat includes all types of fat (saturated, polyunsaturated, and monounsaturated). The total fat, saturated fat and cholesterol content are all important in relation to heart disease and it is wise to look for lower fat choices.

- The saturated fats for the entire day should be under 10% of the total calories per day. This would mean under 200 calories from saturated fat or under 22 grams (nine calories per gram).

- †The percent of daily values for fat, carbohydrate, and protein are listed here based on a 2,000-calorie daily intake. More active people will need more calories, in which case, these amounts make up a smaller percentage of total daily allowances.

Nutrition Facts

Serving Size 1.0 Cup (120g)
Servings Per Container   8

Amount Per Serving

Calories 130   Calories From Fat 60

% Daily Value †

Total Fat 6.5g	10%
Saturated Fat 2.5g	12%
Cholesterol 30mg	10%
Sodium 240mg	10%
Total Carbohydrate 15g	5%
Dietary Fiber 2.5g	10%
Sugars 3g	
Protein 3g	6%

Vitamin A 10%		Vitamin E 5%	
Calcium 15%		Iron 5%	

†Percent Daily Values are based on a 2,000-calorie diet. Your daily values may be higher or lower depending on your calorie needs:

	2,000	2,500	3,200
Calories:	2,000	2,500	3,200
Total Fat (g)	65	80	107
Sat Fat (g)	20	25	36
Cholesterol (mg)	300	300	300
Sodium (mg)	2,400	2,400	2,400
Total Carb (g)	300	375	480
Fiber	25	30	37

Calories per gram:

Fat 9   Carbohydrate 4   Protein 4

Ingredients: Whole wheat, oat bran, raisins, gelatin, malt, flavoring, vitamins, and minerals.

- For those who count carbohydrates, one helping of this cereal has 15 grams of carbohydrate, which is one carbohydrate choice (or count). If one cup of white milk (any type) is added, then one additional carbohydrate choice must also be added, so that there would be a total of two carb choices. The sugars include those found naturally in the food, as well as those added to the food. Both are included in the grams of "Total Carbohydrate." Dietary fiber is also included, but because it is not absorbed, most people who count carbs subtract it from the total carbohydrate.

- The recommended daily amounts for cholesterol, sodium (salt), and fiber stay the same for the 24-hour period for the three caloric intakes.

- The ingredients are also usually included on the label (in the order of the amount present).

FAST-FOOD RESTAURANTS

It is difficult to eat at fast-food restaurants and not eat foods high in animal fat, calories, and salt. Eating at fast-food restaurants goes against good nutrition principles and may be bad for the heart. In addition, meals are usually low in vitamin-containing fruits and vegetables. Some fast-food restaurants are now trying to provide healthier food choices (salads, leaner meat, and deep-frying in vegetable oils rather than animal fat). However, eating at fast-food restaurants should be limited.

ALCOHOL

We hesitate to discuss alcohol under normal nutrition. It is, of course, illegal for children and adolescents to use alcohol prior to reaching the legal drinking age in a particular state or country. We do not condone alcohol use for children or adolescents. However, exposure often begins prior to the legal drinking age. Education is important, regardless of the age.

Blood sugars may initially be elevated after drinking alcohol; beer, for example, contains a fair amount of carbohydrate. However, the more dangerous effect of alcohol is the lowering of the blood sugar level (as much as 6-12 hours later). The alcohol prevents the other foods stored in the body from being converted to blood sugar. Some general rules, if alcohol consumption is to occur, are listed below.

- Use alcohol only in moderation. Sip slowly and make a drink last a long time.

- Eat when consuming alcohol. Never drink on an empty stomach.

- A low blood sugar is the main worry—and a bedtime snack (solid protein and some carbohydrate) must be taken after drinking in the evening, even if the bedtime blood sugar level is high.

- The next morning, get up at the usual time, test blood sugar, take insulin, eat breakfast, and then go back to bed if you feel ill. "Sleeping-in" can result in a bad reaction.

- NEVER drink and drive. Ask a friend who has not been drinking to drive, or call someone to come and get you.

A college student, helping to teach our College Workshop course to newly-graduated high school seniors, had a useful recommendation regarding college parties. He noted that if he had a cup in his hand, no one tried to push further drinks. In contrast, if his hands were empty (no glass), he received a lot of pressure. The answer was to hold the same cup all evening and to just have fun!

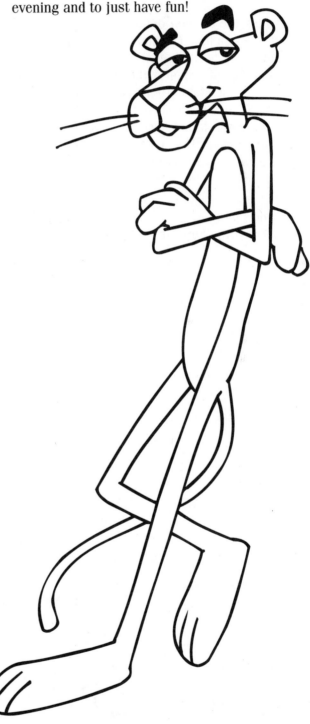

APPENDIX TO CHAPTER 10
THREE-DAY FOOD RECORD FORM

Instructions for completing food record form:

1. Please write down everything you eat or drink for three days. This includes meals and snacks. Often it's easier to remember what you eat if you record your food intake at the time you eat it.

2. Include the amount of food or beverage eaten. Also include the method of preparation (baked, fried, broiled, etc.), as well as any brand names of products (labels can also be enclosed). Use standard measuring cups or spoons. Record meat portions in ounces after cooking. If you do not have a scale, you can estimate ounces. The size of a deck of cards is about equal to three ounces of meat.

3. Be sure to include items added to your food. For example, include salad dressing on salad, margarine or butter on bread.

4. Include any supplements you take (vitamin, mineral, or protein powders). Write down the name of the supplement, what it contains and the amount taken. Include a copy of the label, if possible.

5. Please include meal and snack times, blood glucose values, amount of insulin, type of food, amount of food, grams of carbohydrate, and any activity or exercise.

The following is an example of how to complete your food record. Please record what you eat on the forms on the following page. The forms can then be faxed or mailed to your diabetes care provider. An example for the start of a day follows:

Time	Blood Glucose	Insulin	Food (include amounts)	Carbs	Activity
8:00	170	4R/10N	Cheerios-3/4 cup	15 gms	
			Skim milk-1/2 cup	6 gms	
			Orange juice-1 cup	30 gms	
9:00					Jog-20 min.

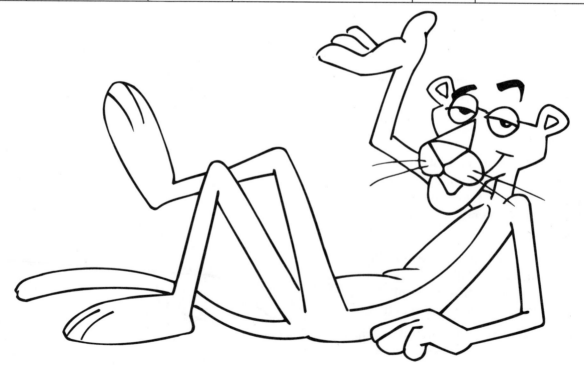

   Chapter 10: Normal Nutrition

THREE-DAY FOOD RECORD FORM

Name:_____ Home Phone: _____

Date: _____ Work Phone: _____

Dietitian: _____ Best time to be reached: _____

Time	Blood Glucose	Insulin	Food (include amounts)	Carbs	Activity

This page may be copied as often as desired. (Record three separate days of records.)

DEFINITIONS

Acesulfame-K: An artificial sweetener which does not need insulin to be absorbed by the body.

It is available in foods such as Sunnette or as Sweet-One when used as a sweetener at the table.

Artificial sweetener: A very sweet substance (usually 100-200 times sweeter than table sugar) used in very small amounts (and thus having almost no calories) to make foods or drinks taste sweet.

Aspartame: An artificial sweetener which does not need insulin to be absorbed by the body. It is available as a tablet or powder called "Equal" or "NutraSweet."

Calorie: A measurement of the food taken into the body for energy.

Caloric intake: Refers to the energy from foods that are eaten.

Carbohydrate: One of the main energy nutrients. It supplies energy for the body and is further divided into sugars and starches. Carbohydrates are found in all fruits and vegetables, all grain products, dried beans and peas, milk and yogurt. Carbohydrates include:

Starch: Complex carbohydrates such as vegetables, pasta, whole grain breads and cereals.

Sugar: Simple carbohydrates such as table sugar, honey, the four sugars listed below, and others.

Fructose: The type of sugar found in fruit. It does not require insulin in order for the body to use it.

Glucose: The main type of sugar found in the blood and urine. It is this sugar that is elevated in people with diabetes. Table sugar is half glucose.

Lactose: The main sugar found in milk. It needs insulin to be used completely.

Sucrose: Table sugar or "granulated sugar"—the body breaks it down to glucose and fructose. The glucose needs insulin to be used.

Cholesterol: A fat present in foods from animals. It is also made in our body. Our blood cholesterol level results from our own body's production (85%) and from the animal products we eat (15%). A high blood cholesterol (>200 mg/dl) results in a greater risk for heart attacks.

Cup (c): A measure of volume of eight ounces or 240cc (ml). Two cups equal one pint. Four cups equal one quart.

Dextrose: Another name for glucose.

Dietetic: This just means that at least one part of the food has been changed (e.g., salt, sugar, or fat). It does not necessarily mean the sugar has been removed!

Exchange: Division of foods into six groups. Each exchange within the six groups contains a similar amount of carbohydrate, protein, fat, and calories.

Fats: One of the energy nutrients. Total fat includes:

Polyunsaturated fats: Fats found mainly in vegetable oils.

Saturated fats: Fats found mainly in animal foods.

Monounsaturated fats: Fats that have one double bond. It is high in olive and canola oils. When large amounts (3 Tbsp) are consumed each day, blood cholesterol levels will be lower.

Cholesterol and Triglyceride: Fats present in foods and in our bodies. High cholesterol and triglyceride blood levels for many years are a cause of "clogged" blood vessels and heart attacks.

Fiber: The parts of plants in food that are not absorbed by the body.

Gram (gm): A unit of weight in the metric system; 1000 grams is equal to 1 kg. There are 448 grams in one pound. Carbohydrate, protein, and fat in foods are measured as grams. Information can be obtained from label reading. One gram of carbohydrate provides four calories. One gram of protein provides four calories. One gram of fat provides nine calories.

Ounce (oz): A unit of weight equivalent to 28 grams. It is also equal to 30cc (ml) of water.

Mannitol: A sugar alcohol that is used in foods to give a sweet taste. It does provide calories, but doesn't increase the blood sugar as much as sucrose. Too much will cause diarrhea or an upset stomach.

Protein: One of the energy nutrients. It is found in meat, eggs, fish, milk products and, in lesser amounts, in vegetables and other non-meat products.

Registered Dietitian (R.D.): A person trained to help you with your diet. He or she has a minimum of a four year college degree in nutrition or a related area, has completed an internship, and has passed a national exam.

Saccharin: An artificial sweetener (e.g., Sweet'N Low) which needs no insulin and provides no calories.

Sorbitol: A sugar alcohol that is used in foods to give a sweet taste. It does provide calories, but does not increase the blood sugar as much as sucrose.

Tablespoon (Tbsp): A measure of 3 tsp or 15cc (ml). It is equal to 15 grams (1/2 oz) of water. There are 16 tablespoons of sugar (sucrose) in one cup.

Teaspoon (tsp): A measure of 5cc (ml). It is also equal to five grams of water.

QUESTIONS (Q) AND ANSWERS (A) FROM NEWSNOTES

Q. What is fiber and what is its value in the diabetic diet?

A. Fiber is generally defined as the part of food that is not able to be broken down by the enzymes in the intestine. In the past 50-100 years, the food industry has moved toward the purification of foods, leaving out the parts our bodies cannot absorb and assuming they were of no value. It was forgotten that man had developed over millions of years eating much fiber in his foods. Then in the 1960s, two British epidemiologists noted that African natives had little or no problem with appendicitis, cancer of the colon, obesity, gallstones, adult diabetes, hemorrhoids, constipation, diverticulitis, gallbladder disease, and several other diseases which were fairly common in industrialized countries. They developed the "fiber hypothesis" and gave reasons why each of these diseases could be related to lack of fiber intake.

Some of the physiological effects of fiber are to prolong the time it takes food to leave the stomach, to shorten the transit of food through the rest of the intestine, to reduce fat absorption, and to increase stool weight and bulk. Pressure in the colon is generally reduced.

The effect of fiber in the diabetic diet primarily relates to the delay in food leaving the stomach. For example, sugar (such as in sugar pop) eaten with a high-fiber food (such as whole wheat bread) might slowly trickle from the stomach for slow absorption with a mild increase in the blood sugar. When the same food (sugar pop) is consumed alone, it all passes immediately into the intestine for immediate absorption. (We measured one boy's blood sugar after consuming sugar pop alone, watching it rise from 250 to 450 mg/dl [13.9 to 25 mmol/L] in 30 minutes.)

Although fiber sounds like a blessing for the diabetic diet, it has been more useful in adult-onset (type 2) diabetes than in type 1 (childhood or insulin-dependent) diabetes. So many things affect the person with type 1 diabetes, particularly insulin dose and exercise, that altering one part of the diet (fiber) and expecting miraculous changes in diabetes control has not been realistic.

Increasing fiber intake should still be a goal for all children and young adults. The high-fiber foods are mainly vegetables, bran or whole grain cereals, whole wheat or rye bread, and fruits. Approximately one cup of vegetables (two vegetable exchanges) and five fruit exchanges (e.g., 2 1/2 bananas, or 2 1/2 medium apples) should be aimed for in all our diets, just to meet the "Prudent American Diet." At least twice this many fruits and vegetables, plus all whole wheat and rye bread and daily exchanges of beans, would be required for the high-fiber, high-carbohydrate diet.

It is unrealistic to think of requiring our teenagers to eat the high-carbohydrate, high-fiber diet when one survey showed that half of all U.S. teenagers eat less than one helping of fruit or vegetable per day. They are not even near the eight "exchanges" of fruits and vegetables (combined) currently recommended for all teens, much less the higher quantities required for the high-fiber diet. The question, "Where's the beef?" missed the point entirely for our teenagers. They eat too much hamburger already! The real question is, "Where are the fruits and vegetables?"

Fortunately, children with diabetes do far better than most teenagers. This is because of the teaching they regularly receive in the diabetes clinic, and meeting with the dietitians on a regular basis. Families who come to clinic and do not take advantage of this opportunity for their youth to learn about good nutrition are missing a unique opportunity.

Q. Why do you check the blood cholesterol levels each year on the people seen at the Clinic?

A. Blood cholesterol levels (and when possible, triglyceride and lipoprotein levels) are one of the best predictors of who will have heart problems in later life. When someone with diabetes becomes older, this becomes an important concern. The two other big risk factors for coronary artery disease are cigarette smoking and high blood pressure. Needless to say, no one with diabetes should smoke—and blood pressures should be checked at regular clinic visits.

Research from the Clinic was among the first to show that children with diabetes have an increased problem with elevated blood cholesterol levels. When the high levels are found, the first concern always relates to the diabetes control. If the control is poor (high hemoglobin A_{1c} level), the high cholesterol may be secondary to the poor diabetes control. If the diabetes control is good and the blood cholesterol level is still high, the next thing to consider is diet. Although most people immediately think of eggs and cholesterol

intake, it is even more important to reduce the animal fat (saturated fat) and to increase the vegetable fats, fowl, and fish (sources of polyunsaturated and monounsaturated fats) in the diet than it is to reduce the cholesterol intake. We call the ratio of polyunsaturated to saturated fat intake the P/S ratio. It is also important to reduce total fat intake and possibly to increase the intake of monounsaturated oils.

Q. More has been in the newspapers of late about the dangers of NutraSweet (aspartame). Do we need to stop using it?

A. A recent news article mentioned a five-year-old boy who became "inconsolably and wildly emotional" after drinking NutraSweet products. We have not heard of similar instances in our Clinic, although a few people have complained of headaches and stomachaches after high NutraSweet intake. Children with a rare inherited condition (phenylketonuria) cannot consume NutraSweet because it contains phenylalanine. We have only one known patient in our Clinic with both diabetes and phenylketonuria, so this is fortunately a rare combination.

As emphasized by our dietitians in an earlier issue of NEWSNOTES, moderation is probably the answer for now. We generally suggest restricting the diet pop to no more than two per day. Common sense should also be used in watching the number of other foods consumed each day which contain NutraSweet. However, if you think you or your child has specific symptoms after consuming NutraSweet products, you should share this information with your dietitian.

Chapter 11

FOOD MANAGEMENT AND DIABETES

Key ideas of this chapter:

🐾 Realize that the ideal food plan for a person with diabetes is a healthy food plan from which all people would benefit.

🐾 Be aware of the principles of food management for a person with diabetes.

🐾 Be aware of the different types of food plans which are used in diabetes management.

🐾 Become familiar with the carbohydrate content of different foods.

Food is one of the four major "external" influences (along with insulin, exercise, and stress) on blood sugar levels in people with diabetes. As discussed in Chapter 2, the body (particularly the liver and muscle) also makes sugar (internal sugar), which adds to the blood sugar. Other sugars (external sugar) come from the food we eat. Recommendations for the use of sugars for people with diabetes have changed from complete avoidance to allowing sugar within the context of a healthy meal plan. As discussed in Chapter 10, the right amount and types of food are essential for normal growth and health. **TYPE 1 (INSULIN-DEPENDENT) DIABETES CANNOT BE TREATED WITH DIET ALONE.** In contrast, type 2 (adult-onset) diabetes sometimes can be treated with diet (and exercise) alone.

The objectives of food management in diabetes are:

🐾① to help keep the blood sugars as close to normal as possible;

🐾② to keep the blood fats (e.g., cholesterol and triglycerides) at normal levels;

🐾③ to improve the overall health by maintaining the best possible nutrition;

🐾④ to help avoid long-term complications;

🐾⑤ to help attain normal growth and development for children and appropriate weight for adults; and

🐾⑥ to help prevent severe hypoglycemia.

In regard to these objectives, it is amazing how often we hear parents comment, "My child with diabetes is the healthiest in our family BECAUSE HE/SHE EATS THE BEST." Although this is not proven, it may be true. As stressed in the previous chapter, good nutrition for a person with diabetes is really just a healthy diet from which all people would benefit. It should be obvious that all family members need to eat similarly to the person with diabetes.

Views on food management for people with diabetes have changed considerably. There was a time when some diabetes care providers believed every family should rigidly be given an ADA (American Diabetes Association) exchange food program. In 1994, the Position Statement of the ADA stated:

"Today there is no one 'diabetic' or 'ADA' diet. The recommended food program can only be defined as a dietary prescription based on nutrition assessment and treatment goals. Medical nutrition therapy for people with diabetes should be individualized, with consideration given to usual eating habits and other lifestyle changes."

We are pleased to say that this has been the philosophy of the past eight editions of this book over the last 24 years.

The DCCT (Diabetes Control and Complications Trial), mentioned in many chapters of this book also contributed to our knowledge about food and diabetes. In the DCCT, six main nutrition factors were found that contributed to better sugar control (lower HbA_{1c} levels). The six were:

1. following a meal plan of some sort;
2. avoidance of extra snacks;
3. avoidance of over-treatment of low blood sugars (hypoglycemia);
4. prompt treatment of high blood sugars when found;
5. adjusting insulin levels for meals; and
6. consistency of night snacks.

The DCCT did **NOT** report that one type of meal plan was any more effective than another type.

Three of the major meal planning approaches which we use to help people manage insulin-dependent diabetes will be discussed later in this chapter. All three programs have some advantages. There is no proof that one of the three is better than the other. Some families will prefer one plan, and other families another. Some families will change from one plan to another, or use a combination of plans that works for them. The 11 principles listed below are important in all three plans. They would be beneficial for any person to follow.

PRINCIPLES OF FOOD MANAGEMENT FOR A PERSON WITH DIABETES

1. EAT A WELL-BALANCED DIET
2. KEEP THE DAY-TO-DAY INTAKE CONSISTENT
3. EAT MEALS AND SNACKS AT THE SAME TIME EACH DAY
4. USE SNACKS TO PREVENT INSULIN REACTIONS
5. MANAGE CARBOHYDRATE INTAKE CAREFULLY
6. AVOID OVER-TREATING LOW BLOOD SUGARS
7. REDUCE CHOLESTEROL AND SATURATED FAT INTAKE; REDUCE TOTAL FAT AND TRANS-FATTY ACID INTAKE
8. MAINTAIN APPROPRIATE GROWTH AND WEIGHT FOR HEIGHT; AVOID BECOMING OVERWEIGHT
9. INCREASE FIBER INTAKE
10. AVOID FOODS HIGH IN SALT (SODIUM)
11. AVOID EXCESSIVE PROTEIN INTAKE

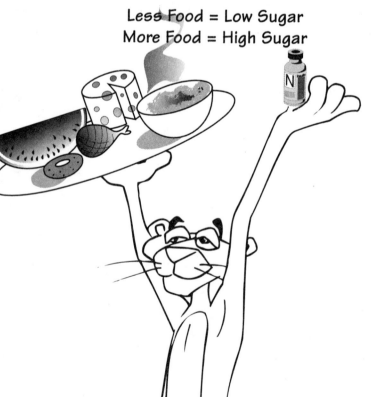

Less Food = Low Sugar
More Food = High Sugar

Eat a Well-balanced Diet

A well-balanced meal plan is a step toward good health for everyone in the family. It is particularly important in supporting the growth of children. If you understand normal nutrition, as outlined in Chapter 10, you can help your family have a well-balanced meal plan. Most people have a period of weight loss prior to being diagnosed with diabetes. Starting insulin treatment allows the body to regain weight. Usually the individual's appetite is ravenous for about one month as the body returns to its usual growth pattern. The appetite then returns to normal. Most individuals can then self-regulate their caloric intake without a set number of calories being prescribed for each day. If excessive weight gain does become a problem, the dietitian can suggest a set number of calories. The exchange food program can help in following a recommended caloric intake.

A well-balanced meal plan is currently considered to contain 10-20% of calories from protein, 50-60% from carbohydrate and 25-30% from fat. Meals should be balanced and contain a rich source of carbohydrates (fruits, vegetables, and whole grains), a moderate amount of protein (milk, cheese, yogurt, meat, poultry, fish, egg white, nuts and seeds), and a limited amount of fat (butter, egg yolk, animal fat, etc.). An excess of animal fat may result in higher blood fats and a greater likelihood for heart disease in later life. A high-protein diet is harmful to the kidneys for people who have either early or advanced kidney damage from diabetes. It is wise to work with the dietitian to help assure intake of the recommended balance of foods.

Keep the Day-to-day Intake Consistent

Your energy comes primarily from the food you eat, or your caloric intake. If your caloric intake is the same from day-to-day, the insulin and the food will be balanced. If you eat less one day, you may have too much insulin and low blood sugar reactions. If you eat more one day, you will have too little insulin and have high blood sugars (see the picture of Pink Panther balancing food and insulin). You should also try to eat similar amounts of carbohydrate, fat, and protein each day. Your body will need more or less insulin as more or less carbohydrate is eaten. IT IS IMPORTANT TO BE CONSISTENT IN EATING ABOUT THE SAME AMOUNT OF FOOD AT THE SAME TIMES EACH DAY. For people on a relatively constant insulin dose, the constant carbohydrate and the exchange food programs both help to keep the daily intake consistent. **CONSISTENCY IS ONE OF THE MOST IMPORTANT PRINCIPLES IN ALL OF DIABETES MANAGEMENT.**

Eat Meals and Snacks at the Same Time Each Day

The insulin you inject will be working to lower the blood sugar whether you eat or not. Therefore, it is important never to miss meals and to eat at approximately the same time each day to prevent low blood sugar reactions (hypoglycemia). **EATING MEALS AND SNACKS ON TIME IS HELPFUL IN MANAGING YOUR DIABETES.** Low blood sugar reactions can be a problem when school buses are delayed or when meals are delayed. It is important to carry snacks for emergencies, such as a late bus. If a family member is late arriving home for a meal, it is wise for the child with diabetes to go ahead and eat. Eventually, as the child with diabetes grows older, he/she can take responsibility for eating when the normal family routine is broken. Avoidance of extra snacks was one of the factors in the DCCT which resulted in better sugar control. People who snack constantly will usually have constantly elevated blood sugar levels.

Use Snacks to Prevent Insulin Reactions

Snacks help to balance the insulin activity. Peaks in insulin activity vary from person to person, and you will learn from experience when you need a snack. It may be before lunch, in the late afternoon, or at bedtime. Discuss your need for snacks at your clinic visits. Young children often use a mid- or late-morning snack, although teens and adults may not always need a morning snack. Mid- or late-afternoon snacks are also needed by most people with diabetes. Almost everyone with diabetes needs a bedtime snack. Once it is decided which snacks you need, TRY TO BE CONSISTENT AND NOT SKIP SNACKS. Suggestions for daytime and bedtime snacks are given in Tables 1 and 2.

Table 1

HEALTHY DAYTIME SNACKS

Snacks, besides being fun to eat, help prevent low blood sugar levels and provide energy between meals. Typical snacks are usually 1-2 carbohydrate choices or 15-30 grams of carbohydrate. Below are some low-fat snack ideas to try.

15 grams of carbohydrate or one carbohydrate choice

1 medium apple or orange
2 popcorn cakes
3 cups air popped or low-fat microwave popcorn
8 oz or 1 carton light yogurt
5-6 saltine crackers
1/2 cup low-fat ice cream
1/2 cup unsweetened applesauce
1 fruit roll-up

18 small pretzel twists
1/2 small bagel with fat-free cream cheese
4-5 vanilla wafers
1 1/2 graham crackers
2 Tbsp raisins
1/2 cup sugar-free pudding
1 fruit juice bar

30 grams of carbohydrate or 2 carbohydrate choices

1 small bagel with fat-free cream cheese
1 low-fat granola bar
4 oz individual fruit cup and 1 cup skim milk
1/4 cup dried fruit
1 cereal bar
14 animal crackers and 1/2 cup skim milk

1 oz baked tortilla chips with 1/4 cup salsa
1 large banana or 2 pieces of fruit
1 cup Cheerios with 1/2 cup skim milk
2 caramel corn cakes
15 baked potato chips
2 fig cookies and 1 cup skim milk

SPECIAL SUGGESTIONS

- Encourage fresh fruit rather than juice as a routine snack (unless blood sugar is low)

- Sugar-free flavorings (e.g., sugar-free cocoa or milk flavorings) can be added to milk, if needed

- If the child is still hungry after the snack, offer water, popsicles made using diet pop or Kool-Aid, or sticks of sliced fresh carrots or celery placed in a dish with cold water and ice cubes

- Don't make issues of "food jags" or eating "crazes"; they usually pass (if not emphasized)

TWO GOOD SUMMER DAYTIME SNACKS

Yogurt creamsicles

Combine:
1/2 cup plain skim milk yogurt (1/2 carb)
1/2 cup fruit juice concentrate, undiluted (3 carbs)

Freeze in popsicle molds until solid.
The total mixture = 3 carb choices

Fruit popsicles

Blend:
1 cup fresh fruit: berries, peaches, or bananas (2 carbs)
1/2 cup apple juice concentrate, undiluted (3 carbs)
Freeze in popsicle molds until solid.
The total mixture = 5 carb choices

Table 2

POSSIBLE BEDTIME SNACKS

Bedtime snacks play an important role in blood sugar control for people with type 1 diabetes. A snack which includes food sources of carbohydrate and protein is helpful in maintaining blood sugar levels throughout the night. A typical snack includes 15 grams of carbohydrate and 7-8 grams of protein, but this can vary depending on age, blood sugar levels and activity throughout the day. Most protein also contains some fat, which results in food staying in the stomach longer. Examples of foods containing 15 grams of carbohydrate and 7-8 grams of protein are listed below:

<ins>15 grams of Carbohydrate</ins>	**plus**	<ins>7-8 grams of Protein</ins>
1 slice of bread		2 Tbsp peanut butter
1 6 inch tortilla		1/4 cup grated cheese
6 saltine crackers		1 string cheese
3 cups popcorn		1 oz of meat or 1 egg
12 small pretzels		2 Tbsp sunflower seeds
3/4-1 cup cereal		1/4 cup peanuts
5 vanilla wafers		1 cup milk*
		8 oz of no-sugar-added yogurt*

Yogurt and milk provide about 15 grams of carbohydrate as well as protein

🐾 We prefer some solid food at bedtime—which will "churn-around" in the stomach prior to passing to the intestine where most food is absorbed. Thus, milk or yogurt alone might pass rapidly through the stomach, but milk and cereal or yogurt and crackers might pass through more slowly.

Adjustments in carbohydrate amounts can be made based on what the blood sugar is at bedtime. Here are some guidelines to follow:

- If blood sugar is 150-200 mg/dl (8.3-11.1mmol/L), have **15-20** grams of carbohydrate and 7-8 grams of protein.

- If blood sugar is 100-150 mg/dl (5.5-8.3 mmol/L), have **25-30** grams of carbohydrate and 7-8 grams of protein.

- If blood sugar is less than 100 mg/dl (5.5 mmol/L), have **30-45** grams of carbohydrate and 7-8 grams of protein.

Table 3 gives possible recipes for cornstarch snacks.

The type of snack is also important. Sugar from fruits will last only one or two hours. Fruits are good for a morning or afternoon snack. Proteins with fat, such as cheese or meat, convert to sugar more slowly and delay absorption. A SOLID SNACK CONTAINING PROTEIN, FAT, AND STARCH IS BEST FOR BEDTIME, as it will be more apt to last through the night. Cornstarch is believed to be broken down slower than other carbohydrates and helps some children to prevent lows during the night. Two possible cornstarch recipes are given in Table 3. Your dietitian can suggest other cornstarch recipes, or you can buy cornstarch snack bars (usually $1.00 each) from several companies. When eating cheese, use reduced or low-fat cheeses. String and mozzarella cheeses often are low-fat cheeses.

Use lean sources of animal proteins, such as chicken, turkey breast or fish when possible. Avoid eating large amounts of luncheon meats, which are very high in saturated fats and often in sodium, too. Solid foods are digested more slowly than liquids and are better for the bedtime snack.

🐾 Manage Carbohydrate Intake Carefully

It is recommended that about half of the food we eat be carbohydrate, and as insulin must be available to utilize most carbohydrates, it is important to learn to manage carbohydrate intake carefully. Tables 4 and 5 both deal with learning the carbohydrate contents of different foods. As discussed in the previous chapter, it is now known that the rise in blood sugar after

Table 3

TWO CORNSTARCH RECIPES TO USE FOR BEDTIME SNACKS*

Corny "O"s**

1/2 stick butter or margarine
1/2 cup chocolate chips
1/2 cup peanut butter
5 cups Cheerios
1 cup cornstarch
1/2 cup powdered sugar

1. Melt butter and chocolate chips, add peanut butter

2. Pour mixture over Cheerios

3. In a paper sack, combine cornstarch mixture with Cheerios mixture and shake it until Cheerios are completely covered with cornstarch

Quantity:	10 servings
Serving size:	1/2 cup
Carb	34 gms/serving
Protein	5 gms/serving
Fat	14 gms/serving

*Developed by Michelle Hansen, MS, RD, CDE

** Not for children under 2 years old

"Corny Cookies"

12 Tbsp (3/4 cup) peanut butter
3 Tbsp honey
1/4 cup cornstarch
2 cups cornflakes

1. Stir together peanut butter, honey and cornstarch

2. Form into balls, about 1 Tbsp size, and roll in crushed cornflakes

3. Flatten balls with a tumbler and chill

Quantity:	1 dozen
Serving size:	2 cookies
Carb	26 gms/2 cookies
Protein	8 gms/2 cookies
Fat	16 gms/2 cookies

Serving Size	1 cookie
Carb	13 gms/1 cookie
Protein	4 gms/1 cookie
Fat	8 gms/1 cookie

eating is dependent upon the total amount of carbohydrate eaten and not the form of carbohydrate (simple or complex). It was pointed out that **"a carbohydrate, is a carbohydrate, is a carbohydrate..."** We now know that the more important factors are: A) **how much** carbohydrate is eaten; B) **when** the carbohydrate is eaten; C) **with what** the carbohydrate is eaten; and D) having **adequate insulin** available when carbohydrate is eaten. Each will be discussed in more detail.

A. How much carbohydrate is eaten

Concentrated sources of sugar (e.g., a can of sugar pop) contain a large amount of carbohydrate in a small portion or quantity (approximately 10 tsp or 40 grams). This can be consumed rapidly by a thirsty person in the summer. Three small-to-medium apples would contain about the same amount of carbohydrate. However, due to the bulk (fiber), it is unlikely anyone would eat the three apples all at once—or at least in the same time taken to drink the sugar pop. The can of sugar pop would contain three times as much carbohydrate as one apple and would raise the blood sugar much more. If sugar pop were to be consumed by a person with diabetes at a meal, it would require leaving out similar amounts of carbohydrate from other foods (e.g., one glass of milk, one baked potato, and one apple could be eliminated and they would have about the same carbohydrate content as the sugar pop). The other nutrients from the milk, potato, and apple would then be missed. We do not recommend making this kind of substitution. The carbohydrate counts of some high-carbohydrate foods are shown in Table 4.

B. When the carbohydrate is eaten

Restriction of large amounts of carbohydrate between meals is important, unless additional insulin is given to manage additional carbohydrates. An extreme example is, once again, having the sugar pop (40 grams of carbohydrate) as a morning or afternoon snack.

One boy with diabetes brought a can of regular sugar pop (10 tsp of sugar, see Table 4) to our clinic with him—freely admitting that he still drank regular pop. We measured his blood sugar before drinking the pop (180 mg/dl or 10 mmol/L) and one hour later (450 mg/dl or 25 mmol/L).

When concentrated carbohydrates are eaten, it is best to eat them with a meal (or right after) and to either eliminate other carbohydrates that would normally have been eaten (see above), take extra Humalog or Regular insulin, or do extra exercise. As discussed in section A, eliminating other carbohydrates may result in eliminating important nutrients and should not be done on a regular basis.

C. With what the carbohydrate is eaten

Research done at our Center on children with diabetes, who came in on four consecutive Saturday mornings, evaluated four different breakfasts varying in sugar or protein and fat content. The blood sugars peaked later and remained higher for a longer time when the protein and fat were added (whether extra sugar was added or not). Although most research on the effect of carbohydrates on blood sugar levels is done by giving the carbohydrate by itself, the effects of other foods are very important. The best way to find out the effect of an added carbohydrate is to check the blood sugar, eat the food and/or meal, and check the blood sugar again after two hours. Then, compare the blood sugar to the same meal on another day without the added carbohydrate. When extra carbohydrate is to be eaten, it is best to eat it with a meal. Then, extra insulin can be taken or other carbohydrates can be reduced.

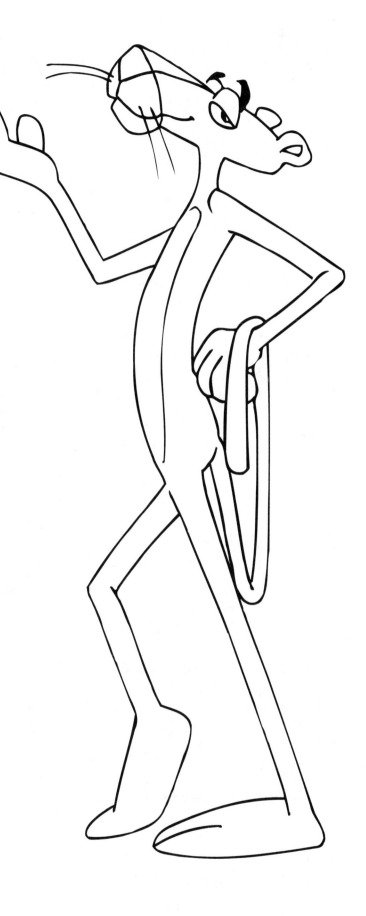

SUGAR CONTENT OF SOME
HIGH-CARBOHYDRATE FOODS

Food Item	Size Portion	Sugar Content in Teaspoons*	"Carb" Counts
Beverages			
Cola Drinks	12 oz can	10	3
Rootbeer	12 oz can	7	2
7-Up®*	12 oz can	9	3
Grape, orange, or apple juice	6 oz can	5	1.5
Dairy Products			
Sherbet	1 scoop	9	3
Ice Cream Cone	1 scoop	3 1/2	1
Chocolate Milk Shake	10 oz glass	11	4
Milk	8 oz glass	4	1
Chocolate Milk	8 oz glass	9 1/2	3
Fruit Yogurt	8 oz cup	9	3
Cakes and Cookies			
Angel Food Cake	4 oz piece	7	2
Chocolate Cake, plain	4 oz piece	6	2
Chocolate Cake, w/frosting	4 oz piece	10	3
Cupcake, w/frosting	1	6	2
Brownies, no frosting	1 oz piece	3	1
Sugar Cookie	1	1 1/2	1/2
Oatmeal Cookie	1	2	1
Donut, plain	1	3	1
Donut, glazed	1	6	2
Desserts			
JELL-O	1/2 cup	4 1/2	1 1/2
Pastry	4 oz piece	4	1
Apple Pie	1 slice	7	2
Berry Pie	1 slice	10	3
Chocolate Pudding	1/2 cup	4	1
Candies			
Chocolate Candy Bar	1 1/2 oz	2 1/2	1
Chewing Gum	1 stick	1/2	-
Fudge	1 oz square	4 1/2	1 1/2
Hard Candy	4 oz	20	7
LIFE SAVERS®	1	1/3	-
Marshmallow	1 piece	1 1/2	1/2
Chocolate Creme	1 piece	2	1
Miscellaneous			
Jelly	1 Tbsp	4-6	2
Strawberry Jam	1 Tbsp	4	1
Brown Sugar	1 Tbsp	3	1
Honey	1 Tbsp	3	1
Chocolate Sauce	1 Tbsp	3	1
Karo Syrup®	1 Tbsp	3	1

*3 tsp = 1 Tbsp = 1 "carb" count = 15 grams of carbohydrate

Make sure you eat a bedtime snack including protein and fat.

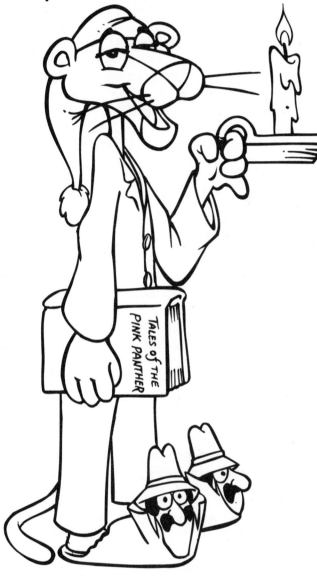

TALES of THE PINK PANTHER

D. Having adequate insulin activity when the carbohydrate is eaten

As in the example in section A, eating extra high-carbohydrate food can be done along with adding extra Humalog or Regular insulin, or by removing a similar amount of carbohydrate foods that would normally be eaten. Either way, when carbohydrate is eaten, it should be when adequate insulin is acting to allow the resulting sugar to pass from the blood into the body's cells. It is wise to measure the blood sugar two hours after the meal to see if the method used was appropriate to use again on the next similar occasion.

On special occasions, such as birthday parties, the child with diabetes can consume a high-sugar food. Extra sugar **will not make the person ill and will not cause acidosis.** It may result in higher than normal blood sugar and more frequent urination as the sugar passes into the urine. Often the extra activity or excitement at the party balances the extra sugar intake.

It is generally healthier to allow the child to fit in a sweet food on an "as-needed" basis rather than to have the child sneaking candy or treats. This can be planned for a time prior to exercise, which will then help burn any excess sugar, or preferably with a meal. We encourage the entire family to get used to eating foods without a "sugary" taste. Most people find that after a while they don't miss this taste at all! **To allow for better nutrition, avoid having high-sugar foods (Table 4) such as donuts, cookies, cake, etc. in the home. If they are there, they will be hard to avoid.** This will result in better nutrition for the entire family.

There are several alternatives for handling holidays and parties where there are a great number of concentrated sweets. Halloween focuses on candy and is thus a special problem for young children. If a child does go trick-or-treating, he/she can bring home the foods containing sugar, select a few for his/her regular treats, and either give or throw the rest away. As discussed above, if sweets are to be eaten, it is best to eat them when insulin is working rather than removing other carbohydrates in the meal, or increase the dose of Humalog or Regular insulin for that meal. Taking the treats to a sick friend or a child in the hospital is a nice option. Another option is to "sell" each piece of candy for a set amount of money to the parents. The money is then spent to purchase something the child desires.

It is important not to become upset with a child if he/she does eat extra sweets. The stress of the parent being upset can raise the sugar more than the sweets (see Chapter 16 on Family Concerns). Instead, discuss the incident with the child and try to find compromises.

🐾 Avoid Over-treating Low Blood Sugars

As noted above, avoidance of the over-treatment of low blood sugars (hypoglycemia) was one of the factors found in the DCCT to relate to better sugar control (a lower HbA$_{lc}$ level). The problem is how to accomplish this. Only a person who has had a truly low blood sugar can know the feeling of being "ravenously hungry" and wanting to eat everything in sight (and so the person does). For many years, people thought "rebounding" to be the cause of the high blood sugar after hypoglycemia, whereas only in recent years was it realized to be primarily due to excessive eating after the low blood sugar. Chapter 5 discusses the treatment of hypoglycemia and emphasizes: 1) checking the blood sugar to see how low the value is, and repeating this at 10-minute intervals to see if the value is rising; 2) drinking one cup of milk (8-10 oz) 1/2 cup of juice, or four ounces of sugar pop, or taking 1/2 tube of instant glucose (e.g., 15 grams of carbohydrate or one "carb" count). Then wait 10 minutes and do the second blood sugar level. If the value has not risen, repeat the process using 15 grams of carbohydrate or one "carb" choice every 10 minutes until a rise does occur. If the blood sugar is rising after 10 minutes and is above 60 mg/dl (3.2 mmol/L), eat solid food, such as two or three crackers with peanut butter or cheese. Or, if it is close to mealtime, just eat the next meal. Not eating too much, but enough to raise the blood sugar is tricky and can vary from person to person or from one time to another for the same person. Careful monitoring of blood sugar levels is essential.

🐾 Reduce Cholesterol and Saturated Fat Intake; Reduce Total Fat Intake and Trans Fatty Acid Intake

Cholesterol and triglyceride are two of the major fats present in our blood. Cholesterol is found in many foods, but is particularly high in egg yolks, organ meats, and large portions of high-fat red meat (e.g., prime rib). Cholesterol is found in animal products only; fruits, vegetables, cereals, grains, beans, nuts and seeds have no cholesterol. The eating of saturated fat in meat may raise blood cholesterol levels even more than eating high cholesterol foods. This is discussed in more detail in the previous chapter on normal nutrition. Blood cholesterol and triglyceride levels can also be high if blood sugar levels are too high.

The blood cholesterol level should be checked once a year (fasting is not necessary). If a high level is found, the dietitian can make suggestions to help lower it. The average American now eats 400-450 mg of cholesterol per day. This should gradually be reduced to about 300 mg per day. Table 1 in the previous chapter gives the cholesterol content of some common foods. Each egg has about 213 mg of cholesterol. Egg white is a good source of protein. Some people now just eat the whites, which have no cholesterol. If your doctor has not checked your blood cholesterol level, you could request that this be done.

Triglyceride levels for a given person tend to be variable. They are related to the diabetes control at the time, the amount of exercise in the previous week and other factors. It is necessary to be fasting for accurate triglyceride and lipoprotein (LDL and HDL) determinations. Fasting is sometimes dangerous for people with diabetes (e.g., driving across town with no food intake). We now usually draw a "lipid panel" once yearly when it has been 3-4 hours since the last meal.

🐾 Maintain Appropriate Growth and Weight for Height—Avoid Becoming Overweight

Normal growth is important for children and teenagers. An important part of clinic visits is to make sure the height and weight are increasing appropriately. Research at our Center has shown that if sugar control is poor in the teenaged years, final adult height will be lower.

It is much easier to stay healthy if you are able to maintain a normal weight range for your size. This book is written mostly for young people who require insulin. Fortunately, people with insulin-dependent diabetes are usually not obese. People who develop diabetes after age 40 years (usually adult or type 2 diabetes) are often overweight and may not require insulin. Weight loss may be their main treatment.

THE ONLY WAY YOU CAN BE OVERWEIGHT IS

IF YOU EAT TOO MUCH FOOD OR IF YOU DON'T GET ENOUGH EXERCISE. If you eat less and exercise daily, you will always lose weight. Exercise is even more important for people with diabetes than for other people (see Chapter 12). People with diabetes should avoid fad diets and diets for rapid weight loss. An overweight person should work with a dietitian to find a balanced diet for gradual weight loss. As discussed earlier, reduction of fat in the diet is often the best long-term solution (along with adequate exercise). The insulin dosage may have to be reduced if food intake is decreased or exercise is increased. **It is better to stay at an appropriate weight and not become overweight at all, as it is difficult to lose excess weight!**

We discourage the use of quick weight loss diets and diet pills. They do not teach a person to eat correctly and, when the fad is over, the weight is almost always regained. It is much wiser to work with the dietitian to learn correct eating habits and to develop a plan to gradually reduce weight. It is important for parents to be careful not to be critical or to emphasize a child's weight gain. It will only make the problem worse and can lead to eating disorders or missed shots. If a parent has concerns, it might be better to express them to the dietitian or to other diabetes team members.

Increase Fiber Intake

Fiber is the roughage in our food that is not absorbed into the body. Many of us don't have enough fiber in our diets. Adding fiber may blunt the rise in blood sugar levels for children with diabetes. Thus, the blood sugar may not be as high two hours after eating an apple (one carb choice) as it is two hours after drinking 1/2 cup (four ounces) of apple juice (one carb choice). Extra fiber is good for people, particularly in helping to avoid constipation. Raw fruits, vegetables, legumes, high-fiber cereals, and whole wheat breads are the most effective high-fiber foods. The fiber content of some common foods is shown in Table 4 in the previous chapter.

Avoid Foods High in Salt (sodium)

If a person has a tendency toward high blood pressure, a high salt intake may bring out this tendency. People who have early kidney damage seem to be more likely to have an increased blood pressure from high salt intake. Some people who are asked to not flavor foods with sugar may instead use more salt in flavoring. Also, people who eat at fast food restaurants tend to have high salt intake. As increased blood pressure is an important risk factor for both the eye and the kidney complications of diabetes, it is important not to eat large amounts of salt. Some health authorities recommend that all people eat under 3,000 mg of sodium (1 1/4 tsp of table salt) each day. If the blood pressure is elevated, 2,400 mg (approximately 1 tsp of table salt) or less per day is recommended. This can be discussed with the dietitian.

Avoid Excessive Protein Intake

It is difficult when one is told not to eat excessive amounts of simple sugar, animal fat, salt, and also that an excess of protein should be avoided. Many teenagers eat 4-6 times the quantity of protein they need. Once again, this is particularly true for those who frequently eat or snack at fast-food restaurants. Athletes should not consume protein (amino acid) supplements. Only exercise builds muscle—not protein supplements. We know that extra protein is bad when kidney damage is present, as it presents an extra load for the kidneys to handle. Information is not yet available to know whether higher protein intake might help cause the kidney complications of diabetes. The best method to reduce protein intake is to eat less red meat. Spaghetti, pasta, and casseroles that do not have a lot of meat are healthier than a hamburger, steak, or other meat. Protein can be eliminated from breakfast (except milk) and the morning and afternoon snacks. However, we recommend that the bedtime snack includes carbohydrate, protein and fat, as they help to keep the blood sugar at a reasonable level throughout the night.

TYPES OF MEAL PLANNING APPROACHES

Different types of meal planning approaches have been used for people with diabetes for about 4,000 years. They are talked about in an ancient scroll called the "Ebers Papyrus," which was written about 2000 B.C. In 1993 the DCCT showed that people with diabetes who followed a dietary program had better sugar control than those who didn't. There are now many types of food management plans for people with diabetes. The three approaches used most commonly in our Clinic are:

 CONSTANT CARBOHYDRATE

 CARBOHYDRATE ("CARB") COUNTING

 EXCHANGES

When a child is initially diagnosed to have diabetes, the clinic caring for the child may prefer one type of meal planning approach over the others. It may then be unnecessary to read about the other approaches, at least initially.

Any of the three can work. No single approach has been proven better than any other in achieving good blood sugar control. It is up to each family to eventually decide which approach works best for them. Some families will switch from one approach to another or combine parts of each to fit their needs. It is important to meet with a registered dietitian to develop a meal plan that meets your lifestyle.

Constant Carbohydrate Meal Plan

CAREFUL MANAGEMENT OF CARBOHYDRATE INTAKE MUST BE PART OF ANY OF THE PROGRAMS. IT IS IMPOSSIBLE TO EAT VARYING AMOUNTS OF CARBOHYDRATE (WITHOUT CHANGING THE INSULIN DOSAGE) AND KEEP THE BLOOD SUGAR ANYWHERE NEAR NORMAL. Thus, all of the meal plans place emphasis on knowing how much carbohydrate is being eaten. In this meal plan, the amount of insulin (usually two shots per day) is kept relatively constant from day-to-day to match relatively consistent food intake. **The amount of carbohydrate (types can vary) is kept about the same for each meal and each snack from one day to the next. CONSISTENCY IS THE KEY.** The constant carbohydrate food program is formed around the 11 principles discussed earlier in this chapter. The amount of food eaten at a meal or snack can vary with factors such as expected exercise, insulin taken, and blood sugar level. More food may be needed for activities such as sports, hiking, and farming. However, the normal eating pattern of the child and the family should stay the same as much as possible. The constant carbohydrate food program is not to be confused with a "regular" or "free" diet that does not consider the importance of snacks, timing of meals, keeping the amount of carbohydrate relatively consistent from day-to-day, or any of the other 11 nutrition principles.

Carbohydrate ("Carb") Counting (Choices)

Carbohydrate counting is both similar to and different from the other two food programs. It is similar to the Constant Carbohydrate Meal Plan in that emphasis is placed on carbohydrate intake and on keeping protein and fat relatively consistent. (Protein and fat may also influence the blood sugar levels.) It is different in that it presumes that carbohydrate intake (and insulin dose) will vary, thus providing more flexibility and greater safety from hypoglycemia. It is similar to the Exchange Meal Plan in that similar sized "exchanges" of carbohydrate are used, but different in that protein and fat exchanges are not used. Tables 5 and 6 give summaries of foods equaling one carb choice (count), which is the amount of each food equal to 15 grams of carbohydrate. It may be helpful to copy Table 5 initially and carry it in a wallet or purse.

Carbohydrate counting is simply counting the grams of carbohydrate to be eaten and then matching it with an amount of insulin. It was greatly aided by the food labeling laws (Chapter 10), which require that the grams of total carbohydrate be given on the label of most every food. (Fiber is included in total carbohydrate and some people subtract the grams of fiber, as it is not absorbed into the body.) More detailed quantities of various foods equaling one carb count or choice; (e.g., 15 grams of carbohydrate) are given in Table 6. The total grams of carbohydrate to be eaten are divided by 15 to get carb counts (15 grams of carbohydrate equals one carb count). The units of short-acting insulin (Humalog or Regular) are then adjusted prior to every meal to fit the carb counts (counts of 15 grams of carbohydrate), as well as to the amount of exercise expected and the blood sugar level.

Every person is different in their need for Humalog or Regular insulin, and the same person may vary from one time of day to another. Some people can do fine using one unit of short-acting insulin per 15 grams of carbohydrate (one carb count) for all meals and snacks. Others might use one unit of insulin for each 15 grams of carbohydrate intake at breakfast, one unit of insulin for every 30 grams of carbohydrate (1/2 unit per 15 grams carbohydrate) at lunch, and possibly one unit of insulin per 10 grams (1.5 units per 15 grams carbohydrate) at dinner. After calculating the dose of insulin for the "carb" counts, the final dose must be adjusted considering planned exercise and the blood sugar level. Some people subtract a unit if the blood sugar is below 70 mg/dl (3.9 mmol/L) or add a unit if the blood sugar is above 200 mg/dl (11.1 mmol/L). Careful record keeping for the first one or two weeks is essential (possibly using Table 3 in Chapter 25 to record the blood sugar, carb count and insulin dose). Checking blood sugars two hours after meals allows one to see if the insulin to carbohydrate ratio used for a given meal resulted in the correct insulin dose. It is then important to review the records with the dietitian and physician to decide the best insulin ratios to use at different meals.

Some degree of thinking (just like the "thinking scales" in Chapter 20) is obviously necessary for "carb" counting. However, once the best dosages are determined, the process becomes very automatic. Most people who use an insulin pump use carb counting to determine the bolus of insulin to be taken with any food intake (see Chapter 25). Use of "carb" counting allows people to better observe the relationship between factors affecting the blood sugar and insulin dosage. In England (and the entire U.K.), carbohydrate counting (using 10 gram "carb" counts) has been used successfully for many years. A summary of 15 gram carbohydrate equivalents in foods frequently eaten is given in Tables 5 and 6. In the exchange meal plan below, the starch/bread list, the fruit list, and the milk list all contain approximately 15 grams of carbohydrate. For those wanting more detailed information on carb counting or on carbohydrate quantities in foods, there are now entire books written on these subjects.

Carbohydrate Counting Resources:

1) *Counting Carbohydrates*, by Brackenridge, B.P., Fredrickson, L., and Reed, C. Available from MiniMed Technologies, 12744 San Fernando Road, Sylmar, CA 91342 (1-800-933-3322)

2) *Calories and Carbohydrates* (11th Edition), by Barbara Kraus, 1995

3) *The Complete Book of Food Counts* (4th Edition), by Corinne Netzer, 1997

4) *Food Values of Portions Commonly Used* (17th Edition), by Pennington and Church, 1998

5) *The Diabetes Carbohydrate and Fat Gram Guide*, by Lea Ann Holzmeister, 1997

6) *Nutrition In the Fast Lane*, Eli Lilly and Co., 1999

An Exchange Meal Plan

If you/your child is newly diagnosed and your dietitian has already met with your family and recommended a different food management plan, it may not be necessary to spend time on this section.

In the exchange food program, foods are grouped into one of six food lists, with foods in each of the six lists having similar numbers of calories. Then the foods within a group can be traded for one another because they all have similar caloric, protein, carbohydrate, and fat content.

The exchange food program was initially developed for weight control and is still often effective for this purpose. Many families in which someone has just been diagnosed with diabetes will initially learn the exchange food program to gain a feeling for how much of which foods to eat. As they feel more comfortable with their eating, they may then gradually change to the constant carbohydrate meal plan. In the exchange food program, the number of calories to be eaten each day is initially chosen. Examples of how many of each of the six types of exchanges to eat each day for the number of calories are shown in Table 7. A brief summary of the three food groupings is given in Table 8. Foods in each sub-group contain similar numbers of calories and similar amounts of carbohydrate, protein, and fat. In the exchange food program, a caloric level that is appropriate for the age, size, and activity of the person is prescribed. Most children under age 14 years need 1,000 calories per day plus 100 calories for each year of age. For example, a five-year-old would need 1,500 calories:

five years x 100 = 500 cal/day
500 + 1,000 = 1,500 cal/day

The dietitian changes the calories into exchanges, which are then divided into meals and snacks as shown in Table 7. This meal plan allows both consistent carbohydrate intake and a variety of foods. In addition to working with the dietitian, if you are going to use the exchange food program we suggest you buy the ADA booklet "Exchange Lists for Meal Planning" (see Table 8 for ordering address).

In Canada, the Good Health Eating Guide (GHEG) was developed by the Canadian Diabetes Association to have six food groups. They are slightly different from the U.S.: fruits and vegetables are combined into one group and each serving is equivalent to 10 grams of carbohydrate and one gram of protein. The sixth food group is the extras (free foods).

ONE CARBOHYDRATE (CARB) COUNT OR CHOICE*

1 Starch = 1 Fruit = 1 Milk = 15 grams carbohydrate = 1 "CARB" Choice

Food Group	Carbohydrate Content	Portion Sizes
Starch/Grains	15gms	1 slice bread 1/2 cup pasta 1/2 hamburger bun 1/2 cup peas or corn 1 small potato 1/3 cup rice 1/3 cup cooked dried beans
Fruit	15 gms	1 piece fruit, medium sized 1/2 cup canned fruit 1/2 cup fruit juice 1/4 cup dried fruit 1 cup berries or melon
Milk	15 gms	1 cup skim, 1%, 2% or whole milk 8 oz plain yogurt

These are not exact but are close enough for most people.
Note: *This half-page may be copied and carried in the wallet as needed.*

CARBOHYDRATE "CARB" COUNTING

Examples of 15 gram (1 "carb") carbohydrate "choice" or "count":

A. **Starch/Bread group**	**Amount to equal 1 "carb" count**
bread	= 1 slice
bagel	= 1 half
1/2 hamburger or hot dog bun	= 1 (a whole is 2 "carb" counts)
cereal	= 1/3 to 1 cup (see label on box)
noodles	= 1/2 cup
popcorn	= 3 cups
crackers	= 4
graham cracker squares	= 2
saltines	= 6
pancake or waffle	= 1 (5 inch diameter)
potato (or corn) chips	= 15
corn	= 1/2 cup or one ear
potato	= 1 small baked or 1/2 cup mashed
rice	= 1/3 cup cooked (2 Tbsp uncooked)
sweet potatoes or yams	= 1/4 cup
green peas	= 1/2 cup
squash	= 1/2 cup
lima beans	= 1/2 cup

B. **Other vegetables**	
raw	= 3 cups
cooked	= 1 1/2 cups

C. **Fruits**	
small orange, pear, peach or apple	= 1
banana (large)	= 1/2
raisins	= 25 gms (check weight on box) or 2 Tbsp
canned fruit (not in sugar)	= 1/2 cup
cantaloupe or watermelon	= 1 cup
juices	= 1/2 cup orange, grapefruit, or apple
	= 1/3 cup of others

D. **Dairy**	
milk	= 1 cup (8 oz) regardless of fat content
yogurt	= 1 cup (8 oz) plain

E. **Italian foods**	
pizza	= 1/6 of a small pizza
pasta	= 1/2 cup
spaghetti	= 1/2 cup (about 30 strands or a "small" helping)
lasagna	= 1 square or a "small" helping

F. **Soups**	= 1 cup if milk or broth-based
	= 1/2 cup if bean-based

G. **Casseroles**	= 1/2 cup

H. **Desserts** (also see Table 3 in this chapter)	
fruit (apple) pie	= 1/2 piece (1 piece is 2 "carb" counts)
cake (chocolate, etc.)	= 1/2 piece (1 piece is 2 "carb" counts)
sugar (for baking)	= 3 tsp

I. **Free foods**	Lettuce, carrots, celery, coffee, tea, diet pop, and other foods with few calories

NOTE: Meats and fats do not contain carbohydrate, but do affect the blood sugar levels so intake should be kept constant.

CHOOSING A MEAL PLAN APPROACH

One type of meal plan has not been shown to be better for people with type 1 diabetes than another. The best meal plan for your family is the one that fits your lifestyle. All three programs work. You could take parts of each program and develop a meal plan suitable for your eating habits and lifestyle. Many families change from one type of program to another to fit their needs at the time. **HOWEVER, THERE MUST BE SOME PROGRAM OF FOOD MANAGEMENT.** Initially, after evaluating your family's eating patterns, it may be wise to let the dietitian help choose the best food program for your family.

A proper meal plan, combined with insulin therapy, exercise, and smooth handling of stress (see Chapter 13) are all very important in the day-to-day management of diabetes. **A PERSON WITH DIABETES WILL FOLLOW ANY FOOD PROGRAM BETTER IF THE WHOLE FAMILY HAS GOOD NUTRITION PRACTICES.** In this way, the entire family will be eating healthier.

SUMMARY

CONSISTENCY is the key to food management and diabetes, and the entire family must help in attaining this. It is now known that there is no difference in the effect of a simple sugar compared to a complex carbohydrate as far as the rise in blood sugar is concerned. Almost any food can be eaten by a person with diabetes in moderation if it is worked into the meal plan. Thus, foods with simple sugars in them can be eaten by a person with diabetes. However, they should be eaten at a meal when insulin is taken beforehand, and either extra insulin, a reduction in intake of other carbohydrates or extra exercise should be considered. More frequent blood sugar testing (e.g. two and four hours after eating various foods) is encouraged in order to know how a given food affects any individual. Blood sugar testing with insulin reactions is important in helping to know how low the blood sugar is. The excessive eating with a hypoglycemic reaction (or just the psychological feeling of hunger) is a major problem in controlling blood sugar levels. Remember that **food management for people with diabetes does not mean a restrictive diet, but rather a healthy eating regimen that family and friends can also enjoy.**

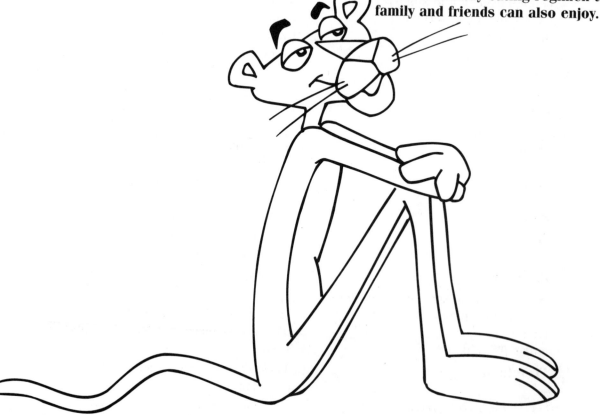

Table 7

EXAMPLES OF EXCHANGES FOR DIFFERENT CALORIC DIETS

Calories:	1200	1500	1800	2000	2200	2500	2700	3000	3500
BREAKFAST									
Meat	0	0	1	1	1	1	1	1	1
Bread	1	1	2	2	3	2	3	4	5
Fat	0	0	1	0	0	1	1	1	1
Fruit	1	2	2	2	2	2	2	2	2
Milk	1	1	1	1	1	2	2	2	2
LUNCH									
Meat	1	1	1	2	2	3	3	3	5
Bread	2	2	2	3	3	3	4	4	6
Vegetable	0	0	1	1	1	1	1	1	1
Fat	1	1	1	1	1	1	2	2	2
Fruit	1	1	2	2	2	2	2	2	2
Milk	1/2	1	1	1	1	1	1	1	1
DINNER									
Meat	2	2	2	3	3	3	3	4	5
Bread	1	2	2	3	3	3	3	4	6
Vegetable	1	1	1	1	1	1	1	1	1
Fat	0	1	1	1	1	1	1	1	2
Fruit	1	1	1	1	1	2	2	2	2
Milk	1/2	1	1	1	1	1	1	1	1

Snacks (also to be eaten to reach the number of calories shown at the top of the table)

10:00 a.m.	fresh fruit (small apple, orange, small or half a medium banana)
3:00 p.m.	1200-2400 cal: 1 bread, 1 fruit
	2500-3500 cal: 2 bread, 1 fruit
9:00 p.m.	1200-2400 cal: 1 bread, 1 meat
	2500-3500 cal: 2 bread, 1 meat

These plans are all 30% fat or less

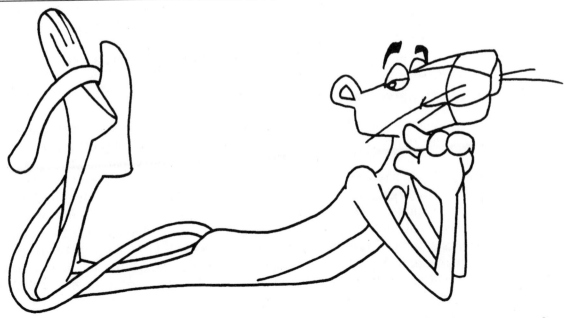

SUMMARY OF EXCHANGE LISTS

The purpose of this food list is to give examples of food exchanges and the concept of the "exchange food program." A more complete reference is "Exchange Lists for Meal Planning," 1999 update published by the American Diabetes Association and the American Dietetic Association, P.O. Box 930850, Atlanta, GA 31193. The cost is $1.75, plus $4.99 for shipping and handling (or less if purchased in quantities). In general, the idea of the exchange food program is to develop "equivalents" in each food group that are similar to each other in amounts of sugar and in calories. Nutrition teaching should be given by a dietitian or nutritionist. The food groups, with examples of foods that have similar values in each of the groups, are listed on the following pages.

CARBOHYDRATE GROUP

Starch/Bread List: One bread exchange contains about 15 grams of carbohydrate and three grams of protein (80 calories). Examples are: one slice of bread, 1/2 hamburger or hot dog bun, 3/4 cup of unsweetened cereal, 1/2 cup noodles, three cups popcorn, crackers (six small saltines, two squares of graham crackers, three of most other crackers), one pancake or waffle (5 inch), or 15 potato or corn chips.

The vegetables included in the bread exchanges are: corn (1/2 cup or one ear), white potato (one baked or 1/2 cup mashed), yam or sweet potato (1/4 cup), green peas (1/2 cup), squash (1/2 cup) and lima beans (1/2 cup).

Fruit List: One fruit exchange contains about 15 grams of carbohydrate (60 calories) and essentially no fat or protein. Examples of one fruit exchange are: grape juice (1/3 cup), apple or pineapple juice (1/2 cup), orange or grapefruit juice (1/2 cup), one small apple, orange, pear or peach, 1/2 banana, 1/2 cup berries, 1/3 of a small cantaloupe, or one cup of watermelon.

Milk List: One milk exchange is the quantity equal to about eight grams of protein or 32 calories, and 12 grams of carbohydrate or 48 calories (with a trace of fat for a total of 90 calories). Examples of one milk exchange are: one cup of skim or non-fat milk, one cup of 1% milk (also includes 1/2 fat exchange), one cup yogurt made from skim milk, one cup of yogurt from 2% milk (also includes one fat exchange), or one cup 2% milk (also includes one fat exchange).

Vegetable List: One-half cup of most vegetables (cooked or raw) has about 5 grams of carbohydrate and two grams of protein (25 calories) and is considered one exchange. Raw lettuce may be taken in larger quantities, but salad dressing usually equals one fat exchange. Some raw vegetables are higher in carbohydrate, equal to 15 grams carbohydrate and two grams protein, and should be considered equivalent to one bread exchange in quantity. These include corn and potatoes and are listed in the Bread Exchanges.

MEAT AND MEAT SUBSTITUTE GROUP

These are divided into **Very Lean** and **Lean** meats, **Medium Fat** meats and **High Fat** meats. One ounce of the lean meats contains seven grams of protein and three grams of fat (55 calories). The best of the **Lean Meats** are poultry (chicken and turkey without the skin) and fish, although lean pork, USDA Select or Choice grades of lean beef and 1/2 or 1% fat cottage cheese have also been placed in this group. The **Medium Fat** Meats group equals one protein and one fat exchange (five grams) and includes one ounce of ground beef, most cuts of beef, pork, lamb or veal, one ounce of low-fat cheese or one egg. It includes seven grams of protein and five grams of fat (75 calories). The **High Fat** Meats group (one protein, eight grams fat) includes sausages, spare ribs, most regular cheeses, and sandwich meats. It includes seven grams of protein and eight grams of fat (100 calories).

8
Table

FAT GROUP

Fat is necessary for the body and is particularly important during periods of fasting (overnight), when it is very slowly absorbed. One fat exchange contains five grams of fat (45 calories). The polyunsaturated fats are better for us than saturated fats, with one exchange equaling 1 tsp margarine or 1 tsp of any vegetable oil (except coconut). One exchange of saturated fat includes: 1 tsp butter, one strip of bacon, or 2 Tbsp of cream.

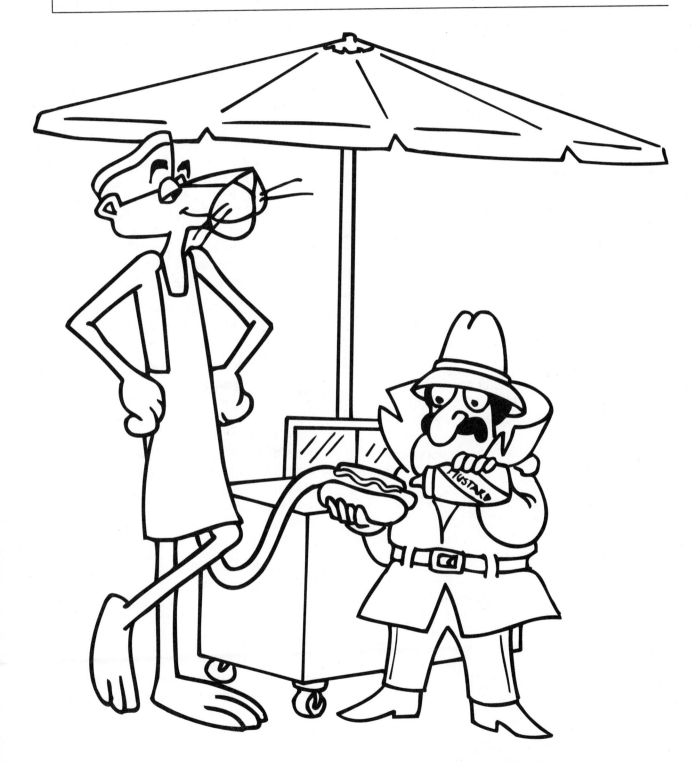

Good nutrition is important for your heart.

DEFINITIONS

ADA: American Diabetes Association.

"Carb Count" (or Choice): 15 gram equivalent (in the U.S.) of carbohydrate used to determine the units of short-acting insulin to be taken.

Carbohydrate ("Carb") Counting: A meal plan in which counting the units of carbohydrate to be eaten (and considering the blood sugar level and any planned exercise) is used to adjust the dosage of Humalog or Regular insulin to take prior to meals. A "carb count" in the U.S. is 15 grams of carbohydrate.

Cholesterol: One of the two main blood fats. High levels are related to a greater chance for heart attacks in later life.

Constant Carbohydrate Diet: A meal plan in which the amount of carbohydrate is kept consistent from day-to-day to match a relatively consistent dose of insulin.

DCCT: Diabetes Control and Complications Trial, which ended in June, 1993. It showed that good glucose control helped to prevent the eye, kidney, and nerve complications of diabetes.

Exchange Diet: A meal plan in which foods are grouped into one of six food lists having similar nutritional composition. Caloric intake and number of exchanges are set, but foods within a food group can be exchanged with one another.

Tablespoon (Tbsp): A measure of 15cc (ml) or three teaspoons. It is equal to 15 grams (1/2 oz) of water.

Teaspoon (tsp): A measure of 5cc (ml). It is also equal to five grams of water.

Triglyceride: One of the two main blood fats. High levels are believed to be related to a greater risk for heart attacks in later life for people with diabetes.

QUESTIONS (Q) AND ANSWERS (A) FROM NEWSNOTES

Q. Is there any way to know if the pop received at fast-food restaurants, theaters, and other places is truly "sugar-free" or the regular sugar-containing pop?

A. This question is asked frequently and the answer is "yes." Probably the cheapest way to test is by using the Test-Tape®, a roll of yellow tape from which a piece can be dipped into the pop. It turns green if there is sugar in the pop. The Diastix® (the sugar-only part of KetoDiastix®), or the distal sugar block on KetoDiastix will also change color if there is sugar present. Unfortunately, it is more common for the wrong pop to be served than most people realize, probably in the range of 20% of the time (one glass in five). As sugar pop is one of the most concentrated sources of sugar (approximately 10 teaspoons per can), it usually raises the blood sugar level to the 200 to 400 mg/dl (11.1 to 22.2 mmol/L) level. This is especially true if it is consumed without other foods, which slow the absorption of the sugar, or at a time when Humalog or Regular insulin is not taken to allow the sugar to enter the cells.

Q. Why does fructose sometimes cause an increase in blood sugar whereas at other times it does not?

A. This is a complex question, but it is again related to the hormone insulin. When adequate insulin is available throughout the day, the insulin "turns off" many metabolic pathways, such as those for making ketones, glycogen (sugar from stored sugar), and sugar from other foods (like protein). It also turns off the pathway which allows fructose to be metabolized to blood sugar (glucose).

Thus, people who are in good sugar control (low HbA_{1c}) will have the pathway "turned off" to make sugar (glucose) from fructose and can generally tolerate more fructose than people who are in poor sugar control (high HbA_{1c}).

It follows the adage that "Good control breeds good control, whereas poor control breeds poor control." It is obviously advantageous to be in good sugar control.

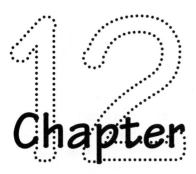

Chapter 12 EXERCISE AND DIABETES

Key ideas of this chapter:

🐾 Know the importance of regular exercise.

🐾 Recognize how to exercise safely without frequent low blood sugars.

Many of the people with the best controlled diabetes are those who exercise regularly. Exercise should be a normal part of life for everyone. We strongly encourage regular exercise for anyone who has diabetes, even if this means making a special effort to plan daily exercise. Young people from our Clinic have participated in almost every sport: football, baseball, golf, track, swimming, wrestling, dancing, skiing, basketball, soccer, weight lifting, horseback riding, jumping rope, jogging, and tennis. In the figure in Chapter 13, Diabetes and Blood Sugar Control, **EXERCISE** is listed as one of the "Big 4" factors to help attain good sugar control.

Many former and present professional athletes have diabetes. Professional baseball players with diabetes include Bill Gullickson (pitcher) and Ron Santo (third base). Professional football players include Kenny Duckett (wide receiver), Johnathon Hayes (tight end), Wade Wilson (quarterback) and Jay Leuwenberg, who was an All-American center for the University of Colorado in the 1990s. In the U.K., Gary Mabbott has type 1 diabetes and is a star football (American soccer) player. Hockey player Bobby Clarke, a former player of the Philadelphia Flyers, developed diabetes

 Table 1

THE IMPORTANCE OF EXERCISE

🐾 1 Exercise helps burn excess sugar

🐾 2 Exercise helps people feel better

🐾 3 Exercise helps keep the body in good shape

🐾 4 Exercise helps keep the heart rate (pulse) and blood pressure lower

🐾 5 Exercise helps keep blood fat levels normal

🐾 6 Exercise helps make people more sensitive to insulin

🐾 7 Exercise may help maintain normal blood circulation in the feet

at age 15. He won the award for outstanding player in the National Hockey League twice. Billy Talbert began playing tennis at age 12, two years after he developed diabetes. Because of the diabetes, he had been told by his doctor that he could no longer play baseball. He became one of the best tennis players in the world, winning 37 national tournaments and being captain of America's winning Davis Cup Team and a member of the Tennis Hall of Fame. When he was in Denver to instruct youth with diabetes about tennis, we asked Billy why he felt he had no complications after over 40 years with diabetes. He replied, "I have gotten some exercise every day of my life in which it has been possible."

THE IMPORTANCE OF EXERCISE

Exercise is important and helps people with diabetes in the following ways (Table 1):

1 Exercise Helps Burn Excess Sugar

Physical exercise helps the body burn more sugar. Insulin is still needed to allow the sugar to be burned, but the insulin is more effective during periods of exercise. As more blood flows to exercising muscles, these muscles take more sugar from the blood to use for energy. As blood flow increases in the arms and legs during exercise, more insulin is absorbed into the blood. The increased sugar and insulin flowing in the blood to the muscles during exercise causes more sugar to be burned. The old belief that people should not exercise if they have high blood sugar is wrong. The exercise usually helps lower the blood sugar. IT IS ONLY WHEN URINE KETONES ARE PRESENT THAT PEOPLE SHOULD NOT EXERCISE.

2 Exercise Helps People Feel Better

There is a feeling of "well-being" and pride that comes from being in good physical condition. Many people just seem to feel better when they exercise daily. They tend not to tire as easily. Some people even say they are happier.

Teenagers get much of their support from friends. Friends often are made during sports activities. Exercise can give people the opportunity to mix with others.

Sometimes people feel sorry for themselves. When they do this, they become stressed and produce adrenaline that can raise the blood sugar level. Other people like to watch TV and eat snacks that raise the blood sugar level. Exercise is a good way to improve a bad mood and to change a bad habit. In this way, exercise serves a double purpose.

3 Exercise Helps Keep the Body in Good Shape

Exercise is important, not only for people with diabetes, but for everybody. For thousands of years, people had to hunt for food and were very active. In the last 100 years, modern machines have made it possible for people to live with almost no exercise. This lack of activity has led to new health problems such as obesity and heart trouble. THE ONLY WAYS TO PREVENT OBESITY ARE TO EXERCISE AND NOT TO OVEREAT. Exercise helps burn excess calories and prevents obesity. A person who keeps a normal weight is less likely to have a heart attack in later life.

4 Exercise Helps Keep the Heart Rate (pulse) and Blood Pressure Lower

The heart is helped by exercise for many reasons. The heart of a person who is in good physical shape can do the same work with fewer heartbeats. An average heart rate (pulse) is 80 beats per minute. Many people who exercise regularly will have values in the 60s. Blood pressure tends to be lower in people who exercise. Thus, the heart doesn't have to pump as hard. Lower blood pressure helps prevent heart attacks in later life. It is also important in preventing the eye and kidney complications of diabetes (see Chapter 21 on complications). Exercise tends to build extra blood vessels in the heart. This lets more blood flow to the heart.

5 Exercise Helps Keep Blood Fat Levels Normal

We have discussed the importance of reducing cholesterol and saturated (animal) fat in the diet in Chapter 11. Many children with diabetes have high levels of the blood fats, cholesterol, and/or triglycerides. These high blood fat levels can lead to early aging of blood vessels. Exercise and good blood sugar control are the best ways to reduce blood triglyceride levels. One study showed that triglyceride levels could be reduced greatly after only four sessions of running 40 minutes a day. Exercise also may help remove cholesterol from blood vessel walls by increasing HDL (high density lipoprotein). Lowering the blood fat levels improves the health of blood vessels (including those supplying blood to the heart) and lessens the risk of heart attacks.

Exercise Helps to Make People More Sensitive to Insulin

The only way humans can increase insulin sensitivity is by exercising. The number of insulin receptors, the places where insulin attaches to cell membranes to allow sugar to pass into the cell, actually increases as a result of regular exercise. As a result, the person is more sensitive to insulin, the insulin can work more efficiently, and usually a lower daily dose is required. Regular exercise (and weight loss) allows many people with type 2 (adult-onset) diabetes to stop medications.

Exercise May Help Maintain Normal Blood Circulation to the Feet in Later Life

Data from the Pittsburgh Diabetes Registry showed that when boys with diabetes played in high school sports, they were more likely to keep normal foot circulation in later years. It is likely that the boys who were active in high school were also more apt to be active in later years. The same findings likely apply to females, although in the 1950s, when this study was begun, not many high school athletic programs were available for girls. It is important to get boys and girls with diabetes started in a sports activity at a young age so that they will be good enough to make a sports team (whether they are a star or not) as a teenager. Most younger children are constantly active so that exercise is not a problem in the younger age group.

MANAGING EXERCISE IN PEOPLE WITH DIABETES

Now that you know seven of the many reasons why exercise is important for a person with diabetes, you should ask yourself some questions.

Which Kinds of Exercise are Best?

THE BEST EXERCISE IS THE ONE YOU LIKE. Different strokes for different folks! If you hate to jog or swim, but do it because you are told to, you probably won't exercise regularly. Swimming five days a week in an outdoor pool is fun in the summer, but it is often impossible to do in the winter. You may have to choose a different exercise, such as jumping rope or riding an exercise bicycle, in the winter.

Only aerobic exercises help heart fitness. Aerobic exercises include most continuous activities (such as jogging, walking, swimming, or bicycling) that are done for a period of 25 minutes or longer. Many training programs use machines at health spas that feature continuous aerobic activity rather than short bursts of activity followed by a rest (a non-aerobic activity). When activities such as weight lifting are done in short bursts with rests in between, they are considered strength-building, but not aerobic.

Boxing is the only activity in which we have

Insulin Receptors

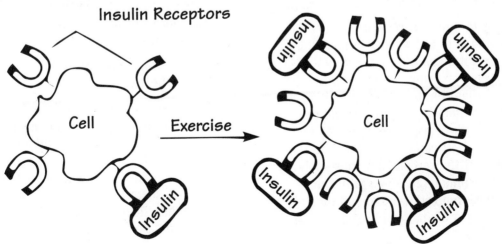

asked youth not to participate. The high incidence of eye injuries is not needed by a person who has diabetes (which can also cause eye problems). In addition, the high incidence of brain damage makes boxing dangerous for people with or without diabetes.

Careful diabetes management to prevent low blood sugar levels (as discussed in this chapter) is important in all sports, but is particularly important for those in which there is an associated danger (e.g., scuba diving). Fortunately, dangerous activities are not generally used for daily aerobic activity.

When Should I Exercise?

The best time to exercise will vary with your schedule. Think ahead and make changes in insulin doses and snacks to help prevent low blood sugars. Children like to play after school, and most organized sports activities take place then. This is the time that most intermediate-acting insulins are having their main effect so that extra care to prevent low blood sugar is important. When possible, pick an exercise time, preferably the same time each day, and adjust the snacks and insulin dose to fit the exercise. YOUR DIABETES MANAGEMENT CAN BE ADJUSTED TO SUIT YOUR LIFESTYLE. YOUR LIFESTYLE DOES NOT HAVE TO BE ADJUSTED TO FIT YOUR DIABETES.

When Should I Not Exercise?

If your urine ketone level is large or moderate, exercise can raise the sugar or ketone level even higher. Thus, it is not good for you to exercise when you have urine ketones. Remember to check urine ketones before exercising if you are not feeling well.

How Should I Get Started?

The best way to make exercise a part of everyday living is to begin early in life. Older children may not be as willing to begin a regular exercise program. Exercise should be part of the normal routine. Many people prefer TV or computer games to exercise, and the parent may have to encourage a change in attitude. The parent can reward the child for good behavior with exercise activities such as skating and swimming. It is helpful if the parent can have fun with the child in the activity. Jogging, walking, or jumping rope is

good for parents too! Whenever a child has a parent's attention and company, that time quickly becomes a reward. A child of any age will soon pick up the parent's attitude toward exercise. The parent needs to be a good example by exercising regularly, even if it is not with the child.

When beginning a new exercise program, it is always best to START SLOWLY and gradually extend the time and amount of exercise. This will result in fewer sore muscles and a better chance to continue the program.

How Often and How Far?

How often should the child with diabetes exercise? TWENTY-FIVE MINUTES OF AEROBIC EXERCISE, AT LEAST THREE TIMES PER WEEK, IS ENOUGH TO IMPROVE THE HEALTH OF THE HEART. The more exercise a person gets, the more fat that is "burned." Some people burn more calories with their exercise than others. This is partly related to how hard the person exercises. For example, a person who runs at a rate of seven minutes per mile burns 300 calories in 30 minutes. However, if the person runs at 11 minutes per mile, only 200 calories are burned in 30 minutes. If weight loss is one of the goals, it may be necessary to work harder or for a longer period to reach the desired goals.

It is wise to check the pulse immediately (for 10 seconds, and multiply by six) after stopping the activity. If the pulse is more than 160 beats per minute, the exercise has probably been too strenuous.

How Can I Prevent Low Blood Sugar (hypoglycemic) Reactions During Exercise?

It is essential to prevent low blood sugar reactions during exercise. This can be done in several ways.

Check blood sugars before, during, and after the exercise

The best way to know how any exercise affects a person is to check blood sugars before, during (when possible), and after the exercise. Once a pattern is detected (e.g., "swimming always makes my blood sugar fall" or "softball doesn't seem to affect my blood sugar"), then more intelligent insulin and food changes can be made. Sometimes blood sugars go up with exercise. This may be because of output of the hormone adrenaline (epinephrine), which is a normal response in people with or without diabetes. The adrenaline causes sugar to be released from muscle and liver stores and raises the blood sugar for varying periods of time. Keeping good records is important so that when a similar exercise is done at a similar time of the day (with the same insulin peaking) and with a similar starting blood sugar level, the best plans for insulin changes and food can be made. A suggested exercise record is shown in Table 2.

Some people become frustrated with the "ups and downs" of blood sugars during exercise. It is important to remember that **"DIABETES IS A COMPROMISE."** One must put up with the changes in blood sugars in return for the better health of the heart, blood vessels and the entire body.

Eat before heavy exercise

If you are going to exercise around mealtime, you should eat the meal first. When possible, allow a half-hour for digestion. Liquids such as milk and juices are absorbed most rapidly and generally prevent low blood sugar reactions for the next 30-60 minutes. Solid foods, such as those eaten at mealtime, are digested more slowly and usually provide protection for at least 2-3 hours. When it is possible to choose the exercise time, try to begin the exercise 30-60 minutes after a meal or snack (and omit usage of Humalog).

Have extra snacks available during exercise

THE PERSON WITH DIABETES MUST ALWAYS HAVE A SOURCE OF SUGAR AVAILABLE. Parents have sewn pockets in basketball shorts, jogging pants, and other clothes to hold a sugar packet, sugar cube, or a glucose tablet for a possible emergency. Joggers' wallets on shoes work nicely. A sandwich or similar snack should be available nearby, as a sugar packet may last only a few minutes. It is helpful for the coach or instructor to have a tube of instant glucose or some other emergency source of sugar.

It is often difficult to guess the amount of a snack necessary for a particular activity. If the exercise is in the hour after a meal, an extra snack may not be needed. If a person is physically unfit, the blood sugar may drop more rapidly than if the person is physically fit. It is very useful to monitor the blood sugar to determine what the correct snack is for each child. If the blood sugar is low (e.g., below 100 mg/dl or 5.5 mmol/L), a larger snack is needed than when the blood sugar is high. **IN FACT, EXERCISING CAN BE A VERY EFFECTIVE WAY TO LOWER A HIGH BLOOD SUGAR (AS LONG AS URINE KETONES ARE NOT PRESENT).** Blood sugars may actually increase slightly during the first hour of exercise because the body releases the excitatory hormone, adrenaline. Blood sugars may then decline. The type of snack can be varied depending on the expected length of the activity. IN GENERAL, THE MORE RAPIDLY ABSORBED CARBOHYDRATES, SUCH AS MILK OR JUICE, ARE USED FOR SHORT-TERM ACTIVITIES. More food is added, such as crackers or bread, if the activity is to last longer. THE SNACK THAT KEEPS THE BLOOD SUGAR UP THE LONGEST IS ONE THAT INCLUDES PROTEIN AND FAT ALONG WITH THE CARBOHYDRATE. This might be a cheese or meat sandwich with a glass of juice. It is wise to check the blood sugar after the activity to help decide what to use for a snack the next time. Experience is the best teacher!

Extra foods taken during the exercise period can help keep blood sugars in the normal range (see Table 3). Extra water may also be important, particularly during hot weather. A general rule is to drink eight ounces of fluids for every 30 minutes of vigorous activity. Liquids such as milk, Gatorade, and fruit juices help replace water, salts, and carbohydrates. Drinking Gatorade (or other sports drinks) at half-hour intervals during strenuous exercise works well for many people. It is a good idea to keep packets of cheese and crackers in the glove box of the car to eat before or after an activity. This is especially important if the distance is great between home and the activity.

"DELAYED HYPOGLYCEMIA" refers to low blood sugars several hours after the exercise is over. It is quite common and can occur as late as 6-8 hours after heavy exercise (and can result in an insulin reaction in the middle of

EXERCISE RECORD

Day and date	Type of exercise	Insulin dose (time)	Time of day (start/end)	Pre-exercise blood sugar	Snack(s) eaten (time)	Blood sugars during or after the exercise (and time)	Any hypoglycemic episodes (and when)

This page may be copied as often as desired.

Table 2

the night). It happens because the sugar that was "burned" by the muscle goes from the blood back into the muscle. Hormone changes with sleep (e.g., lower adrenaline levels) may also be important. It is best prevented by:

i) Extra carbohydrate at the next meal or snack (even when the blood sugar is above-range)

ii) A longer-lasting snack (including solid carbohydrate, protein, and fat) at bedtime

iii) Reducing the insulin dose (see below)

EXTRA FOOD TO COVER EXERCISE*†

Expected length of exercise	Blood sugars mg/dl mmol/L		Examples of foods
A. Short (15-30 minutes)†	<80	<4.4	8 oz Gatorade or milk** or 4-6 oz juice**
	80-150	4.4-8.3	A fresh fruit (or any 15 grams carbohydrate **)
	>150	>8.3	None
B. Longer (30-120 minutes)†	<80	<4.4	8 oz Gatorade or milk** or 4 oz juice plus 1/2 sandwich
	80-150	4.4-8.3	8 oz Gatorade or milk plus fresh fruit
	>150	>8.3	1/2 sandwich**
C. Longest (2-4 hours)*†	<80	<4.4	Juice or Gatorade, whole sandwich
	80-150	4.4-8.3	Fruit, whole sandwich
	>150	>8.3	Whole sandwich

*Remember to also drink water, Gatorade, or other fluids (one, two or three 8 oz glasses for A, B, or C above, respectively) before or during the exercise to prevent dehydration. The exercise for this table is assumed to be of moderate degree (e.g., walking, bicycling leisurely, shooting a basketball, or mowing the lawn). If more vigorous exercise (e.g., jogging, bicycle race, basketball game, or digging in the garden) is undertaken for a similar period of time, then more food may need to be added. Amounts vary for different people and the best way to learn is to do blood sugars before and after the exercise and keep a record of the blood sugar values (see Table 2).

**Each of these represent 15 gms of carbohydrate which will last for about 30 minutes of moderate exercise. A sandwich with meat or other protein lasts longer.

†May also need to reduce insulin dosage.

❖ Reduce the insulin dosage

Before trying an activity for the first time, discuss any changes that might be needed in insulin dosage with your diabetes care provider. The insulin dose is easy to decrease if you know which insulin is having its main effect during the time of exercise. If on two shots per day, the day is divided into four periods, and one of the insulins is most active in each period (see Chapter 20, Adjusting The Insulin Dose). You should reduce the insulin that is most active during the period of heavy exercise. The figures in Chapter 7 show which insulin acts during each of the four periods.

If extra morning exercise is planned, you can reduce or leave out the morning Humalog or Regular insulin. If late afternoon exercise is planned, you can reduce the morning NPH or Lente insulin by 10-20%. NPH or Lente insulin is never left out entirely. People reduce insulin by different amounts. **EXPERIENCE IS THE BEST TEACHER**.

You should reduce the insulin that is active during the period of exercise. Suppose you are receiving 30 units of NPH insulin in the morning and you have a soccer game in the afternoon. You might reduce the dose by 10-20% (3-6 units). You would then receive 24-27 units of NPH insulin.

If strenuous exercise is planned for all day, both the morning NPH and the short-acting insulins can be reduced. The evening insulin dose may also need to be reduced to prevent "delayed hypoglycemia." If strenuous exercise is planned for the evening, the evening Humalog or Regular insulin can be reduced or omitted. One reason the evening NPH might be decreased is for overnights at friends' homes, when a child may be staying up later than usual. More activity and excitement burn more sugar, and less insulin may be needed. You may have to try a few times before you find the best way to reduce your insulin for activities. Keep careful records and discuss them at clinic visits. Blood sugar tests before and after exercise can help you make these decisions.

❖ Changing the short-acting insulin

Most low blood sugars from Humalog occur in the first 90 minutes after injection. Thus, if exercise is planned in the first hour after eating, it would be better to use Regular insulin only (no Humalog) if a pre-meal shot is being taken. In contrast, if heavy exercise (e.g., a soccer game) is to occur two to four hours after eating (when Regular insulin is peaking), it would be better to use only Humalog as the short-acting insulin. It is OK to use Humalog insulin on one day and to use Regular insulin at the same time on another day. It is important to THINK AHEAD as to which insulin might be better on a given day.

❖ Change the injection site

The choice of where you inject the insulin can help prevent low blood sugars. Exercise increases blood flow into the part of the body that is moving. The increased blood flow takes up more insulin. When a person with diabetes exercises, the blood insulin level may increase, whereas insulin levels decrease in non-diabetics during exercise. If you inject insulin into an arm or leg that you will use heavily during exercise, your body may absorb the insulin too rapidly. If you are going to run, don't inject insulin into the leg. If you are going to play tennis, avoid the tennis arm. The abdomen is a good site for most strenuous exercise days.

❖ Make sure others know

It is important that coaches and teammates are aware of the diabetes. A team manager may be a good person to carry extra sugar snacks. It is helpful if the coach can have at least some awareness of the diabetes and know the symptoms and treatment of low blood sugar. A letter is included at the end of this chapter that you are welcome to copy as often as you like to share with coaches. Remember that when a low blood sugar occurs during a sporting event, it is important to rest for at least 10 minutes to let the blood sugar rise. The coach should be aware of this.

Table 4

SUGGESTIONS FOR EXERCISING SAFELY

- Eat before heavy exercise
- Have extra snacks available during exercise; some people use Gatorade, 4-8 oz, for every 30 minutes of vigorous exercise
- Always carry sugar
- Reduce the insulin dose
- Change the injection site
- Change the type of short-acting insulin
- Check blood sugars before and after exercise to learn the best insulin adjustment for the activity
- Wear an ID bracelet or necklace
- Try to exercise with a friend who knows about low blood sugar reactions
- Make sure coaches know about low blood sugars (see letter at end of this chapter)
- Do not exercise if ketones are present
- Drink plenty of water, especially in hot weather
- If delayed hypoglycemia occurs frequently, an extra carbohydrate should be taken with the next meal or snack
- Have fun

NUTRITION FOR EXERCISE

We frequently have adolescents ask us, "Can I take a protein supplement and/or should I take amino acids?" The answer to these questions is "No." Taking extra protein or amino acid supplements will NOT build muscles. The only way to build muscles is to do the physical exercise necessary to expand the muscle mass. The foods to eat are described in Chapters 10 and 11. There is no better food plan for building muscles than the plan described in those chapters.

AGE AND EXERCISE

Adults are advised to discuss plans to begin a new exercise program with their diabetes care provider first. As with everyone, starting slowly and gradually increasing the amount of exercise is important. Proper stretching (5-10 minutes) **BEFORE and AFTER** the exercise will help prevent cramps and stiffness that may otherwise discourage further exercise. Finally, if diabetes complications are present, or if someone is over the age of 20 and has had

diabetes for 10 years or longer, it is wise to check with the diabetes care provider prior to beginning a new exercise program. Strenuous activities, including weight lifting and jogging, are discouraged for people who have severe eye changes of diabetes (proliferative retinopathy). This should be discussed with the diabetes eye specialist. Similarly, people with neuropathy should discuss the pros and cons of exercise with their diabetes care provider. When peripheral neuropathy is severe, weight-bearing exercise should be limited. With both severe eye changes and neuropathy, exercises that involve straining, jarring or causing increased pressure on the eyes or feet must be avoided. It is sometimes wise to have a "baseline" electrocardiogram (ECG) done prior to beginning a new exercise program. Other tests are then possible if there are any suggestions of abnormalities. People may ask their diabetes care provider to review with them the ADA guidelines for exercise that were published in December, 1997 (*Diabetes Care* 20, p. 1908).

SUMMARY

Exercise is important for all people, but especially for a person with diabetes. Choose exercises that you enjoy. If possible, the amount of exercise and the time of day should be fairly **CONSISTENT**. You can change the diabetes management to fit the exercise. It is not necessary to change the exercise to fit the diabetes. Suggestions for exercising safely are summarized in Table 4. You can plan the exercise after a meal, reduce the insulin dosage, or take extra snacks to help prevent low blood sugars. YOU SHOULD CARRY A SOURCE OF SUGAR AT ALL TIMES AND YOU SHOULD ALWAYS HAVE A LONGER-LASTING SNACK AVAILABLE NEARBY. Remember, it is wise to THINK AHEAD about what the day's schedule will bring and plan accordingly.

DEFINITIONS

Abdomen: The area around the belly button. The fatty tissue of the abdomen can be used as an injection site.

Adrenaline (epinephrine): The excitatory hormone. This normally increases early in exercise and may result in an initial rise in the blood sugar.

Aerobic: A continuous exercise usually lasting 25 minutes or longer.

Buttocks (seat): What a person sits on. The fatty tissue of the buttocks can be used as an injection site.

Delayed hypoglycemia: Low blood sugars occurring 4-12 hours after heavy physical exercise. This usually occurs as sugar leaves the blood to replace depleted muscle sugar stores.

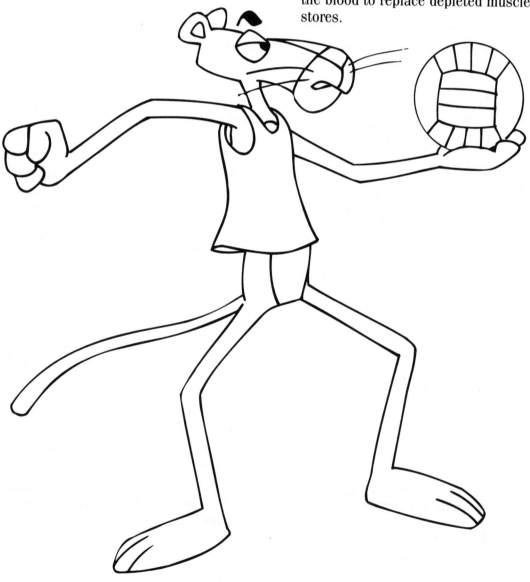

QUESTIONS (Q) AND ANSWERS (A) FROM NEWSNOTES

Q. My daughter just started swimming practices everyday from 3:30-5:30 p.m. Her pre-dinner blood sugars are over 200 mg/dl (11.1 mmol/L) when she gets home. However, she has awakened at 3:00-4:00 a.m. the past two mornings feeling shaky. Is that possible?

A. Your daughter has the classic "delayed hypoglycemia," which is not uncommon. Her blood sugar is high when she gets home from swimming as she has put out adrenaline (epinephrine), the excitatory hormone, during the exercise. All people, with or without diabetes, normally do this. The adrenaline causes breakdown of the stored sugar in muscle (glycogen) to help keep the blood sugar up during the exercise. It is a safety mechanism.

At a later time, the sugar goes back into the muscle—often 4-12 hours later. When this happens, the blood sugar falls and she awakens feeling shaky. This is less apt to happen if the evening NPH insulin dose is decreased, and it is often necessary to decrease the dose by as much as 2-6 units to prevent delayed hypoglycemia.

Q. Our doctor has told us not to reduce the insulin dose on heavy exercise days, but just to eat more food. We were told on one of the Children's Diabetes Foundation's ski days to also reduce the insulin dose. We are now confused.

A. An important part of managing exercise with diabetes is to prevent low blood sugars or "insulin reactions." Planning ahead is very helpful. Some children can just eat more food and will do fine. Many teenage girls are watching their diets, and when told to eat more food, will refuse to do so. Severe reactions can then result. Reduction of insulin dosage is the only way to prevent reactions in such cases. Often a combination of some reduction in insulin dosage and eating extra snacks turns out to be the best solution.

Q. How does exercise make a person more sensitive to insulin?

A. It is currently believed that exercise increases the number of insulin receptors on a cell. It is thus easier for the insulin to attach to the surface of the cell, allowing sugar to move across the cell membrane into the cell. Exercise is the only way known to increase the number of insulin receptors on a human cell.

(You may copy the letter on page 125 as often as you wish.)

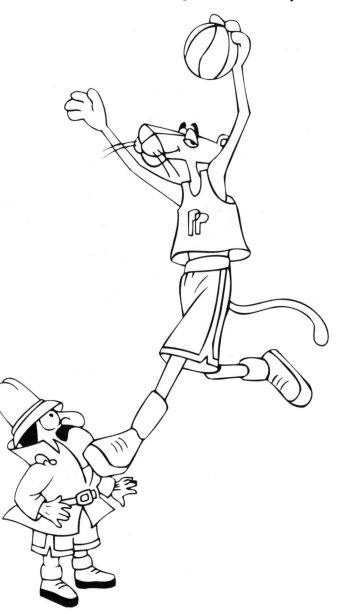

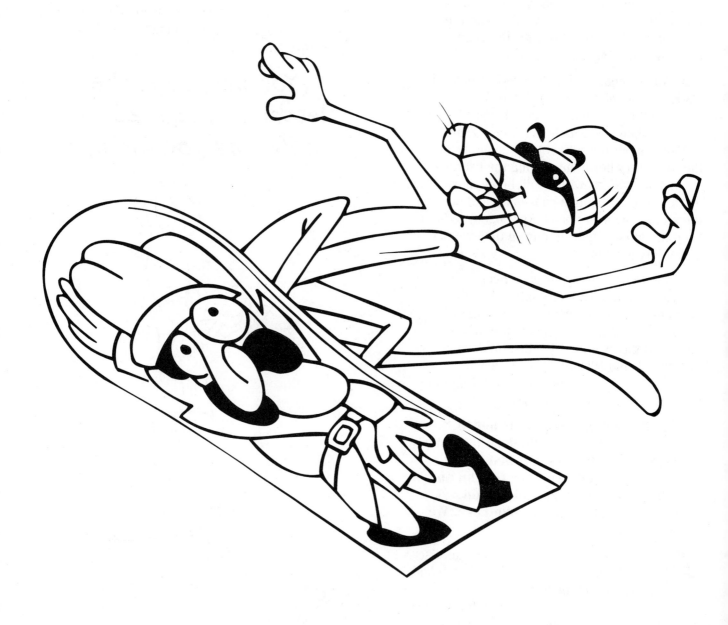

Dear Coach,

This letter is on behalf of _____ who is participating in
_____ this year. Although we do not want to single out people with
diabetes, there are things that you need to be aware of to help _____'s
performance and enjoyment of the sport.

Exercise is very important for children and adolescents with diabetes. The overall effect
of exercise is to lower blood sugar. We hope _____ will take the right amount
of insulin and eat according to the anticipated activity for the day. However, even when
these things are done, there may be times, especially with increased activity, when
he/she may have an "insulin reaction," a low blood sugar, a condition requiring
immediate attention. The symptoms of an insulin reaction include one or more of the
following: shakiness, dizziness, sweating, rapid onset of extreme hunger or tiredness,
and paleness. Some people complain of double vision and headaches. You may also
notice _____'s performance to suddenly become very poor, or his/her
overall mood may change to being very crabby or emotional.

If a low blood sugar occurs, a can of fruit juice, 8 oz of Gatorade, or two teaspoons of
sugar followed in 5-10 minutes by solid food (fruit, cheese and crackers, or a sandwich)
will help correct this condition. He/She should rest for a minimum of 10 minutes to let
the blood sugar return to normal. However, some children will still have a headache and
may not feel like continuing. We encourage families to be prepared for insulin reactions
at all times by having the proper foods available.

Many people with diabetes will change their insulin dose on days they anticipate a
practice or game. The scheduling (or cancellation) of these events ahead of time helps
the person (and parents) to be prepared.

Again, it is very important for youth with diabetes to be involved in sports. It helps with
their sugar control and allows their insulin to work more effectively. A person with
*diabetes **should not be and does not want to be** treated differently because of having*
diabetes. Please do not hesitate to call if you need more information or have any
concerns. Our phone number is _____.

Sincerely,

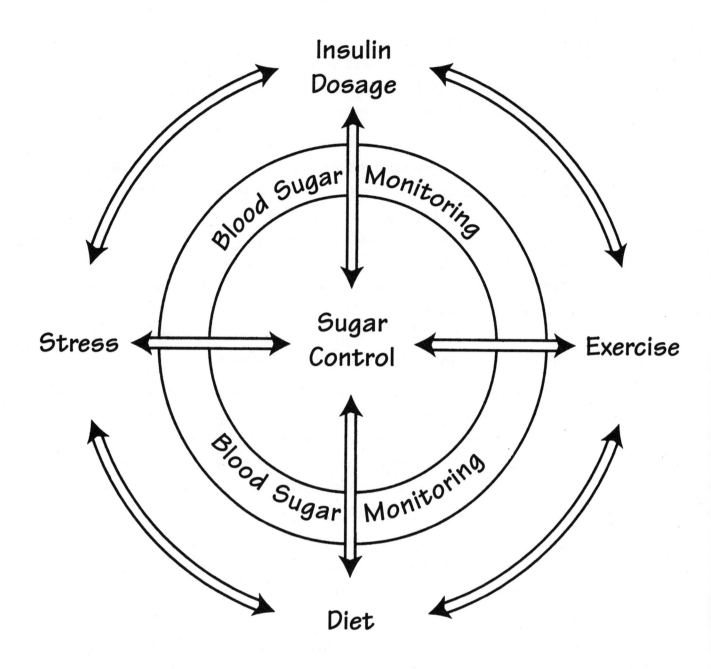

Four of the major influences on blood sugar control. All four must be in balance for the best sugar control. Blood sugar control is measured by daily blood sugar levels and by Hemoglobin A_{1c} (HbA_{1c}) levels done every three months.

Chapter 13

DIABETES AND BLOOD SUGAR CONTROL

Key ideas of this chapter:

❀ Understand how blood sugar control is measured.

❀ To help people realize the importance of good blood sugar control (a low HbA_{1c}).

The term "sugar control" is used in diabetes to describe how close the blood sugar is kept to normal limits. "Good sugar control" refers to blood sugar levels that more closely approach the normal sugar levels of someone without diabetes. In contrast, a person with constant high blood sugar levels is considered "in poor sugar control." This person may have such side effects as frequent thirst, frequent urination, weight loss, or episodes of acidosis.

It is important to have a reliable method to measure "overall" blood sugar control. It is obviously not possible to measure the blood sugar level every second of the day. Advances were made in the late 1970s to make the measurement of "overall" sugar control possible. This is done using the hemoglobin A_{1c} (HbA_{1c}) test. The glycohemoglobin, glycated hemoglobin, or hemoglobin A_1 (HbA_1) tests are names for similar tests. These tests all reflect how often the blood sugars have been high every second of the day in the past 90 days and will be discussed later in this chapter.

THE DCCT

In 1993, the Diabetes Control and Complications Trial (DCCT) proved that good sugar control helped to prevent the eye, kidney, and nerve complications of diabetes. People receiving **"intensive management"** (insulin pumps or 3-4 shots of insulin per day along with at least four blood sugar levels per day) had better sugar control (lower HbA_{1c} values) than people receiving **"conventional management"** (1-2 shots of insulin per day with 0-2 blood sugars per day). The intensive management group had a lower chance for the eye, kidney, and nerve complications than did the conventional management group.

SUGAR CONTROL

Good blood sugar control is the result of balancing the correct insulin dosage, regular exercise, good dietary habits, avoiding stress, and monitoring blood sugar levels. Each of these factors is discussed elsewhere in this book in more detail. Perhaps the most important of the four is the correct insulin dosage. Blood sugar control will remain poor if insulin is lacking, even if the other three factors are in balance. Thus, it will not help to do extra exercise if the person is not receiving the correct insulin dosage. However, any one of the four factors can result in poor sugar control. For example, if the other three factors are normally in balance, but the person decides to constantly drink sugar pop (10 tsp of sugar per can), good blood sugar control will likely be lost. Similarly, with a lot of stress, the adrenaline (excitatory hormone) levels will be high and will raise the blood sugar levels. Finally, exercise is important both for "burning" extra sugar and for making people more sensitive to insulin. Thus, all four of these factors must be in balance to result in the best sugar control possible for any person. The regular monitoring of blood sugar levels (Chapter 6) is essential to understand the effects of these four influences for any given person so that appropriate adjustments in the insulin dose can be made.

HOW IS SUGAR CONTROL MEASURED?

It is not always easy to decide whether a person has good or poor blood sugar control. Some helpful things that reflect sugar control are the following:

Control of Symptoms of Diabetes

A person who goes to the bathroom very frequently (particularly if a person is getting up two or more times per night) or who is often thirsty has obvious symptoms of high blood and urine sugar. This person usually needs more insulin, less sugar in the diet, or more daily exercise.

Occasionally, blurred vision may occur as a symptom of poor sugar control. High sugar levels in the lens of the eye pull water into the lens; this makes it difficult to change the shape of the lens to focus for clear vision. The blurred vision usually stops when blood sugar control improves. People should not be fitted for glasses unless blood sugar levels are stable. If the blurred vision does not improve when blood sugar control improves, the eye doctor should be contacted.

Vaginal yeast infections are more common in females with diabetes, particularly if the blood sugar levels have been high. This may be because yeast grows well in a high-sugar environment. When antibiotics are taken for bacterial infections, yeast also tends to grow as the bacteria disappear. If vaginal itching or burning is noticed, the diabetes care provider should be contacted.

Normal Physical and Emotional Growth

Children and adolescents who have poor blood sugar control sometimes have poor gains in height or weight. Even the difference between "fair" and "excellent" control can change the rate of growth in height. One study showed an average growth rate of two inches per year during the adolescent growth spurt when the HbA_{1c} averaged 12.4%, but a gain of 3.3 inches per year when the HbA_{1c} averaged 8.4%. Research reported in 1995 from our Clinic showed that final adult height was more apt to be taller if blood sugar control was good during adolescence. Following the height and weight every three months is an important part of the diabetes clinic visit.

Some people feel poorly when they have high blood sugar levels. They may be tired constantly, have a bad temper, or have any of a variety of symptoms. When better sugar control is achieved, they often are surprised to realize how well they feel—and to realize how poorly they had previously felt. Feeling tired and poorly over a long time does not allow for normal emotional growth.

Blood Glucose (Sugar) Measurements

BLOOD GLUCOSE TESTS ARE THE BEST WAY TO MEASURE SUGAR CONTROL ON A DAY-TO-DAY BASIS and are discussed in detail in Chapter 6. As noted in a previous section, the intensive treatment group in the DCCT tested at least four blood sugar levels each day. All families with someone with diabetes must have a method in the home for measuring blood sugars and must know how to do the tests accurately. Studies have shown that checking blood sugars and using the test results are as important for good sugar control as is the method of giving insulin (two shots per day, an insulin pump, or more than two shots per day). The blood sugar levels (fasting or anytime food has not been eaten for two or more hours) that we consider representative of good sugar control vary with the person's age. Thus, for a person:

Age	Desired Range
under 5 years	80-200 mg/dl (4.4-11.1 mmol/L)
5-11 years	70-180 mg/dl (3.9-10.0 mmol/L)
12 years and older	70-150 mg/dl (3.9-8.3 mmol/L)

If good sugar levels are achieved 50-60% of the time, the glucose control is usually good. If more than 50% of values are consistently above the desired range or if more than 10% of values are below these levels, the sugar control is not good and the diabetes care provider needs to be contacted. **It is important not to be unhappy with a blood test result, but instead to always be pleased that the test was done.** Hopefully, the results will be used to help attain better sugar control. Blood sugar monitoring was discussed in detail in Chapter 6.

In contrast to blood sugar testing at home, blood sugar measurements in a doctor's office may be of little value. There may be stress in coming in for the clinic visit, or the drawing of blood through an arm vein may lead to stress. The adrenaline output with stress may cause the blood sugar level to be high in the office.

Hemoglobin A_{1c} (HbA$_{1c}$), Glycohemoglobin (HbA$_1$), or Glycosylated (or Glycated) Hemoglobin

These names are used for slightly different forms of the same test. **THIS TEST IS THE MOST VALUABLE WAY TO MONITOR BLOOD SUGAR LEVELS OVER TIME.** Hemoglobin is the protein in the red blood cells that carry oxygen to the various parts of the body. If the blood sugar is high, sugar attaches to the hemoglobin and remains there for the life of the red blood cell (an average of 2-3 months). For the purposes of this book, we will call hemoglobin with sugar attached hemoglobin A_{1c} or HbA$_{1c}$. The HbA$_{1c}$ reflects how often the blood sugars have been high for every second of the past three months (for the past 7,776,000 seconds). No one could do that many blood sugars. **The HbA$_{1c}$ represents the forest while the daily blood sugars reflect the trees.** The HbA$_{1c}$ and glycated hemoglobin tests have been used routinely since the late 1970s and have been called the "answer to a prayer" for people with diabetes and their doctors. Previously there was no good test to monitor long-term blood sugar control. No one really knew if they were in good sugar control or not. The HbA$_{1c}$ test solved that problem.

The HbA$_{1c}$ test can be done at the time of the clinic visit and the person does not have to be fasting. Many clinics now do the test by finger poke and may have the result done in 10 minutes. THE TEST IS NOT ALTERED BY ANYTHING THE PERSON DOES ON THE DAY THAT THE TEST IS DRAWN. Other tests, such as a blood sugar level, can be affected if eating, exercise habits, or emotions are changed on the day of the test. The main disadvantage of this test is that an illness may make the level go up quickly by as much as one to two points. After the illness, the HbA$_{1c}$ value comes down much more slowly.

There are now several methods that are used for determining the HbA$_1$. Unfortunately, normal values and desired ranges for the different methods of doing the test vary from test to test. Three of the more common methods with normal and desired ranges (for different aged people with diabetes) are shown in the following table.

Table **NORMAL AND ACCEPTABLE HbA$_{1c}$ AND HbA$_1$ VALUES**

	HbA$_{1c}$		HbA$_1$
Normal (Non-diabetic):			
Test Type:	Hemoglobin A$_{1c}$	Hemoglobin A$_{1c}$	Glycated Hemoglobin
Company:	Miles (DCA 2000)	Biorad	Isolab
	Values up to 6.2%	4.3-6.2%	4.0-8.0%
Desired ranges for someone with diabetes:			
≥21 years	<7.5%	<7.5%	<9.6%
12-21 years	<7.8%	<7.8%	<10%
5-11 years old	<8.5%	<8.5%	<11%
below five years old	7.5-9.3%	7.5-9.3%	10-12%

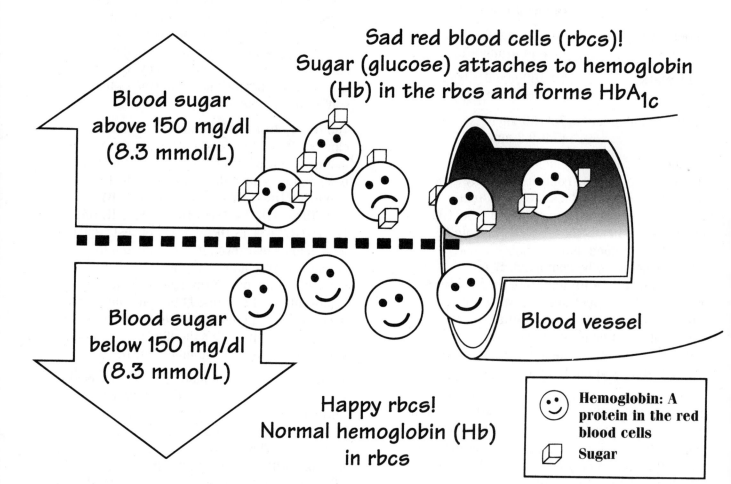

Sad red blood cells (rbcs)!
Sugar (glucose) attaches to hemoglobin (Hb) in the rbcs and forms HbA$_{1c}$

Blood sugar above 150 mg/dl (8.3 mmol/L)

Blood sugar below 150 mg/dl (8.3 mmol/L)

Blood vessel

Happy rbcs!
Normal hemoglobin (Hb) in rbcs

Hemoglobin: A protein in the red blood cells

Sugar

We encourage different ranges for different ages. We want people 12 years old and above, when complications are more likely to develop, to be in better sugar control. The pre-teens do not have the same risk for complications, so their values do not have to be as low. Finally, low blood sugars are more dangerous for preschoolers, as the brain continues to grow for the first four years after birth and low blood sugars are dangerous to a growing brain. Thus, preschoolers' blood sugar values should **not** be kept as low as older children's. The lower the HbA_{1c} value, the greater the chance for low blood sugars. After age 20 years, growth has decreased and life (hopefully) starts to become more consistent so that an even lower HbA_{1c} can be a goal (see Table in this chapter). The American Diabetes Association (ADA) Standards of Care (see Chapter 19) recommends this test be done every three months for a person with type 1 diabetes. IT IS THE ONLY WAY TO KNOW HOW A PERSON WITH DIABETES IS DOING EVERY SECOND OF THE DAY. We consider it the single best test for measuring long-term diabetes control. The desired ranges shown in the table are achievable and families should continue to strive to reach these goals.

Fructosamine (or Glycosylated Albumin) Test

This test measures the amount of sugar attached to the main serum protein, albumin. It reflects the blood sugars every second of the day for the past 2-3 weeks (whereas the HbA_{1c} reflects the past two or three months). It is often helpful to know how someone is doing more recently (in contrast to the past three months). The test is also helpful for someone who is changing treatment (more shots, an insulin pump, etc.) A commercial meter, the Duet®, is now available which measures either blood sugar or fructosamine in the home setting. This home meter may be particularly helpful to families who are unable to have an HbA_{1c} determined every three months when attending a diabetes clinic.

Blood Cholesterol and Triglyceride Levels

High blood fat (triglyceride or cholesterol) levels in some children with diabetes are related to poor sugar control. Other children may have high blood fat levels from eating poorly or it may be because they inherited a tendency to have high blood fat levels. As high blood fat levels can lead to earlier blood vessel aging, this may be a link between high blood sugar levels and later changes in blood vessel walls. We generally recommend that the total cholesterol level (or preferably, a lipid panel including triglyceride, LDL and HDL levels) be measured once a year (if normal). The total cholesterol value should be under 200 mg/dl (5.2 mmol/L). The triglyceride levels vary by age, but fasting levels should be below 130 mg/dl (1.5 mmol/L) for children and young adults. Cholesterol and triglyceride levels are also discussed in Chapters 11 and 21.

DEFINITIONS

Bacteria: Microscopic (only able to be seen with a microscope) agents that cause infections such as "strep throat."

DCCT: The Diabetes Control and Complications Trial. A very large research trial which showed that better sugar control reduced the likelihood of eye, kidney, and nerve problems in people over age 13 years with type 1 diabetes.

Emotions: How one feels psychologically (e.g., happy, sad).

Fructosamine: A test that measures the sugar attached to the albumin in the blood, which reflects how often the blood sugars have been high over the past two or three weeks.

HDL: High Density Lipoprotein. This is the "good" cholesterol protein which is believed to carry cholesterol from the blood vessel wall. Thus, a higher value is good.

Hemoglobin A_{1c} (HbA_{1c}, glycated or glycosylated hemoglobin): Hemoglobin protein in the red blood cells with sugar attached to it. This is used as a measure of sugar control over the previous three months.

LDL: Low Density Lipoprotein. This is the "bad" cholesterol protein which is believed to carry cholesterol into the blood vessel wall. An aim is to have LDL levels below 130 mg/dl (3.35 mmol/L (or below 100 mg/dl [2.6 mmol/L} for people at high risk for heart attacks).

Lens: The structure in the front of the eye that changes shape to allow the eye to focus on near or distant objects (see picture in Chapter 21).

SBGM: Self Blood-Glucose Monitoring. The measurement of blood glucose (sugar) levels by the person with diabetes (or their family).

Serum: The clear part of the blood when the blood cells are removed.

Symptoms: The complaints of a person; how they are feeling.

Yeast: A fungus that grows more readily when blood sugar levels are high and can cause an infection.

QUESTIONS (Q) AND ANSWERS (A) FROM NEWSNOTES

Q. Does the hemoglobin A_{1c} really give the average blood sugar over the past three months?

A. No, it reflects how often the blood sugars have been high over the past three months. When the blood sugar is high, the sugar attaches to all body proteins (including the red blood cell hemoglobin) and then stays attached to the hemoglobin (as hemoglobin A_{1c} or HbA_{1c}) until the red blood cell is replaced 2-3 months later. To represent the "average blood sugar," the sugar molecule would also have to detach from the protein when the blood sugar is low. This does not happen. Thus, the test only reflects how often the blood sugar has been high. The test is still far superior to any test in the past which reflects blood sugar control. It should be done on all people with type 1 diabetes every three months. In our research, reported in the *Journal of The American Medical Association* in 1989, higher hemoglobin A_{1c} values correlated with a greater likelihood of developing the eye and kidney complications of diabetes.

Q. Is it possible to get AIDS or other diseases as a result of having a blood test?

A. NO. Only sterile syringes and needles that have not been previously used are utilized in a doctor's office or a hospital setting. Drug users who share the same needle from one person to another without proper sterilization techniques can pass diseases between themselves.

However, this is not something that can happen as a result of having blood drawn in a doctor's office.

Q. Our daughter's HbA_{1c} has not reached the desired level. With all the concern from the DCCT on preventing complications, could you please make any suggestions on ways to achieve better control?

A. I have six suggestions:

1. This question was addressed in relation to the idea of doing an afternoon blood sugar after school and judging the afternoon snack and/or insulin supplement on the value at that time. This can be helpful in lowering the HbA_{1c}.

2. The use of Humalog insulin rather than Regular insulin often results in some improvement.

3. One of the biggest keys to better control, which was reported in the DCCT, was more frequent blood glucose monitoring, along with making good use of the results. All subjects did a **minimum** of four blood glucose levels each day. An unfortunate trend in recent years has been to not record results as they are all recorded in the meter. When this is not done, trends for high and low values are often missed and insulin adjustments may not be made. We prefer using the data sheets, either one or two weeks of values (see Chapter 6), and faxing the results to your diabetes care provider if more than half of the values at anytime of day are "above range" for the age. Be sure to include a fax and/or phone number where you can be reached.

4. Strangely enough, preventing low blood sugars is often important in achieving better control. Low blood sugars often result in excessive eating and sending the blood sugar up to 300 or 400 mg/dl (16.7 or 22.2 mmol/L). Although excessive eating is probably the major cause of the subsequent high blood sugars, output of balancing hormones (rebounding) likely plays a secondary role in some people.

5. I do think that "turning off" the liver's production of glucose (sugar) in the early morning is important in relation to keeping liver glucose production "turned off" all day

long. For many people, the human NPH insulin just does not last long enough from pre-dinner to arising the next morning to fulfill this function. It may be necessary to take the evening NPH at bedtime to have it successfully last through the night. An alternative that sometimes works is to use Ultralente insulin at dinner, as this sometimes lasts longer than NPH insulin.

Last but not least, a word must be said about missed insulin shots. One shot missed per week results in upsetting balancing hormone equilibrium and secondarily having very high HbA$_{1c}$ values. It is essential not to miss insulin injections.

The following were the questions Dr. Chase was asked to answer while addressing the Billings, Montana American Diabetes Association meeting during the May, 1987, Outreach Clinic.

Q. How do the following affect blood sugar?

Exercise?

A. This varies according to the duration and difficulty of the exercise, as well as the person. Most people release epinephrine (adrenaline) during exercise which initially makes the blood sugar rise. However, if the insulin was injected in an exercising extremity, the insulin levels may also increase as more blood flows through the extremity and more insulin is absorbed from the injection site, which lowers the blood sugar. Different people release different amounts of epinephrine during exercise to keep the blood sugar higher for varying time periods.

Another important variable is the blood sugar level prior to starting the exercise. If the level is low prior to starting, the person will be more apt to have a reaction during the exercise.

Keep good records the first time the exercise is done so that this information can be used in the future. It should be remembered that the sugar goes back into the muscle in the 2-12 hours following the exercise, and low blood sugars **(delayed hypoglycemia)** can occur at any time in this "after-exercise" period.

Illness?

A. Blood sugars most frequently increase with illnesses. Remember that urine ketones must also be checked. Some people who still make some of their own insulin may have a lower blood sugar with illness. Also, if vomiting or diarrhea is a problem, there will be less food in the stomach to maintain the blood sugar and low sugars may be a problem. If there is a question regarding the insulin dose, the diabetes care provider should be phoned.

Alcohol?

A. Alcohol, or other liquids consumed with alcohol, may initially increase the blood sugar. However, this is temporary and the main effect of alcohol will be to block the release of sugar from the liver and to lower the blood sugar level (up to 12 hours later). It is important to have the protein bedtime snack even if the blood sugar is high. It is also important to get up at a reasonable time the next morning to get food and insulin into the body.

Stress?

A. Stress usually results in epinephrine (adrenaline) release and an increase in blood sugar.

Excitement?

A. Young children react by burning more sugar and lowering the blood sugar. Older children may increase their blood sugar. The reason for the difference in response is unknown.

Good Weather?

A. Children tend to play outside for longer hours in good weather and the blood sugars are generally lower. The insulin dose may have to be reduced. This is especially true of the evening Humalog or Regular insulin when children are active after supper in the summer months.

Tobacco?

A. There has been some evidence that nicotine (smoking or chewing) can increase the blood sugar. People report a "buzz" after either, and this may resemble the feelings of low blood sugar. People with (or without) diabetes should not smoke or chew tobacco.

Q. Changes in our daughter's insulin dose have confused me and my wife. Initially she was on a low insulin dose which you increased after reviewing her blood sugars and seeing that her HbA$_{1c}$ was high. She got into good sugar control, but now her dose is coming back down again. This doesn't make sense to us.

A. This is quite common, and follows an old adage that: **"Good control breeds good control; poor control breeds poor control."** Thus, for someone in poor sugar control, when the liver is making sugar at a very high rate, it takes very little (stress, infection, etc.) to make even more sugar and it may take a lot of insulin to get the liver's sugar production machinery turned off. This may also be the case for a newly-diagnosed person.

However, once the liver's pathways for making sugar are turned off, it may not take as much insulin to keep them turned off. Also, stress and infections will not have as great of an effect in a person in good sugar control. This may be part of the reason for the "honeymoon" period in the newly diagnosed person.

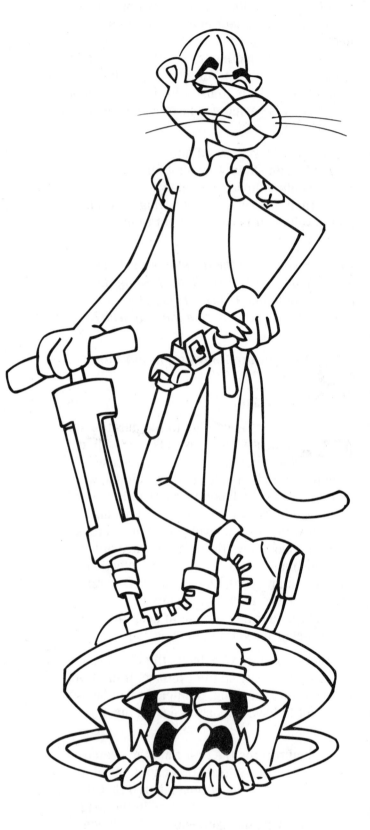

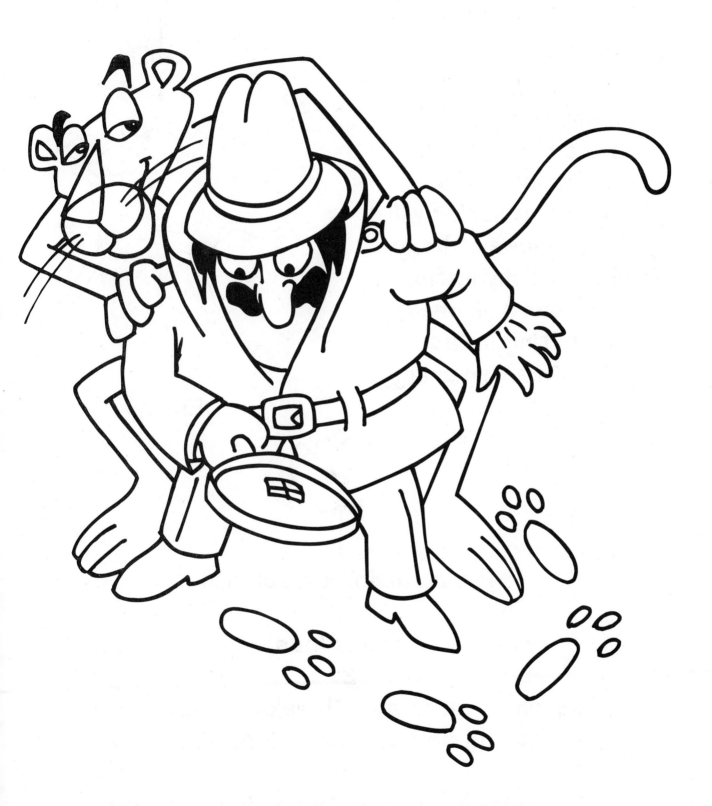

DIABETES

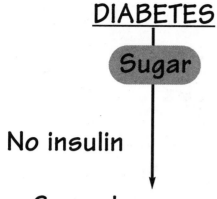
Sugar

No insulin

Sugar becomes high in the blood. Sugar spills into urine. Frequent urination will result in loss of body fluids or dehydration. Sugar can't be used, resulting in fat breakdown as an energy source.

NORMAL

Sugar

Insulin

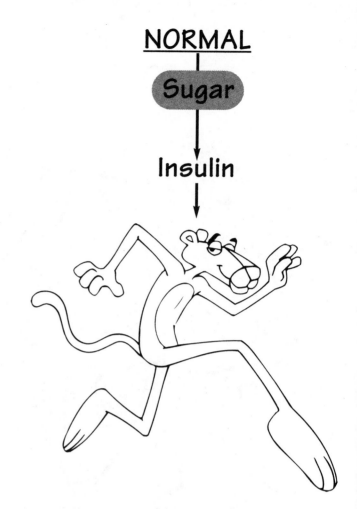

Energy

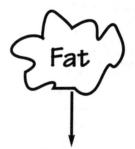
Fat

Fat breakdown results in:
1.
Weight loss
2.
Ketones, which are a breakdown product of fat and appear in the blood and urine
3.
Too many ketones in the body = acidosis

KETONURIA AND ACIDOSIS (DIABETIC KETOACIDOSIS OR DKA)

Chapter 14

(Note: This chapter is complex and we advise reading it after other basic concepts are learned.)

Key ideas of this chapter:

* Understand what ketones and acidosis (ketoacidosis) are.

* Know the danger of acidosis (ketoacidosis).

* Know the steps to take to deal with urine ketones (ketonuria) in order to prevent acidosis.

CAUSES OF KETONURIA AND ACIDOSIS

One "emergency" in diabetes, low blood sugar (hypoglycemia), was discussed in Chapter 5. The other emergency is ketonuria, the appearance of moderate or large ketones in the urine, which can develop into acidosis. The measurement of urine ketones is very easy (a dipstick) and was discussed in Chapter 4. The lack of knowledge about when to measure urine ketones and what to do when they are positive, and not having ketone sticks which have not expired available in the home, are the most common deficiencies in families referred to our center. These deficiencies can result in a serious episode of acidosis.

"Large" ketones are usually present in the urine for at least four hours before the total body's acidity is increased (acidosis). Acidosis is very dangerous and people can go into a coma or die from it. It is the cause of 85% of hospitalizations of children with known diabetes. The good news is that it is 98% preventable if people follow the instructions in this chapter and always remember to take their insulin shots. It is possible, with good knowledge and by following the instructions in this chapter, to never have an episode of · acidosis. **Acidosis can be prevented in a child who is known to have diabetes.**

Ketonuria and acidosis are due to there not being enough insulin available to meet the body's needs. The three main causes are: 1) **illnesses, 2) forgetting to take an insulin shot, 3) not enough insulin** (see Table 1). With an illness, extra energy may be needed by the body. This cannot be made unless extra insulin is available to make the extra energy from sugar. If a shot is forgotten, insulin is not available to the body. A lack of insulin could

Table 1

MAIN CAUSES OF ACIDOSIS

1. **Infection**
2. **Missed Insulin Injections**
3. **Not Enough Insulin**

happen in a person coming out of the "honeymoon" period who has not had insulin dosages adequately increased.

Remember the statement from Chapter 2: **I MUST TAKE MY INSULIN EVERY DAY FROM NOW ON. IF I FORGET MY INSULIN, MY DIABETES WILL GET OUT OF CONTROL. THERE IS ABSOLUTELY NO WAY I WILL NOT NEED INSULIN EVERY DAY FROM NOW ON.**

In Chapter 2, the importance of the role of insulin in allowing sugar to pass into cells was discussed (see Table 2). The second role of insulin, turning off the body's machinery for making sugar, also was discussed. The blood sugar is usually high with ketonuria and acidosis because the second and third functions of insulin are not happening (insulin is not turning off the body's machinery for making sugar and for making ketones). This is because not enough insulin is available. Also, the stress hormones are high with the illness and they act to increase blood sugar and ketone production. The high blood sugar causes sugar to pass into the urine (see Chapter 2) and the person must go to the bathroom a lot (frequent urination). The body may lose too much water and become too dry (dehydration). The tongue may feel dry and furry. Drinking lots of fluids may help prevent this. The main treatment, however, is taking extra insulin to shut off the body's machinery for making sugar and ketones.

It is not high blood sugar that causes ketonuria or acidosis. In fact, eating sugar does not cause acidosis. Ketones come from the breakdown of body fat (see picture at beginning of this chapter). The third role of insulin (see Table 2) is to shut-off fat breakdown. Because enough insulin is not available and because the stress hormones are high, fat begins to break down. The side-product of fat breakdown is ketone production. Ketones are initially passed into the urine (ketonuria). They may start with trace or small levels and gradually build up to moderate and then, to large levels. Once they reach the large level, they may start to build up in the body tissues. They are easier to reverse if treated at the moderate level before building up to large ketonuria. The longer someone has large urine ketones, the more likely they are to build up in the body and to result in acidosis (DKA). Thus, the early detection and reversal by giving extra insulin is critical. There are several reasons why fat is broken down:

- Not enough insulin is available to help the cells burn the needed sugar.

- The body needs more energy (e.g., for illness) and the fat is broken down to provide this energy.

- The stress hormones, steroids, adrenaline (epinephrine) and glucagon have been released, causing fat breakdown.

- Sugar is not available due to vomiting or not eating; thus, fat is broken down for energy. Anytime fat is broken down for energy, ketones (or acetone) are formed.

Table 2

MAIN FUNCTIONS OF INSULIN

1. **To allow sugar to pass into cells where it can be used for energy**
2. **To turn off excess production of sugar in the liver and muscle**
3. **To turn off fat breakdown**

SYMPTOMS OF ACIDOSIS

In any of the above cases, fat is broken down. The ketones are made from the fat. Acidosis usually comes on slowly, over several hours, and has the following symptoms:

- **Upset stomach and/or stomach pain**
- **Vomiting**
- **Sweet (fruity) odor to the breath**
- **Thirst and frequent urination (if the blood sugar is high)**
- **Drowsiness**
- **Deep breathing (indicates need to go to emergency room)**
- **If not treated, coma (loss of consciousness)**

On occasion it may be difficult to know if a person is having difficulty with low blood sugar or with acidosis. Testing the blood sugar and the urine ketones will help identify the correct problem. Table 3 may also be helpful in thinking about the two problems.

PREVENTION OF ACIDOSIS

Acidosis is the cause of 85% of re-admissions to the hospital for someone with known diabetes. Most of these admissions could be prevented if treated earlier. The simple rules outlined in Table 4 will prevent most cases of acidosis. It is a good idea to review this chapter every year. Families may forget the importance of checking urine ketones during any illness. Some people with diabetes who still make some of their own insulin, or who are in very good diabetes control, will have the "machinery" (enzymes) for making ketones effectively "turn off." As a result, they may go several years and never have urine ketones with an illness. As they grow older and a few more islet cells are lost, or they outgrow their remaining islets, they may suddenly find that moderate or large urine ketones are present. The important message is always to remember to check for ketones anytime a person with diabetes is ill, or anytime the blood sugar is above 240 mg/dl (13.3 mmol/L).

The prevention of acidosis is based on being able to detect changes early, when ketones are present in the urine (ketonuria), but before the ketones build up in the body (acidosis). To prevent acidosis, the person with diabetes must have a method in the home to check urine ketones (see Chapter 4). It also depends on the person and/or family being reliable enough to check for urine ketones anytime the person is sick (even with vomiting only one time) or anytime the blood sugar is above 240 mg/dl (13.3 mmol/L). **A low blood sugar can sometimes be present with acidosis, so that urine ketones must be checked with every illness, even if the blood sugar is low.** Another requirement to prevent acidosis is to call the diabetes care provider immediately (night or day) if moderate or large urine ketones are present, and to give extra rapid-acting insulin every two hours (Humalog) or every three hours (Regular) until the urine ketones measure "small" or less. Drinking lots of fluids is also important to help wash the ketones out in the urine. A summary of the instructions is in **bold** print in Table 4.

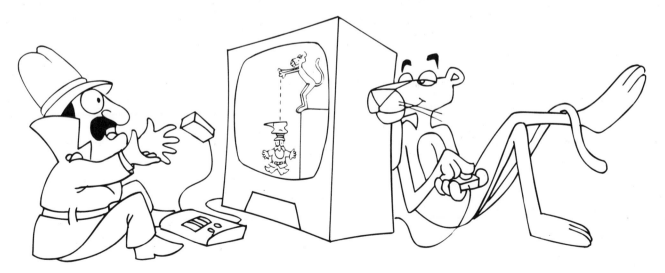

LOW BLOOD SUGAR COMPARED TO ACIDOSIS

	Low Blood Sugar (Hypoglycemia or Insulin Reaction)	Ketoacidosis (Acidosis or DKA)
Due to:	Low blood sugar	Presence of ketones
Time of onset:	Fast—within seconds	Slow—in hours or days
Causes:	Too little food Too much insulin Too much exercise without food Missing or being late for meals or snacks Excitement in young children	Too little insulin Not giving the insulin Infections
Blood sugar: **Urine tests:**	Low (below 60 mg/dl or 3.2 mmol/L) Usually negative urine ketones	Usually high (over 240 mg/dl or 13.3 mmol/L) Usually moderate or large urine ketones

	SYMPTOMS	TREATMENT	SYMPTOMS	TREATMENT
Mild:	Hunger, shaky, sweaty, nervous	Give juice or milk. Wait 10 minutes and then give solid food.	Thirst, frequent urination, sweet breath, moderate or large ketones in urine	Call doctor or nurse. Give lots of fluids and Humalog or Regular insulin every two or three hours.
Moderate:	Headache, unexpected behavior changes, impaired or double vision, confusion, drowsiness, weakness, or difficulty talking	Give instant glucose or a fast-acting sugar, juice, or sugar pop (4 oz). After 10 minutes, give solid food.	Dry mouth, nausea, abdominal cramps, vomiting, moderate or large ketones in urine	Continued contact with doctor. Give lots of fluids. Give Humalog or Regular insulin every two or three hours. Give rectal suppository if vomiting occurs.
Severe:	Loss of consciousness or seizures	Give l/2cc (1/2 mg) Glucagon® into muscle (anterior thigh) or fat and call doctor. Test blood sugar. If no response in 10 minutes, repeat once. If still no response, call paramedics or go to emergency room. May need intravenous sugar.	Labored deep breathing, extreme weakness, confusion, and eventually unconsciousness (coma); large urine ketones	Go to emergency room. May need intravenous fluids and insulin.

Table 3

Table 4

PREVENTION OF KETOACIDOSIS

1. Remember to check urine ketones with any illness (even an upset stomach or vomiting one time) or anytime the blood sugar is above 240 mg/dl (13.3 mmol/L)

2. Call the diabetes care provider immediately (night or day) if moderate or large urine ketones are found

3. Take extra insulin (after checking the blood sugar and urine ketones) every two hours for Humalog or every three hours for Regular insulin until the urine ketones are small or less

4. If the blood sugar falls below 150 mg/dl (8.3 mmol/L) and urine ketones are still moderate or large, drink juice (preferably orange as it replaces potassium), Pedialyte® or sugared pop to keep the blood sugar up so that more insulin can be given to turn off the ketone production

5. Drink lots of fluids to help wash out the ketones

Extra Insulin

When urine ketone spillage (ketonuria) advances to total body acidosis, it is usually because the urine ketones have been present for 4-12 hours (and because the urine ketones have not been checked or extra insulin was not given). Insulin shuts off ketone production; extra insulin must be given if someone has moderate or large ketones. The dose of extra insulin varies for different people, and the diabetes care provider can help decide on a safe dose. For moderate ketones, this extra dose is usually in the range of 5-10% of the total daily dose and is given as Humalog or Regular insulin every two or three hours. For large ketones, 10-20% of the total daily dose (given as Humalog or Regular insulin) is usually given every two or three hours. The blood sugar should be checked before each insulin injection. If the blood sugar drops below 150 mg/dl (8.3 mmol/L), it may be necessary to sip regular sugar pop, juice, or other sugared drinks to bring the blood sugar back up before giving the next insulin injection. Remember, the extra insulin and fluids are being given to clear the urine ketones. The extra insulin may seem like a large dose, but ketones block the normal sensitivity of the body to insulin. Although every person is different, dosages in these ranges are usually needed.

Extra Fluids

In addition to taking extra insulin, drinking fluids (water and fruit juices) is important in the prevention of acidosis. These liquids replace the fluid lost in the urine and help prevent dehydration. The juices also replace some of the salts that are lost in the urine. Orange juice and bananas are particularly good for replacing the potassium that is lost in the urine with ketones. As discussed in the next chapter (Sick-Day Management), Phenergan® suppositories are sometimes used if vomiting is a problem.

When severe acidosis has been present for many hours, coma (loss of consciousness) can follow. This is dangerous. It is much better to prevent severe acidosis than to have to treat it with IV fluids and a hospital admission. The hospital admission is usually in an intensive care unit, which is scary for everyone. Intravenous lines are usually put in both arms (and sometimes the feet). A constant heart-monitoring machine is attached to the patient. The cost is about $10,000. It is better to prevent the episodes. This usually is possible when the rules in Table 4 are followed. Ketoacidosis in patients with known diabetes in our part of the country now rarely occurs in people who attend clinic regularly (fewer than five cases per 1,000 patients per year). When it does occur, it is usually because the directions in Table 4 were not followed.

DEFINITIONS

Acidosis (diabetic ketoacidosis or DKA): What happens in the body when not enough insulin is available. Blood sugar is usually high at this time. Moderate or large ketones (acetone) are present in the urine and then build up in the body. The ketones make the body fluids more acidic resulting in total body acidosis.

Dehydration: Loss of the body fluids. The tongue and skin are usually very dry and the eyes look sunken.

Ketones (or acetone): Fat breakdown products that initially spill into the urine and later build up in the body when there is not enough insulin. They cause acidosis (or ketoacidosis).

Ketonuria: The appearance of ketones in the urine. This comes before acidosis.

Potassium: One of the salts (along with sodium) lost in the urine when ketones are spilled in the urine. Orange juice and bananas contain a lot of potassium and are best to give if urine ketones are present.

QUESTIONS (Q) AND ANSWERS (A) FROM NEWSNOTES

Q. **Please explain what ketoacidosis is and how it can be prevented.**

A. Ketoacidosis (acidosis) is one of the two emergency problems of childhood diabetes (low blood sugar being the other). It is the main cause of children with known diabetes being admitted to the hospital, and is responsible for 85% of hospitalizations. Most of these hospitalizations can be prevented with good family education and with following instructions.

Families can detect ketonuria at home by checking for urine ketones, which should be done ANY TIME THE CHILD IS FEELING ILL OR IF THE BLOOD SUGAR IS ABOVE 240 mg/dl (13.3 mmol/L). Then, if moderate or large ketones are found, the physician should be called immediately and again every 2-3 hours for dosages of Humalog or Regular insulin to inject. After the ketones have decreased to small amounts or have gone away, the extra injections can be stopped.

On any given day, and particularly during the flu season, 5-10 children are being treated for ketonuria by phone by the Barbara Davis Center staff. Fortunately, hospital admissions have gone down dramatically as a result of this treatment and are now infrequent.

The cause of ketonuria is the body's need for energy. The fat tissue under the skin responds by releasing fats, some of which are made into ketones (acetone) by the liver. The fat is broken down because there is not enough insulin or sugar available to use sugar as the main source of energy. Sometimes, such as with an infection, the body needs extra energy and the fat breaks down. As the ketones build up following the fat breakdown, ketoacidosis eventually results. The most frequent symptoms are a stomachache and, eventually, vomiting. Deep breathing is a late sign.

Q. **Why does someone feel sick when the ketones are moderate or large in the urine?**

A. There are at least three parts to the answer to this question. First, the body's acid-base (pH) balance is finely tuned (a bit on the basic side at 7.35-7.45). Acids and bases are difficult to explain, but, for example, soap is an alkaline (base) material while tomatoes are acidic. At any rate, the ketones make the body fluids more acidic as they start to build up (as they really are acids). As the body becomes more acidic, many of the body's machines (enzymes) for metabolism can no longer work effectively. If left untreated, death will eventually follow.

The second reason for not feeling great with ketones is that potassium and sodium, important body salts, are lost with every molecule of ketone going out in the urine. Potassium is important for mobility of the intestine (to move food through). If potassium is depleted, the mobility decreases or stops. Then an upset stomach and vomiting occur. This is the reason that we will often recommend orange juice (high in potassium) and apple juice in addition to water when someone has urine ketones and we are trying to get them washed out. Drinking lots of liquids also helps with keeping good hydration.

Poor hydration would be the third reason for feeling ill. Usually frequent urination due to high blood and urine sugar accompanies urine ketones. This can lead to dehydration. Our bodies are 60% water and if even 10% of body weight is lost as water, it is possible to be very sick. Much fluid can also be lost with the flu (vomiting and diarrhea) so that if fluid is being lost in excess from both the kidneys (frequent urination) and from the gastrointestinal tract (vomiting and/or diarrhea), dehydration can occur even more rapidly.

Q. What is cerebral edema and how does it relate to diabetic ketoacidosis?

A. Cerebral edema refers to swelling of the brain, which is a rare complication of treating diabetic ketoacidosis. The cause is not understood and when it does occur, it is often fatal.

Perhaps we have been lucky, as in 19 years since the Center opened—and in my 32 years of working with children with diabetes—I have seen only two or three cases of cerebral edema in children who had been previously diagnosed with diabetes. (Unfortunately, it is more common in newly-diagnosed children where the ketones have built up over a longer time period.) Part of the reason it is so rare relates to the now relative infrequency of ketoacidosis. Our families diligently check urine ketones with every illness and call when moderate or large urine ketones are detected. This allows extra shots of Humalog or Regular insulin to be given to reverse urine ketones (ketonuria) before ketoacidosis occurs (in one period we had only six cases among 1,200 families in 12 months). This greatly reduces the likelihood of a case of ketoacidosis escalating to cerebral edema. Once again, it is better to prevent ketoacidosis than to deal with its bad effects.

Q. Our son has had diabetes for over two years. Every time he has gotten sick we have checked for urine ketones. The results have always been negative or trace. Can we stop checking now?

A. The answer is NO! This is often the case for someone who still makes some of their own insulin and/or someone who is in excellent sugar control. The machinery (enzymes) for making ketones from fat are so completely turned off that they don't get turned on by the illness. Unfortunately, as your son's insulin production declines, or he outgrows his remaining insulin production, he will probably suddenly have moderate or large urine ketones with an illness. One never knows when this will occur. Thus, the only answer is to keep checking the urine ketones at least twice each day with each illness.

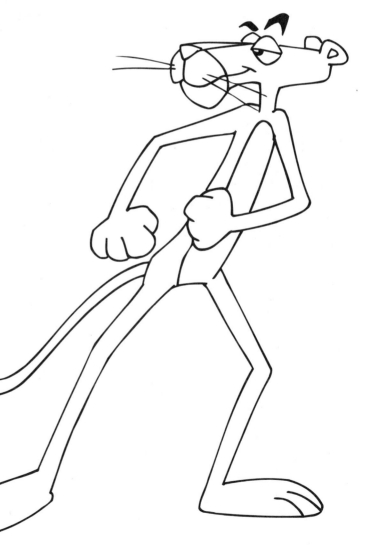

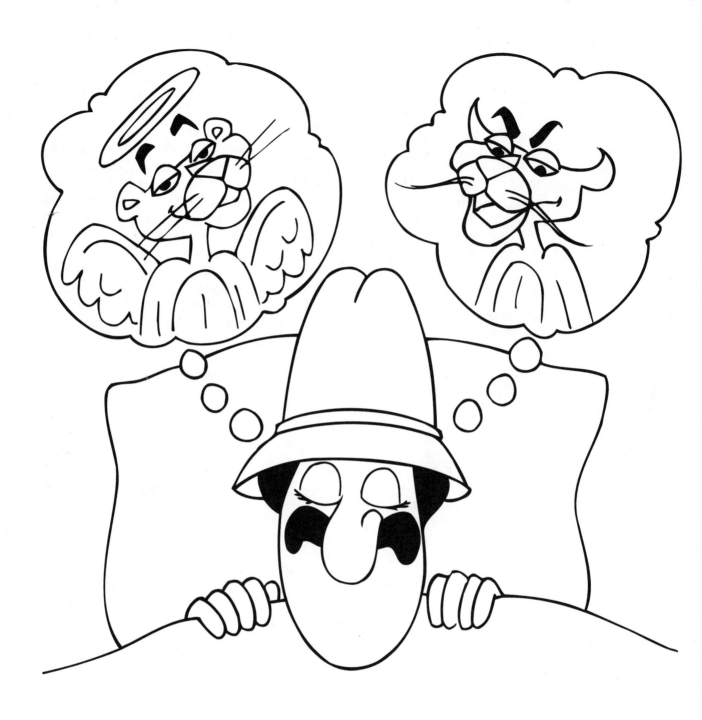

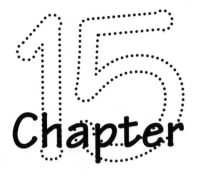

Chapter 15

SICK-DAY AND SURGERY MANAGEMENT

Key ideas of this chapter:

- Know how to manage diabetes in the presence of illness—or when having surgery.

- Appreciate the importance of preventing acidosis (ketoacidosis) or low blood sugar (hypoglycemia) in people with diabetes during illness or when having surgery.

SICK-DAY MANAGEMENT

The person with diabetes can get sick just as any other person does. With proper "thinking ahead" and help from health professionals, the risks from illnesses are not much greater than they are for anyone else. However, there are certain precautions that must be taken. The purpose of this chapter is to review these precautions. If you have a young child with diabetes, just change the "you" to "your child" in your thinking when you read this chapter.

WHAT YOU NEED TO KNOW

When you get sick, the first thing you must do is to get the information you need. This will help you decide if you need assistance from health professionals. They will usually want to know this information. Keep your book open to this page to remind you of the seven things to report when you phone. They are listed in Table 1 and discussed in the following text.

- **Present problem:** Diarrhea, vomiting, bad headache, cold, cough, earache, sore throat, stomachache, or injury. If vomiting or diarrhea are present, note the number of times and when the episodes happen. It is also important to note if there have been any recent illnesses

BEFORE CALLING, KNOW:

1. Present problem
2. Blood sugar level
3. Urine ketone result
4. Signs of low blood sugar or of acidosis
5. Intake of foods and liquids
6. Usual insulin dosage, time, and amount of last dosage
7. Last body weight (if known)

in other family members or close friends. This will help you decide if you have a similar illness.

Fever does not generally occur with diabetes-related problems. Fever is usually a sign of an infection. However, infections can be present without a fever. It is helpful if you are able to take your temperature before calling the diabetes care provider to discuss an illness.

Sick people usually don't feel like doing much. If you are still active, it is usually a good sign.

Blood sugar: As we noted in the chapter on self blood sugar monitoring, you must do even more blood sugar tests than usual on sick days. Both parents and friends should know how to accurately measure blood sugars using test strips or meters in case you are feeling too sick to do the testing. The blood sugar test should always be done before calling your diabetes care provider.

Urine ketones: DON'T FORGET, URINE KETONES (ACETONE) MUST ALWAYS BE CHECKED AT LEAST TWICE DAILY IF A PERSON DOESN'T FEEL WELL (see Table 2). Urine ketones must always be checked if blood sugars are 240 mg/dl (13.3 mmol/L) or more. However, with an illness, ketones can be present even when the blood sugar is lower. It is wise to have some small paper cups in the bathroom. The urine can be left in the cup so that a parent can be certain they agree with the reading (and to make sure the test was really done). **Always do the test before calling your diabetes care provider.** If you don't have the foil-wrapped Ketositx (Chapter 4), check to make sure the Ketostix bottle has not been opened for more than six months.

Signs of low blood sugar and acidosis: These were discussed in Chapters 5 and 14, respectively. Deep, labored breathing or continual vomiting can be signs of acidosis. These indicate that the person should be seen in an emergency room as soon as possible.

Eating and drinking: It is important to know how well you are taking liquids and/or eating. A measuring cup will help you keep track of how much liquid is taken. Often you can look at your tongue in the mirror to see the amount of moisture present. If the tongue starts to become too "dry" (dehydrated), intravenous fluids may be needed.

Insulin dosage: You should know the usual insulin dose and when this was last taken. Were any doses skipped or forgotten? Finally, if you have had a similar illness in the past, it would be helpful for the doctor or nurse to know how much extra Humalog or Regular insulin you took at that time. Did the dose seem to work? If the morning or evening insulin dose has not yet been given and you have moderate or large ketones, **call the diabetes care provider before you give the injection.** Extra short-acting insulin will probably be needed.

Body weight: It is helpful to know the last weight from a clinic visit (within three months) and the present weight (if you have a scale). This will help the doctor choose the right amount of insulin and also know how much weight you may have lost. You might also remind the diabetes care provider the age of your child. Most physicians follow many children and mix-ups can occur.

MOST IMPORTANT

Always check urine ketones with any illness. Even if the blood sugar is low, check for ketones at least twice daily every day you are sick. Call your health care provider if ketones are moderate or large.

Always take some insulin. Never skip a dose entirely. Call your diabetes care provider if you don't know how much to take.

It is particularly important to **check urine ketones if you vomit even ONCE!** Ketones can cause vomiting. If you vomit more than three times, call your diabetes care provider.

CHANGING THE INSULIN DOSAGE FOR ILLNESS

It is important to remember that SOME INSULIN MUST ALWAYS BE GIVEN EACH DAY (Table 2). You cannot skip the injection just because you are sick. Often the body will require more energy during illness to help fight the infection. Hormones other than insulin (e.g., steroids) increase with illnesses and raise the blood sugar level. More insulin will be needed to allow the body to burn extra sugar for energy when the blood sugar is high. Usually only the Humalog or Regular insulin is increased. If the blood sugar is low, the short-acting insulin is not increased and may instead be reduced or omitted. Occasionally the blood sugar will be low but ketones will be present. The ketones form because the body needs extra energy and fat is broken down. Ketones are a by-product of fat breakdown for energy. In this case, you should eat and see if the ketones go away. If vomiting is a problem, and the blood sugar is low or normal, sips of regular pop or of another "high-sugar" liquid may help raise the blood sugar. Sometimes sugar popsicles will help. Once the blood sugar is up, you can then take the insulin to help get rid of ketones (if they are still present).

The best way to know how much insulin is needed is to have kept records from a previous similar illness and to know what insulin dose worked then. It is important and helpful to keep good records. If you do not know about previous illnesses, look at the present blood sugar levels. If the blood sugar is high, check for moderate or large urine ketones. If moderate ketones are present, we usually recommend that you give 5-10% of your total daily insulin dose as Humalog insulin every two hours or as Regular insulin every three hours. If large urine ketones are present, we recommend adding 10-20% of your total daily insulin dose as Humalog (every two hours) or as Regular insulin (every three hours). This is discussed in Chapter 14, Ketonuria and Acidosis. These dosages are in addition to your usual daily dose. When possible, you should call the diabetes specialist to get help with the dose. **You will need to repeat the injections of Humalog or Regular insulin every 2-3 hours, respectively, if moderate or large ketones are still present.** We do not generally give extra shots of insulin unless moderate or large ketones are present and the blood sugar is at least 150 mg/dl (8.3 mmol/L).

GENERAL GUIDELINES: SICK-DAY MANAGEMENT

Generally, the body will require more energy during an illness. More insulin allows more sugar to pass into cells, providing more energy to fight infection. Some insulin is always needed. Important things to remember are:

1. **Ketones:** Always test for ketones in the urine if you feel ill or if the blood sugar is over 240 mg/dl (13.3 mmol/L).

2. **Vomiting:** If you are vomiting and have a low blood sugar, an insulin reaction could occur. At the same time, you may still have ketones. Always test for ketones in the urine if you are vomiting. Vomiting may be due to an infection or due to ketones. Management of vomiting is outlined in Table 3.

3. **Insulin:** Keep a bottle of short-acting (Humalog or Regular) insulin available, even if you don't usually use it. You may need to give the extra short-acting insulin during an illness. Be sure it is not outdated.

4. **Blood Sugar Testing:** All people must have some method of home blood sugar testing available and be ready to do extra testing on sick days (usually every 3-4 hours). This has greatly reduced the need for hospitalizations.

5. **Extra Snacks:** It is important to take in adequate calories on sick days or the body will start to break down fat for energy. If this happens, ketones will appear in the urine (see Chapter 14). Regular sugar pop, popsicles and regular JELL-O® are good to eat if you do not feel like eating regular food and your blood sugar is below 180 mg/dl (10.0 mmol/L). Much of eating is psychologically related and we often suggest you eat whatever you feel like eating on sick days! Also see Table 4.

6. **Past Experience:** Base your judgments on past experience. Refer to your record book to see if this illness has occurred before. See what worked or didn't work in the past.

- **Plan Ahead:** Plan ahead if you are undergoing surgery (e.g., dental surgery). Call the diabetes specialist in advance.

- **Doctor:** Call your pediatrician or family doctor for non-diabetes related problems such as sore throats, earaches, rashes, etc. Unless the diabetes specialist also provides general care, only call him/her if the urine ketones are moderate or large, if you need help with an insulin dose, if hypoglycemia is a problem, or if you need help with other parts of diabetes management.

FLUID REPLACEMENT

If you have difficulty eating or keeping food down and the blood sugar is below 180 mg/dl (10.0 mmol/L), take sugar-containing liquids (see Table 4). These may include fruit juices, popsicles, slushes, tea with sugar or honey, broth, syrup from canned fruit, or even regular pop. Stir pop to get rid of bubbles. If you are vomiting, take a small amount (juice glass size or less) of sugar pop after you vomit. If it stays down 15 minutes, some sugar will be absorbed. If there is no vomiting after 1/2

hour, increase the amount of fluids. If you have ketones and are not vomiting, take at least one cup of liquid every hour. You should have one pint (two cups) to one quart (four cups) of liquid every six hours. The liquids help to prevent dehydration and also to "wash out" the ketones. Specific instructions regarding vomiting are given in Table 3.

FOODS FOR SICK-DAYS

Table 4 suggests carbohydrate-containing foods that might be tried during an illness. Eating carbohydrates is important to provide energy and to prevent the body from breaking down fats (and thus making ketones). Drinking liquids is important to prevent dehydration. Thus, liquids are usually tried first. A general rule of thumb is to offer whatever you/your child like(s) best. You may want to have a "sick-day kit" on hand which could include items such as sugar-containing 7UP®, sports drinks, regular and diet JELL-O or pudding, apple juice in small cans, regular Kool-Aid mix, Cup-a-Soup®, Pedialyte, and any other items you would like to have available.

MANAGEMENT OF VOMITING (NEGATIVE KETONES)

1. Avoid solid foods until the vomiting has stopped.

2. If vomiting is frequent, we recommend giving a Phenergan suppository to reduce vomiting and waiting to give fluids for an hour until the suppository is working. If you do not have suppositories, ask for a prescription for them at the time of your clinic visit.

3. Gradually start liquids (juice, Pedialyte, water, etc.) in small amounts. Juices (especially orange) replace the salts that are lost with vomiting or diarrhea. Pedialyte popsicles are also available. Start with a tablespoon of liquid every 10-20 minutes. If the blood sugar is below 100 mg/dl (5.5 mmol/L), sugar pop can be given. For the child five years of age and over, sucking on a piece of hard candy often works well. If the blood sugar is above 180 mg/dl (10.0 mmol/L), do not give pop with sugar in it. If there is no further vomiting, gradually increase the amount of fluid. If vomiting restarts, it may again be necessary to rest the stomach for another hour and then restart the small amounts of fluids. A repeat suppository can be given after three or four hours.

4. After a few hours without vomiting, gradually return to a normal diet. Soups are often good to start with and they provide needed nutrients.

SICK-DAY FOODS

1. Liquids

   i.   Fruit juice: apple, cranberry, grape, grapefruit, orange, pineapple, etc.

   ii. Sugar-containing beverages: regular 7Up, gingerale, orange, cola, PEPSI®, etc.[1]

  iii. Fruit flavored drinks: regular Kool-Aid, lemonade, Hi-C®, etc.

  iv. Sports drinks: Gatorade®, POWERaDE®, etc. (any flavor)

   v. Tea with honey or sugar

  vi. Pedialyte or Infalyte® (especially for younger children)

  vii. JELL-O: regular (for infants, liquid JELL-O warmed in a bottle) or diet[1]

 viii. Popsicles, regular or diet[1]

  ix. Broth-type soup: bouillon, chicken noodle soup, Cup-a-Soup

2. Solids (when ready)

   i.   Saltine crackers

  ii. Banana (or other fruit)

  iii. Applesauce

  iv. Bread or toast

   v. Graham crackers

  vi. Soup

[1]*Sugar-free may be needed depending on blood sugars (e.g., >180 mg/dl [10.0 mmol/L])*

EXERCISE

The person with moderate or large urine ketones should not exercise. Exercise can further increase the ketones.

CONTACTING YOUR DOCTOR OR NURSE

Keep a card with your doctor's and nurse's phone numbers in a place where you can easily find it. Take the card with you if you are out of town. It is easier to call your own doctor rather than to go to an emergency room and see a new doctor.

Think ahead! You should keep Phenergan or other suppositories on hand in case of vomiting. (Some physicians prefer not to use suppositories.) Before you call the doctor or nurse, be sure you have the necessary information (see the list at the beginning of the chapter). **Always check the blood sugar and urine ketones before calling.** Have the number of your pharmacy available in case the doctor needs it. If you think you have an emergency, see Table 5.

Table 5 tells when to call or get emergency care. Remember to keep regular (sugared) pop, popsicles, and soup available for illnesses.

CLINIC OR EMERGENCY ROOM VISITS

If you do decide to go to a clinic or emergency room, remember to take your hospital card if you have one, your diabetes records, and your insurance information. Take extra clothes in case you must be admitted to the hospital. A relative or friend going with you will need money for food, telephone numbers of people they might need to call, and something to read.

SICK-DAY MANAGEMENT: WHEN TO CALL FOR EMERGENCY CARE

1 If you have vomited more than three times and can keep nothing in your stomach, and urine ketones are not moderate or large, call your primary care physician. If help is needed with an insulin dose, call your diabetes care provider.

2 If moderate or large ketones are present, call your diabetes care provider.

3 If you have difficulty breathing or have "deep breathing," you need to go to an emergency room. This usually indicates severe acidosis (ketoacidosis).

4 If there is any unusual behavior such as confusion, slurred speech, double vision, inability to move or talk, or jerking, someone should give sugar or instant glucose. (Glucagon [Chapter 5] is given only if the person is unconscious or if a convulsion [seizure] occurs.) The health care provider should be contacted if a severe reaction occurs. In case of a convulsion or loss of consciousness, it may be necessary to call the paramedics or to go to an emergency room. Have an emergency number posted by the phone.

SICK-DAY MEDICATIONS

Our general philosophy is that if you need a medicine for an illness, take it! We can handle the problems related to diabetes. The classic example is asthma. With a bad attack, the person will need adrenaline (epinephrine), which raises the blood sugar. Steroids (cortisone) may also be needed which, also raise the blood sugar. For the short time that these medicines are needed, extra insulin can be taken to help control the blood sugar. Short-term elevations of blood sugar are not what we worry about in relation to the complications of diabetes.

Over-the-counter medications can be purchased with care. Look at the label to see if sugar is added. Tablets are less likely to have sugar (and alcohol) than are liquids. Again, the small amounts of sugar in a medicine taken for a short time can be dealt with. We do not endorse any products but do suggest these:

Nasal sprays (e.g., Afrin®): Can be used for colds and allergies. A nasal spray is less likely to affect the entire body than pills or liquid medicines. If these do not work, or if long-term use is anticipated (as with seasonal allergies), antihistamine tablets or liquids such as Chlortrimeton® or Triaminic® might be tried next.

Acetaminophen (TYLENOL®) or Ibuprofen: To relieve fever if a flu is going through the community. Do not give aspirin to children or adolescents.

Pepto-Bismol®, Kaopectate®, or Imodium AD®: These are fine to use for diarrhea. (Lomotil® should NOT be used in children).

DI-GEL®, MYLANTA®, Gelusil®, and Maalox® are all sugar-free antacids.

Cough medications: Use a cold air vaporizer if this relieves the cough. During the day, a cough is often protective to keep material out of the lungs. Thus, we do not give cough medicines. A combined cough and fever means the child should be seen by a physician. If the vaporizer does not stop the cough at night, use sugar-free cough medicines with less than 15% alcohol. Examples: Colrex® Expectorant®, CONTAC Jr.®, Hytuss Tablets®, Queltuss Tablets®, Robitussin CF® liquid, Sorbutuss Syrup®, Supercitin®, Toclonol Expectorant®, Tolu-Sed®, Tolu-Sed DM®, Tussar-SF®.

Sore Throats: A throat culture to rule out a streptococcal (strep) infection should be done because strep can lead to rheumatic fever or nephritis. Salt water gargles (1/4 teaspoon salt in one glass water) may help. Chloraseptic Spray® is sugar-free, as are Cepacol®, Cepastat®, Chloraseptic® mouthwashes or lozenges and N'ICE® lozenges.

FOLLOW THE DIRECTIONS ON THE LABEL FOR ANY MEDICINE YOU USE.

FLU SHOTS

The method of preparing the flu vaccine has improved so that side effects are now less likely. The American Academy of Pediatrics recommends flu shots for all children with diabetes, and we agree with their recommendation. Preventing an episode of flu may prevent an episode of ketoacidosis. It is important to get the shots early in the fall so that the flu shot can be working when the flu season begins.

SURGERY MANAGEMENT

Some general guidelines for diabetes management around surgery are outlined in Table 6. The insulin dose is almost always changed when a person goes to a dentist or to a hospital for elective surgery. The amount of change is extremely variable depending on the person, the type of surgery that is scheduled, and the time of day the surgery is to be done. If possible, surgery should be scheduled early in the morning. In general, it is best to call your diabetes care provider and discuss insulin changes **after** you find out the time of day the procedure is to be done and whether or not food intake will be limited. Sometimes it is also helpful to have the person who is going to do the surgery call the diabetes care provider. This is more apt to be done if the family gives the doctor or dentist a note with the name and phone number of the diabetes specialist. The two of them can then work out the best time for a given patient to have elective surgery.

We frequently receive calls from families related to planned dental surgery. Often this can be done under local anesthesia and, sometimes the patient can eat regular meals prior to and after the surgery. In this situation it is only necessary to reduce the insulin dose slightly in anticipation of some reduction in food intake due to soreness in the mouth.

If the person is going to have a general anesthetic, eating beforehand may be restricted. This is because the person would be more apt to vomit while recovering from the general anesthetic. If vomiting does occur in a person who is still partly under the influence of anesthesia, there is a danger of some of the food getting into the airway. Thus, food restriction is usually necessary if a general anesthetic is to be used. Anytime the amount of food intake is to change, the amount of insulin to be given must also be changed. Different physicians handle the changes in insulin dosage differently. Some physicians reduce the dose of long-acting insulin (often by half) and use supplements of short-acting (Humalog or Regular) insulin only if needed. Other physicians give no long-acting insulin and **must** then give supplements of Humalog or Regular insulin subcutaneously every two or three hours. If the person is going to have a general anesthetic in the hospital, some doctors prefer to give all of the insulin by intravenous infusion. Any of these methods work. **The important thing is the close monitoring of blood sugars! By doing this, low blood sugars can be prevented. It is also wise to check the urine ketones before and after the procedure.** These may increase with changes in the insulin dose and with the stress of surgery. Needless to say, your diabetes care provider must always be notified if the urine ketones are moderate or large following surgery.

Blood sugar monitoring is usually the responsibility of the parent or the patient when procedures are done in the dentist's or doctor's office. If a meter is used for blood sugar monitoring at home, this should be taken along to the dentist's or doctor's office. If the child is being admitted to the hospital, also take the meter along. If the child is to have a general anesthetic, the blood sugar monitoring is the responsibility of the doctor giving the anesthesia or the doctor doing the surgery. The doctor usually orders dextrose, which is glucose (sugar), to be added to the intravenous fluids if the blood sugar is below a certain level (200 mg/dl or 11.1 mmol/L is a safe level to use). Blood sugars are usually measured at regular intervals by the doctor or nurse.

It is also wise to take along urine ketone checking strips. Many doctors or nurses who do not care for people with diabetes on a regular basis may forget the importance of routinely checking for urine ketones. Also take your diabetes care provider's phone numbers with you. If urine ketones are moderate or large, or if you have any other concerns, you may wish to call your diabetes care provider.

GUIDELINES FOR MANAGEMENT AROUND SURGERY

1. Always contact your diabetes care provider if surgery is planned—**AFTER** you find out the time and whether normal food intake will be allowed. You may wish to give the name and phone number of the diabetes care provider to the person doing the surgery.

2. Plan to take your own blood sugar and urine ketone checking equipment.

3. Take your own materials to treat low blood sugar (a source of instant glucose and even glucagon).

4. Always check the urine ketones prior to surgery. Then, if they are present at a later time, it will be known that they were negative earlier. If they are found to be moderate or large, it may be necessary to cancel the planned procedure. Take the urine ketone strips with you to the procedure in case vomiting occurs and you need to do a check. It is also wise to check urine ketones once or twice after the procedure.

5. Take your diabetes clinic's phone card so that you may quickly call the diabetes care provider if needed.

DEFINITIONS

Anesthetic (anesthesia): A medication (such as ether) used to reduce pain or to allow a person to sleep through an otherwise painful procedure.

Dextrose: The name for glucose (sugar) added to an intravenous (IV) feeding to prevent low blood sugar.

Suppository: A medication inserted into the rectum (bottom), usually because liquid, food, or medicine cannot be kept down (as with vomiting).

QUESTIONS (Q) AND ANSWERS (A) FROM NEWSNOTES

Q. In the chapter on "Sick-Day Management" in the Pink Panther book, you state four times that urine ketones must always be checked at least twice daily when someone is ill. Is it necessary to be that repetitive?

A. Forgetting to check urine ketones with an illness is one of the most common errors families make in managing diabetes. As a result, ketones can build up to high levels in the body, which can then be dangerous (and expensive to treat). There is no charge for a few phone calls to a diabetes care provider to receive suggestions for supplemental Humalog or Regular insulin to combat early ketone formation. In contrast, the charge is usually $5,000-$10,000 for one or two nights in an intensive care unit as a result of large ketones building up in the body. As pointed out at the end of Chapter 14 on Acidosis (Ketoacidosis), this charge and the related risk from ketoacidosis can be avoided if families will just check for urine ketones immediately (and twice daily) when the person with diabetes is ill. The diabetes care provider must then be called when moderate or large urine ketones are detected and every 2-3 hours thereafter until the urine ketones are below the moderate level.

Q. Should flu shots be given to children with diabetes?

A. The American Academy of Pediatrics recommends flu shots for all children with diabetes. Flu is a common cause of ketonuria and of acidosis, so the shots may also help prevent ketoacidosis. If you do decide to get them for your child, we would prefer that you go to your primary care physician for this purpose. Call first to make sure the doctor's office has the vaccine. If a young child has not previously received the flu vaccine, it is necessary to get it in two injections, approximately one month apart, and it is best to start during the months of September or October.

Q. Should my child receive the chicken pox vaccination?

A. Yes, if he or she has not had chicken pox! It is recommended by the American Academy of Pediatrics for all children who have not had prior chicken pox infections, and we support that recommendation.

There is an additional factor for children with diabetes who still produce some insulin. Chicken pox is probably one of the many infections that stimulate white blood cells in the pancreas to make toxic particles that cause further islet destruction. This is not proven, but we have heard many times of children being diagnosed with diabetes in the month or two after having chicken pox.

The Varivax is a live, attenuated vaccine. The main side effects are a mild rash (approximately 3%), and/or a temperature elevation (approximately 15%), and/or tenderness at the site (approximately 19%). Ninety-nine percent of people are immune as a result of the vaccination.

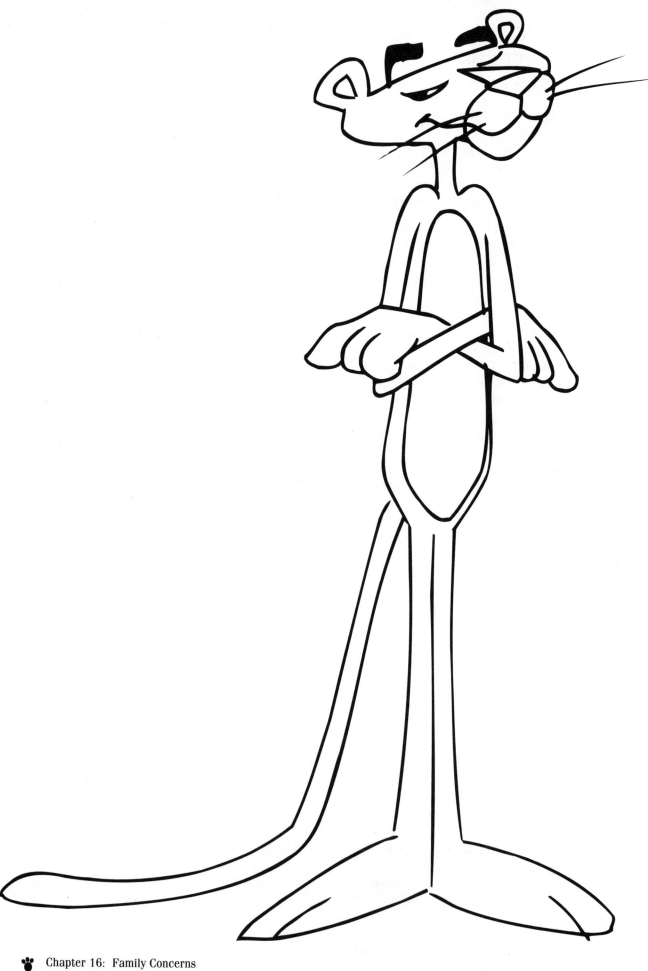

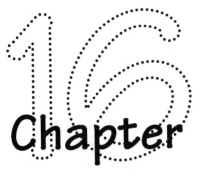

Chapter FAMILY CONCERNS

Key ideas of this chapter:

🐾 Realize the extra stresses that family members may be under as a result of a family member being diagnosed with diabetes.

🐾 Develop methods to deal with the emotions created as a result of the diagnosis of diabetes in a family member.

WORKING AS A FAMILY

The problems a family may have following the initial diagnosis of diabetes include more demands on their time, money, and energy. This is due to the daily routine of the diabetes management and the regular clinic visits. Families must decide among themselves how each new responsibility will be shared so that no one person has too much to do. We particularly request that both the mother and father share the responsibility for the diabetes care. This should include helping to give the insulin injections. It is important for the parents to support one another in such activities as injections, blood sugar testing, exercise, diet, and urine ketone checking. Each parent's interest and investment in care are crucial to the family's adjustment. Each parent should also try to attend clinic visits at least once or twice a year.

Diabetes is a family disease and the family must work together to solve problems and manage the diabetes. Research has shown that the youngsters who do best with their diabetes are those who had help and support from their parents with the tasks of diabetes management. They also reported less conflict in their families. Although every family is different, some plan for family sharing of diabetes-related tasks is important to develop.

SINGLE-PARENT FAMILIES

Approximately one-fourth of children in the U.S. now live in single-parent families. It is important that parents who live separately share vital information when the child with diabetes goes between households. This includes information about blood sugar levels, recent low blood sugars, insulin dosages, and information related to food intake, exercise, and illnesses. GOOD COMMUNICATION AND

COOPERATION ARE ESSENTIAL. The diabetes supplies can be neatly packed in a carrying case to go with the child between households. Many families keep a vial of glucagon and some foil-wrapped urine ketone strips permanently in each household. Hopefully, both parents will be invested enough in the care of their child to put any individual differences aside in dealing with the diabetes and their child(ren).

LEADING A NORMAL LIFE

It is very important to treat a person with diabetes just like any other person. The child should participate in activities for his/her age group just like any other child. It is important for all children to have friends and activities with others away from the family. Teenagers, in particular, get a great deal of support from their friends. Children with diabetes should be disciplined just like any other children. A good rule is to THINK OF THE CHILD FIRST AND THEN THE DIABETES. When children with diabetes are treated differently from other children, they begin to feel different. They sometimes feel alone and unloved and begin to feel sad or depressed. They may begin to use the diabetes to get their own way. Family members then feel powerless and controlled by the child and the diabetes. If the child with diabetes is treated as a normal child, some of these problems can be prevented. Brothers and sisters may be more helpful if they feel the child with diabetes is treated the same way they are.

CONCERNS OF BROTHERS AND SISTERS

When a child first develops diabetes, it is a crisis for the whole family. Often brothers and sisters feel left out because so much attention is given to the child with diabetes. They may have trouble understanding what diabetes is and may fear that their brother or sister will die. They may think they caused the diabetes by having an angry thought against the child with diabetes. It is very important that brothers and sisters be a part of the beginning education. Young children will feel less frightened if they can visit the hospital or clinic.

Brothers and sisters feel it is very unfair if they are punished for some things and their brother or sister with diabetes is not punished for the same things. All children in a family should be treated in a similar way. One sister said she eats a candy bar in front of her brother with diabetes when he gets away with something. She said, "That's how I get even with him."

Some children with diabetes have the opportunity for special activities such as diabetes camp and ski trips. Many brothers and sisters say, "I wish I had diabetes so I could do special things, too." It is important to plan individual time and special activities with all children in a family. A family can prevent future stress if the members understand some of these problems.

SWEETS IN THE HOME

Perhaps no area of diabetes care is argued as much as that of keeping sweets in the home of a child or adolescent with diabetes. Those who argue in favor of allowing sweets in the home will say, "They have to learn to avoid sweets when they are with their friends away from home; they should learn to avoid them at home, too." In our experience, people who say this usually have a sweet tooth themselves and do not want to give up any of their own sweets. Is it fair or reasonable to ask children to do what we are not able to do ourselves?

It is our experience that if sweets such as donuts, cakes, cookies, sugar pop, and candy are going to routinely be in the house, they will be eaten by the person with diabetes just like they are eaten by any other child or teenager. We would argue that if the child or teenager can be taught that these junk foods are not needed at home, they will probably also not need them in the world outside of the home. Trying to avoid them when they are in the home can sometimes result in more stress and high blood sugar levels (particularly if resistance weakens and the person is caught and scolded). Siblings may consciously or unconsciously taunt the child with diabetes, raising both the stress and the blood sugar levels, and creating conflict at home.

Perhaps the most supportive and loving act

that parents, brothers, and sisters can make toward the person with diabetes in their home is to eliminate these foods from the home. They have little nutritional value and everyone's health will be better. If other family members have a need for these products, they should fill the need while at work, school, or away from the child with diabetes. Better sugar control is almost always found when excesses of sweets are eliminated from the home.

DEALING WITH STRESS AND EXCITEMENT

Emotions and stress may have a big effect on diabetes control. Many different kinds of life events can cause stress. These include family problems, arguments with parents or between parents, parent separation, death of a relative, friend or pet, or a move to a new home or school. Other kinds of stressful situations include special events, such as athletic competitions or school exams. Sometimes even a holiday like a birthday, Christmas, or Hanukkah can be stressful for a child. While most older children have high sugars following stress, some younger children will have low sugars during special days or at times of excitement. It is important to think ahead and reduce the insulin dose (or give extra food) and monitor blood sugars at least four times during the day so that young children do not have low blood sugars on days of excitement.

It is necessary for persons with diabetes to lead a normal life and to learn to deal with stress in a healthy manner. Stressful situations help them learn to do this. These persons need to be aware that increased blood sugar may be a result of stress. Sometimes professional assistance in methods of dealing with stress can be helpful.

The diagram in Chapter 13 on Diabetes and Blood Sugar Control shows how the insulin dose, diet, exercise, and stress must be in balance for the best sugar control. This is not possible all of the time for anyone.

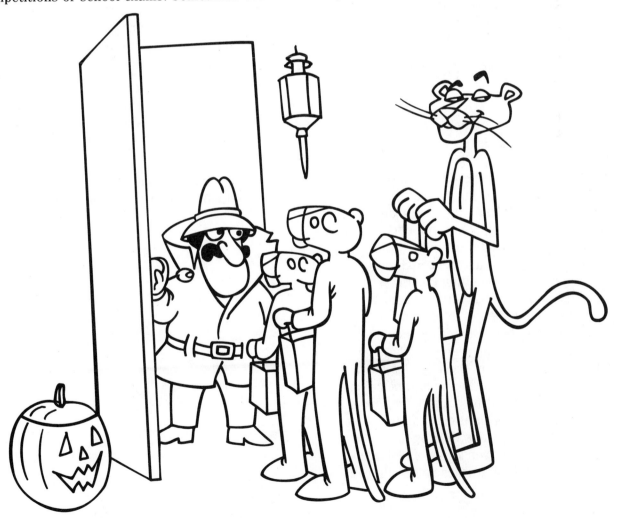

SCHOOL ATTENDANCE

A problem we sometimes see in children with diabetes, as well as in other children, is school absence. If school is missed for a period of time due to illness or hospitalization, the child may be very worried about returning to class. It is not uncommon for the diabetes to remain in poor control when the child is worried about unfinished schoolwork, exams, fellow students, teachers, or other problems. If a child has missed a period of school, the best policy is to encourage returning as soon as possible. Stress can be lessened if the school counselor or teacher can help rearrange the schedule after a long absence. At first, maybe only two or three of the classes will be at school. However, the child needs to return to school full-time as soon as possible. On some occasions, the family may wish to ask members of the diabetes team to help coordinate matters with the school. Sometimes a child may fear how peers will treat him/her. Arranging for a nurse educator or parent to talk to the class about diabetes can be very helpful to the child. It allows for the development of good peer support.

MARRIAGE STRESS FOR THE PARENTS

The diagnosis of any serious condition in a child adds an extra stress to the parents' marriage. If the marriage has already been having difficulty before the diagnosis, the additional stress may make it even worse. It is very important for both parents to talk and share their feelings and plans with each other. They may feel angry and want to deny the diabetes, or one parent may feel angry at the way the other parent is acting. Each person may feel alone because the other reacts to the situation in a different way. Sometimes one parent feels angry because he/she is doing more or less for the child than the other parent. If they don't share these feelings with each other along the way, anger may come out over other family problems. This kind of anger cannot be hidden from children. If all the members of the family talk about their feelings, the problems won't grow and burden the children. The social worker in the clinic can assist families in identifying worries and concerns. On occasion, outpatient counseling or psychotherapy may also be helpful.

CHANGING BEHAVIOR

Sometimes children with diabetes have difficulty with their insulin injections, blood sugar tests at home, the suggested diet, the recommended exercise, or other parts of diabetes management. These "problems" may actually be opportunities to assess what is bothering a child or teenager and to see what can be changed. At these times it may be very helpful to meet with the clinical social worker or psychologist who specializes in working with families. They can help evaluate problems and suggest ways to effect change. Behavioral change takes time, patience, and usually requires help from the whole family. A few visits can often be very helpful to the patient and the family.

DEFINITIONS

Psychologist: A doctor (Ph.D. or Psy D.) trained in helping people with behavior, stress, or feelings that are causing problems or discomfort.

Clinical Social Worker: A person with a Master's degree in social work trained to help individuals or families with emotional or behavioral problems, as well as problems with resources.

Stress: Problems that make people feel worried, afraid, excited, upset, or scared.

QUESTIONS (Q) AND ANSWERS (A) FROM NEWSNOTES

Q. What are the occupational restrictions for a person with diabetes?

A. Restrictions are based on the hypothesis that all people with diabetes are at a greater risk for hypoglycemia. There are indeed some studies to show that hypoglycemia does result in an increased risk for accidents. One study showed that approximately 10% of accident reports in which the accident was due to a medical condition other than alcoholism were said to be due to an insulin reaction.

My own opinion is that restrictions should not be generic—and should be individualized. For example, some people test their blood sugars more often than others and are careful to eat or make sure they are not low before driving a car. Others are less careful. Everyone pays the price from the latter group.

Currently, legal restrictions include working in the military, commercial truck driving, and flying a passenger plane. Some state and local governments may also deny employment in the police or fire fighting forces. Most physicians also recommend that people who have frequent low blood sugars do not work at heights, operate heavy equipment, or handle toxic substances. Working rotating shifts can also result in more difficulty with blood sugar control. Generally, if the rotations are on a monthly or greater basis, it is possible to alter the insulin dosage to cope.

Q. Are psychological problems more or less common in children and adolescents with diabetes compared to people without diabetes?

A. It is a common belief that the presence of any chronic illness increases the likelihood of psychological problems. The presence of pimples or blemishes that make the adolescent feel different from peers can be devastating. We ask youths with diabetes to eat differently than their peers (and not to eat foods generally considered the most tempting), to give two or more insulin shots, and do three or more finger pokes for blood sugar every day of their lives. With this, one might expect lots of psychological problems!

Surprisingly, this in not the case. In the years the Barbara Davis Center has been open, we have had far fewer serious psychological problems (including drug addiction and suicide) than in the general population. Why is this? It is likely related to several factors. One is that "preventive counseling" has been available from the day the Center opened. The psych-social component of the Center has been expensive, and is possible only because of financial support from the Children's Diabetes Foundation and its Guild. When families come for their three-month clinic visits the staff is constantly alert for people who might need some extra help. I often ask teenagers to grade their current stress level from one to ten. An answer of ten (or above) usually means the person is asking for help and that a visit to the psychologist or social worker might be helpful. I strongly believe that the regular clinic visits and the "preventive counseling" have been major reasons for the low incidence of major psychological problems.

Diabetes often results in the entire family focusing on the holistic health of the individual and family, often in ways that might not otherwise have occurred. These often include eating better, getting more exercise, and not smoking. Factors such as these may also relate to the good mental health of the people seen at our Center.

An added factor in the low incidence of serious problems may be the regimentation and seriousness of diabetes care. A number of youths have written in their college applications that having diabetes required them to "grow up" sooner—to learn at an earlier age when they could have fun or when they had to be serious. Good diabetes control and the use of illegal drugs and alcohol do not mix. With the monitoring of diabetes control every three months, any deviation from good control is quickly detected. Preventive counseling can then be introduced before the problem becomes too serious.

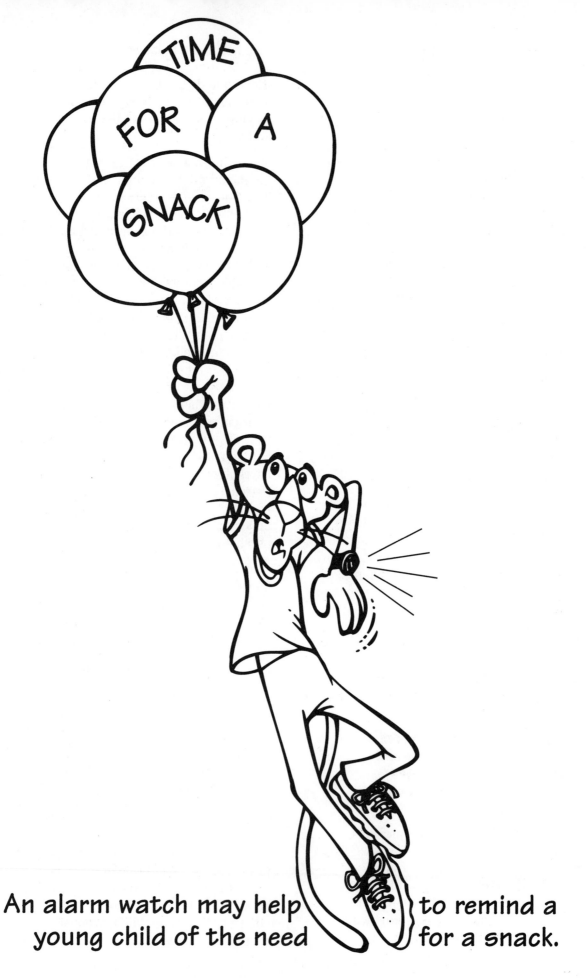

An alarm watch may help to remind a young child of the need for a snack.

Chapter 17

RESPONSIBILITIES OF CHILDREN AT DIFFERENT AGES

Key ideas of this chapter:

🐾 Be aware of different stages in normal development.

🐾 Recognize that responsibilities related to diabetes must depend on the individual child, teenager or young adult and not just on age.

Daily diabetes care has grown more complex in recent years. It is not unusual for families to follow insulin "thinking-scales," mix 2-4 insulins in one syringe, juggle sports and exercise, and to count carbohydrates or follow other food plans. Good sugar control requires the active involvement of parents for many years. The myth that children should be encouraged to do all of their own diabetes care at an early age no longer applies.

Children of different ages are able to do different tasks and to accept different responsibilities. It is important not to expect more from children than they are able to do. If they are not able to do the tasks, they may develop a sense of failure and later poor self-esteem and poor self-care. The ability to do certain tasks may vary from day-to-day and parents must be available to help as needed. And yet, the children should be encouraged to gradually assume care for themselves as they are able. The ability to successfully live independently, both in everyday life and diabetes care, is the eventual goal for all of our children.

The purpose of this chapter is to review "normal" child development and how it relates to diabetes care. Although parts of this chapter may not be important for each reader, they may be helpful to some families. It must be remembered that all children develop at different rates (and our own children are always the most advanced). **Age alone as a guideline does not tell us when an individual child is ready to assume tasks.** There is no such thing as a "magic age" when the diabetes suddenly becomes the responsibility of the child or teenager. Be patient! Independence takes a long time. Thus, the suggestions below may vary for any given child or family. Diabetes is now considered a **"family disease"** and the family must work together, helping each other, rather than expecting the burden of diabetes care to fall entirely on one person.

INFANT UNDER THREE YEARS

Traits and Responsibilities Not Related to Diabetes

This is a time of rapid development of a small, wondrous creature who eats, sleeps, cries, soils diapers, and starts to learn about the world. Motor and brain development are the most rapid of any time in life. Sitting (6-8 months), crawling (6-12 months), walking (12-18 months), and language development open up a new world. Accidents are the infant's major danger. They must be protected from stairs they might fall down, poisons and medicines they might swallow (from cupboards, garages, and purses), auto accidents, and other dangers (including coffee tables with sharp edges). All infants with or without diabetes need love. Parents and care providers need to cuddle and hold infants frequently throughout the day. This is particularly true after shots and blood sugar tests as infants do not understand parents causing pain. Parents must remember that the testing and shots are essential to their infant's life and they must move beyond feelings of guilt (as discussed in Chapter 9). It is also important to remember that much of the fussing around blood sugar tests and shots is due to the interruption in the child's activity rather than being due to pain. Infants develop trust during this period and combining the diabetes care with love will help to make the diabetes care a part of normal life. Young adults often look back with appreciation to their parents for the shots and care they gave them when they were young.

Responsibilities Related to Diabetes

Although babies and toddlers are not able to do any of their own self-care, there are some special features that may help parents. More frequent blood sugar testing is usually done (see Chapter 5) because the babies and toddlers cannot tell if their blood sugars are low. The blood sugar level to aim for is also higher (80 to 200 mg/dl or 4.4 to 11.1 mmol/L;

see Chapter 6) as severe lows may be more dangerous to the infant's rapidly developing brain. Toes are used more frequently as a site for doing the testing. The B-D Ultrafine lancets are smaller and may hurt less.

Shots are sometimes given while the infant is sleeping (if he/she tends to get very upset). The bottom (buttock) is used more frequently as a place to give the shot. Eating is often variable, and we usually advise the parents to wait to give the shot until they see what is eaten (particularly when the rapid-acting Humalog insulin is being used). The Humalog insulin is then reduced if intake is low. Also, the amount of time taken to eat a meal should not be longer than for a child without diabetes. Special treatment may result in eating problems. It is important that the parents stay in control.

The amount of Humalog or Regular insulin is kept low due to body size and due to an apparent increased sensitivity to short-acting insulin. With the insulin syringes currently available, it is not usually necessary to dilute insulins. Most parents learn how to judge 1/2 unit dosages using the 0.3cc insulin syringes.

Low blood sugars can be treated with less carbohydrate than for an older child (usually 5-10 gms due to smaller body size). This amount is found in 1/4 cup of milk, orange or apple juice, or 2-3 oz of sugar pop, although the amount needed may vary from infant to infant. Infants who suck on a bottle of milk or juice frequently during the day or night will tend to have higher blood sugar levels. Overnight sucking on a bottle can also lead to dental decay.

It is important for parents of infants with diabetes to incorporate the diabetes into their everyday lives. Children learn through imitation. If parents have adjusted to the diabetes and can view their child with the same positive feelings they had prior to the diagnosis of diabetes, it will help the child to grow up feeling positive and psychologically healthy. A summary of non-diabetes and diabetes traits for each age group is shown in Table 1.

AGE-RELATED RESPONSIBILITIES AND TRAITS

Table 1

	Non-diabetes-related	Diabetes-related
Ages below 3 years	• developing gross motor skills • developing speech skills • learning to trust • responding to love	• parents must do all care • acceptance of diabetes care as part of normal life • often give shots after seeing what is eaten
Ages 3-7 years	• imaginative/concrete thinkers • cannot think abstractly • self-centered	• parent does all tasks • gradually learns to cooperate for blood sugar tests and insulin shots • inconsistent with food choices—may still need to give shots after meals • gradually learns to recognize hypoglycemia • not much concept of time
Ages 8-12 years	• concrete thinkers • more logical and understanding • more curious • more social • more responsible	• can learn to test blood sugars • at age 10 or 11, can draw up and give shots on occasion, although they still need supervision • can make own food choices • can recognize and treat hypoglycemia • by 11 or 12 years, can be responsible for remembering snacks, but may still need assistance of alarm watches or parent reminders
Ages 13-18 years	• more independent • behavior varies • body image important • away from home more • more responsible • abstract thinking	• capable of doing the majority of shots and blood tests, but still needs some parental involvement and review to make decisions about dosage • knows which foods to eat • gradually recognizes the importance of good sugar control to prevent later complications • may be more willing to inject multiple shots per day

AGES 3-7 YEARS

Traits and Responsibilities Not Related to Diabetes

Children of this age think concretely. Concrete thinking means things are either black or white, right or wrong, good or bad. They do not think abstractly. For example, they are unable to realize that "having a shot of insulin will help me to stay healthy." Instead, a shot may be considered a punishment for doing something wrong. Parents need to repeat over and over that the child hasn't done anything wrong and to try to describe in the child's language why pokes and shots are important.

Sometime in their second or third year of life children start to see themselves as separate individuals from their parents. Children gradually become very curious in the 3 to 7-year-old period. They often want to know how things work. They can annoy parents with the simple words "how" and "why."

Children of this age are also very self-centered. They may progress from playing with a toy alone to gradually learning to share a toy or to share the love of their parents. Primary attachments are to parents and family. Interest in other relationships, such as school peers, begins at 6-7 years of age.

Age responsibilities in children 5-7 years old begin to increase dramatically. They can help pick up their toys, make their bed, or put their dirty clothes in the hamper when guided by the parent. They are capable of fixing simple foods, such as cereal or a sandwich, but still do not understand simple dangers such as putting a knife in a toaster or being careful around boiling water. Thus, they must have much parental supervision.

Children 5-7 years old are learning to read, which opens a whole new world. They are discovering many new things, asking lots of questions, and practicing new skills. They feel more independent and, in some ways, they are. Usually they are cooperative and love to be helpful. However, they still require a good deal of adult supervision.

Responsibilities Related to Diabetes

Children of this age must have the parents do all diabetes related tasks. Fine motor coordination (the coordination of the fingers when handling small items) is not yet fully developed, so they cannot do tasks such as accurately drawing insulin into a syringe.

On the other hand, they can gradually learn to cooperate with their parents (by sitting still for blood sugar tests and insulin shots). They also can feel they are helping by choosing or cleaning a finger for a blood test or by choosing the site for the insulin shot. Children as young as three or four can sometimes recognize low blood sugars. By age 5-7 years this ability is more completely developed—particularly if the parents have encouraged it. They can tell parents when they are hungry. Their complaints may be vague or seem strange to us ("Mommy, my tummy tickles" or "Daddy, I don't feel good.") However, these clues can be very helpful to parents. Helping children verbalize the body sensations of low blood sugars is an important task for family members.

Children of ages 4-7 years may have some concept of which foods they can eat. They can be taught to ask, "Does it have sugar in it?" However, they cannot be expected to always or even very often make the "right" choices over the ones that look or taste good, or to choose foods that are different from what friends or family are eating. They can be expected to have some temper tantrums at being sugar-restricted.

There is not much concept of time at this age. An adult will need to make sure that a snack is taken at a specific time. Sometimes a watch that beeps at a set time can be used as a reminder for a snack.

There is usually no objection to wearing a diabetes ID bracelet or necklace at this age. It is good to get children into the habit of wearing the ID when they are young. This may help them to do this as they get older.

In general, it is important for parents of children in this age group (and in all age groups) to keep a positive attitude. It is important to remember that the blood sugar tests and insulin shots help to keep the child healthy. Playing games around diabetes chores and gradually getting the child to help (even in little ways) may be beneficial. Hugs and kisses will reassure the child that the parents' love continues. Of course, to be able to keep a positive attitude, parents need their own support for their worries and hard work. Friends, family, diabetes support groups, or other sources of support can be extremely helpful.

AGES 8-12 YEARS

Traits and Responsibilities Not Related to Diabetes

Children of this age continue to think in concrete ways. However, they can gradually think more objectively and understand another person's point of view. Fairness and meeting their needs are very important.

Children at these ages are more social and peers begin to play a more important role in their lives. They usually begin to spend nights at friends' houses and have more peer activities than do younger children. They can become involved in some team sports activities (which may be important in getting them to stay involved as they get older). This is an opportune age to do classroom education about diabetes. The more peers understand, it's less likely they will tease and more likely they will become a support to your child. Peer support is important, especially later on during adolescence.

Children can be helpful by learning to take on increased responsibilities. They may help with doing dishes, feeding pets, cleaning their own room and other rooms, or taking out the garbage. Special rewards, such as stars on a calendar, may be helpful in encouraging certain activities.

They are capable of more complex food preparation and can better understand safety and danger issues.

Responsibilities Related to Diabetes

Some children begin to do their own blood sugar testing at ages 8-10 years. At about this age **some** children wish to begin to give some of their own insulin shots. The ability to accurately draw up the insulin is a bit slower in developing, but it is usually present at 10 or 11 years of age. The coordination needed

between seeing something and using the fingers to successfully do the job (eye-hand coordination, fine motor skills) develops during this age. This is an exciting time to watch a child develop. However, adult supervision is **essential** for all of these important tasks. If children begin any of these tasks at too young an age, or have too much responsibility without the parent being available to take over when needed, the child can get "burned out" and be more likely to rebel during the teen years by missing shots or not testing blood sugar levels. In addition, they may have difficulty requesting their parents' help when needed if they are expected to perform self-care tasks alone. Thus, parents must stay involved in diabetes management with this age group!

Children of this age sometimes feel that "life isn't fair," particularly as it pertains to diabetes. It is helpful to just listen to them if they express such feelings.

Children may be able to give their own shots when staying at a friend's house. Their parent can draw the shot ahead of time and put it in a small box, toothbrush holder, or other container and leave it at the friend's home. They may ask the friend's parent to supervise the shot. NPH and Regular insulins can be pre-mixed in a syringe and they will remain as they were. Pre-mixed Humalog and NPH will result in some binding of the Humalog. Regular and Lente insulins cannot be pre-mixed, or the Lente will bind the Regular insulin. However, Humalog and Lente (or Ultralente) can be pre-mixed. As the children are usually very active when staying at a friend's, we often suggest reducing or omitting the dose of short-acting (Regular or Humalog) insulin and reducing the dose of the evening long-acting insulin by 10-20%. It is important to remember to roll the syringe between the hands to re-mix it prior to giving the shot. It is also essential that the friend's parents be informed about hypoglycemia. The handouts in the school or baby-sitters sections (Chapters 22 and 23) may be helpful.

Children of this age can eat lunch at school and make choices to avoid high sugar foods. They can gradually learn to recognize and treat their own hypoglycemic reactions. They are also more aware of time and can learn to be responsible for eating a snack at a set time.

Sports can be very important at this age. A child who learns to enjoy athletics is starting a healthy pattern for controlling diabetes.

In general, parents of the child in this age range must be patient in teaching the child about diabetes and how to do diabetes-related tasks. The parents must still be **very involved** in supervision of the diabetes care. However, they must be secure enough to let the child begin to assume some responsibilities on his/her road to becoming an independent person. Diabetes camp, group ski trips, hikes, or other events allow the children to receive invaluable support from each other, and to realize that they are not the only person in the world with diabetes.

AGES 13-18 YEARS

Traits and Responsibilities Not Related to Diabetes

As teenagers grow older, they gradually develop independence and a sense of their own identity. However, as noted in Chapter 18, Special Challenges of the Teen Years, this age group varies greatly between wanting independence versus needing dependence. Some rebellious behavior may be demonstrated toward parents as teens grow into separate individuals.

Skills increase greatly in this age group. Automobiles can be driven legally and power lawn mowers can (hopefully) be used. Teenagers may take jobs to earn their own money. Activities, in general, are greatly increased.

Body image becomes a major concern. Teenagers worry about how others view them. The slightest pimple may become a catastrophe. Early in this period, friends of the same sex are very important, whereas later on, interest in the opposite sex usually begins. More time is spent with friends. The older teen is away from the home more and stays out later with friends. Experimentation with alcohol at some point is common.

Responsibilities Related to Diabetes

As teenagers grow older, they gradually take over more of their diabetes care. Parents still need to be available to assist with giving a shot from time to time and to take over the diabetes care for a period of time if the youth seems "burned out." Teens generally do better if they get extra help, particularly with insulin dosage. As noted in Chapter 18, A SUPPORTIVE ADULT CAN BE AN ASSET FOR A PERSON WITH DIABETES REGARDLESS OF AGE. Even parents of older teens still need to help with making sure adequate diabetes supplies are available (and paying for them) and making sure that clinic appointments are made and kept every three months. Parents should come to the clinic, although the staff may request to see a teen individually to discuss issues that may be difficult to talk about with parents present.

Many teens dislike the chore of writing blood sugar results in a log book. If the parents agree to do this at the end of each day (with the teenagers' OK), it is a way for the parents to keep tabs on the diabetes. Having values written down (and often faxed to the diabetes care provider) is important in looking at trends and knowing when changes in insulin dosages need to be made.

If experimentation with alcohol happens, it will likely upset the diabetes control (see Chapter 10) and can cause severe hypoglycemia. Experimentation with drugs upsets schedules and diabetes as well. Good peer support in adhering to exercise, a sugar restricted diet, a consistent lifestyle, and not smoking cigarettes (an added risk for diabetic kidney disease and for later heart attacks) are important. Most people who are going to smoke will begin prior to age 20 years. Usually, if the peer group does not smoke, the youth will make a similar choice. Identification with peers is so important in this age group that their support (or lack of it) may greatly affect the teen's diabetes management. A belief in God and church or synagogue activities may help guide the teen, and continued involvement with parents can provide stability, limits, love, and support. Again, support from peers (with or without diabetes) is very important in this age group (see Chapter 18, Special Challenges of the Teen Years).

There is often a feeling of invincibility or "it

can't happen to me." Regular clinic visits at this age may help the teen realize that diabetes care and responsibility are important. Teens with diabetes are faced with more difficult tasks and more serious life issues than their peers. In general, teens with diabetes tend to mature earlier than teens without diabetes, and learn at an earlier age when they have to be serious in life and when they can have fun.

The average ages for mastering tasks as recommended by the American Diabetes Association and by a survey of care providers are shown in Table 2.

The parents' role for the teenager is to be available to help when either forward or backward steps toward adult maturity are taken. Continued support and the provision of stability, limits, and love are essential at this difficult age (as at all ages). **Age alone should not be the primary factor in deciding that a person should assume responsibility for diabetes self-management.** Parents who offer continued assistance and who share the responsibilities with the teen will generally have a teen in better diabetes control.

DEFINITIONS

Eye-hand coordination: The ability to use the hands to finely adjust what is seen with the eyes. This ability usually develops around the age of 10 years.

Fine motor control: The ability to carefully move the fingers with precision (e.g., drawing insulin to an exact line on a syringe). This ability usually develops around age 10 or 11 years.

Self-esteem: How a person feels about himself/herself.

AVERAGE AGES FOR DIABETES-RELATED SKILLS

Age of Mastery (in years)

Skill	Recommended by the American Diabetes Association	Survey of Care Providers*
A. Hypoglycemia		
1) Recognizes and reports	8-10	4-9
2) Able to treat	10-12	6-10
3) Anticipates/prevents	14-16	9-13
B. Blood glucose testing (by meter)	8-10	7-11
C. Insulin injection		
1) Gives to self (at least sometimes)		8-11
2) Draws two insulins	12-14	8-12
3) Able to adjust doses	14-16	12-16
D. Diet		
1) Identifies appropriate pre-exercise snack	10-12	10-13
2) States role of diet in care	14-16	9-5
3) Able to alter food in relation to blood glucose level	14-16	10-15

Abstracted from a survey done by Drs. T. Wysocki, P. Meinhold, D.J. Cox, and W.L. Clarke at Ohio State University and The University of Virginia (Diabetes Care 11:65-68, 1990).

QUESTIONS (Q) AND ANSWERS (A) FROM NEWSNOTES

Q. It seems like every time our eight-year-old son stays at his friend's house or has his friend stay overnight at our house he has low blood sugar the next morning. Should we be making changes?

A. "Overnights" are an important social and developmental step in our society. It is important that children with diabetes be able to participate just like any other child. Overnights are also a step in developing independence and are sometimes the first night spent away from the parents. And yet, it is important that the child be safe in relationship to the diabetes. The children usually run and play a bit harder with their friend on overnights. They also stay up a bit later than normal and use more energy. It is thus generally wise to reduce the insulin dose, both the short-acting (20-50%) and the long-acting (10-20%) insulins, on these nights. A good bedtime snack is also advisable. Remember the "pizza factor," that pizza tends to keep a blood sugar up better than most other foods. If there is a frozen pizza in the freezer, it may be a good night to use it. It is also wise to awaken the child at a reasonable time in the morning and to get a glass of juice or milk down sooner rather than later.

Do remember that if the child is able to do a shot but is not yet old enough to draw it up, the morning NPH and Regular insulin can be pre-drawn. The syringe can be put into a little box or toothbrush holder and just rolled to mix the next morning. (Commercial 70/30 mixtures of NPH and Regular stay the same for three years.) Think about reducing the dose again for the morning shot if it is likely that the two friends will be playing together much of the next day.

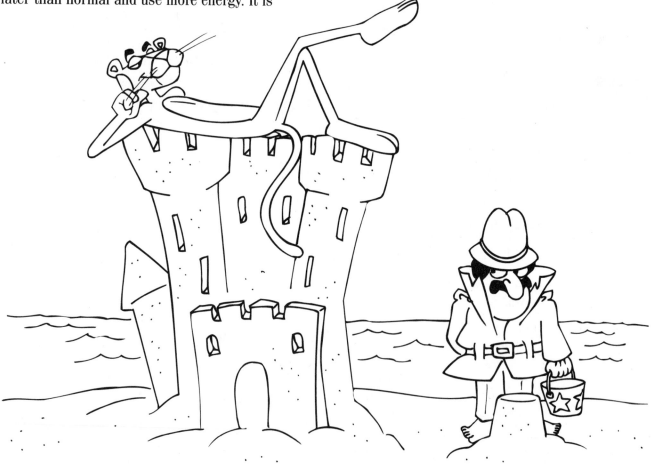

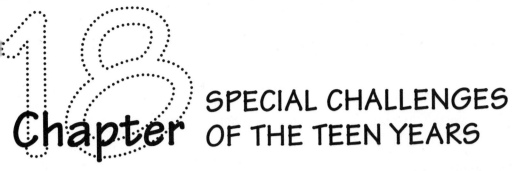

Chapter 18

SPECIAL CHALLENGES OF THE TEEN YEARS

Key ideas of this chapter:

🐾 Appreciate some of the special challenges of the teenage years.

🐾 Develop ideas for dealing with the special challenges of the teenage years.

STRUGGLE FOR INDEPENDENCE

Parents often despair at the thought of their "angelic" child becoming an adolescent. The teen years have been defined as the period in life when one varies between wanting to be a child and wanting to be an adult. These feelings vary from second to second, minute to minute, hour to hour, day to day, week to week, and year to year. The "child" part of the adolescent still wants to be completely dependent on parents and other adults. The emerging "adult" wants to be an entirely independent person. There are many shades between these two extremes that may linger into later life. Hopefully, the variation becomes less with increasing age.

In the past, we believed that children with diabetes should assume their own management at a certain age and that they would suddenly become independent. **We now know that independence is not age specific and is a gradual process.** We think of diabetes as **a family disease** that requires a great deal of parent-child partnership to achieve good sugar control and healthy independence. Parent partnership (involvement) with the teen can be

SPECIAL CHALLENGES FOR THE TEENAGER

🐾 Struggle for independence

🐾 Growth and body changes

🐾 Identity

🐾 Peer relationships, alcohol, drugs, tobacco

🐾 Sexuality

🐾 Consistency (exercise, eating, emotions, and lifestyle)

accomplished in a variety of ways: drawing up and giving injections; keeping a log book to record blood sugars and note trends and problems; faxing blood sugars to the diabetes care team (fax sheets are found in Chapter 6); helping with weekend dosing when teens may want to sleep in and could use some help with shots and a quick breakfast. These not only help the teenager, but also help keep the parent "in the loop" and aware of what is going on with management.

The "child vs. adult" struggle can greatly influence diabetes management during the adolescent years. A teenager may want entire responsibility for the diabetes management at one time—faithfully checking blood sugars, watching food and sugar intake, and taking the responsibility for the injections. At another time, blood sugars will not be checked unless the parent is there to help, injections may be forgotten, or sugar may be consumed in large quantities. Parents can lessen the effects of this variable attitude toward the diabetes care by remaining involved and offering to share these responsibilities with their "child-adult." We believe that **a supportive adult who is readily available, BUT NOT OVERBEARING OR CONSTANTLY NAGGING, can be a help to any person with diabetes, regardless of age.**

Julie is a 16-year-old girl who has had diabetes for seven years. She and her family have always prided themselves on Julie's good diabetes control. Julie is a talented dancer and hopes to become a professional dancer some day. She dances on Mondays, Wednesdays, and Fridays at 5:30 p.m. At a clinic appointment, it is discovered that her diabetes has become out of control with her HbA$_{1c}$ unexpectedly being over 14%. In talking with Julie, she admits to missing evening injections sometimes when she goes to dance class. She says she just doesn't have time to get her homework, blood test and injection done and still get something to eat before leaving for dance class.

PLAN: *Julie's parents volunteered to help with the blood testing and injections on those nights and to make some dinner for her. Julie was relieved to have her parents take over some of the diabetes care, but admitted it was hard to ask for help after being responsible for her own diabetes care for several years.*

Diabetes care is usually NOT the top priority for a teenager. Their main priorities may be their peers, school work, sports, a car, a job, etc. (in varying orders of importance for different teens). Thus, the parents may need to help in keeping a focus on the tasks necessary for good sugar control.

If the teenager's actions (or lack of them) result in possible serious dangers to his/her health, then the parents have no choice but to step back in for a time. This is particularly true when insulin shots are being missed. Hopefully, the next attempt at taking on increased responsibilities will be more successful. Sometimes professional counseling is necessary. However, the majority of teenagers gradually assume adult independence by themselves. In contrast to the parents' worst fears, they do grow up! In fact, the teenager with diabetes may assume adult responsibilities earlier than other teenagers.

The task of how to help children grow to be independent young adults is a challenge for most families. Diabetes complicates that task somewhat. It is normal for parents of children with diabetes to feel anxious about normal separations such as overnights, camp, and school trips. Parents worry about injections, low blood sugars, and whether the schedule and snacks will be remembered. Keep in mind that with good preparation and supervision, these separation experiences are an important part of growing up. They will not only facilitate growing independence, but these experiences are also usually a lot of fun. It is best to start with brief periods of separation, like staying at a relative or friend's house overnight.

Overnights

Staying at a friend's home, even for one night, can be a big step, as can visiting relatives. We generally suggest a small reduction in insulin dosage (short- and long-acting insulins) for overnights (at home or away) as they are up later and tend to burn more energy. (Also, then the parents do not need to worry quite as much about low blood sugars while their child is away.)

Summer Camp

Follow these short visits with longer stays at a diabetes or other summer camp. Children learn that they CAN survive without the parents and the parents learn that their children CAN survive without them! (Re-education for these children and their parents is important.)

Clinic Visits

Teenagers can begin seeing diabetes care team members by themselves at diabetes clinic visits. Parents are still needed at these visits to review plans and problems with their teens and the diabetes care team. As noted in Chapter 17, Responsibilities of Children at Different Ages, **better sugar control usually results if parents stay involved in offering continued assistance and sharing responsibilities with the teenager.**

GROWTH AND BODY CHANGES

The adolescent growth spurt and the development of adult sexual characteristics result in many body changes—probably more than occur at any other single time in life.

Growth Hormone

The gain in height is a result of increased hormone levels (growth hormone, testosterone, and estrogen). Growth hormone partially blocks insulin activity. As a result, insulin requirements increase dramatically and are usually the highest per pound body weight that they will ever be. The insulin requirement usually decreases when growth is completed. If blood sugar control is good during puberty, full growth is usually reached. Research from our Center has shown that better growth (to full adult potential) is more likely with good sugar control.

Sex Hormones

Female sexual development includes breast and hair development, widening of the hips, and the onset of menstrual cycles. These pubertal changes may be slightly delayed in girls with diabetes. Blood sugars may increase during menstruation, and many girls will increase the Humalog or Regular (short-acting)

insulin by one or two units during this time.

Males have enlargement of the testes and penis, and facial and other body hair begins to grow. When body odors become noticeable, for males or females, the use of deodorants is desirable. Acne ("zits") or pimples may develop in either sex, making good skin care important. Tetracycline or other antibiotics are fine to use if acne pustules become a problem. Males may be tempted to try steroid drugs to try to make their muscles larger. Use of these steroid drugs can prevent full height attainment, lead to increased blood cholesterol levels, and an increased risk for heart attacks in later life. They also may cause aggressive behavior, resulting in problems getting along with others. The drugs reduce insulin sensitivity, causing increased blood sugar levels. **Non-prescribed steroid drugs should not be used.**

Thyroid Hormone

The thyroid gland (in the neck) must function properly during this time or growth will not progress normally. As part of the regular diabetes check-up visits, the diabetes care provider will monitor the size and function of the teen's thyroid gland. About half of teenagers with diabetes get some thyroid gland enlargement. This is an "auto-immune" disorder, as is diabetes, and antibodies against the thyroid gland can be measured (although expensive and often not paid for by insurance). A simple test called TSH (**T**hyroid **S**timulating **H**ormone) is usually adequate. Thyroid problems are also discussed in Chapter 21.

Body Image

Teenagers are often very concerned about "body image" (self-consciousness) and a single pimple can be a disaster. It is fortunate that diabetes does not usually result in visible body alterations. Wearing an insulin pump (see Chapter 25) may change this, and is part of the reason why pumps should not be "pushed" on a person until they are ready. However, having diabetes may make teens "feel" different from their peers. The refusal to wear an identification (ID) bracelet or necklace, to wear an insulin pump, or to refrain from eating high sugar foods may relate to not wanting to feel different from peers.

IDENTITY

 Who Am I?

Teens are searching for the answer to the question, "Who am I?" It is important to emphasize the positives about who they are at this stage of their lives (e.g., someone who loves a sport, music, mechanics, school plays, or other interests), and who secondarily happens to have diabetes. The diabetes should not come first. Positive reinforcement should be given when a good attitude toward living with diabetes is demonstrated. Compliments are important. For example, "Good job on getting your blood tests done even with the stress of finals" (even though the stress and not exercising may have resulted in high sugar values). In contrast, it may be necessary for parents to "bite the bullet" and not respond when stress results in blood sugar testing not being done. A cheerful offer to record results or give injections during busy times can be rewarding for both the teen and the parent.

Risk-Taking

The in-the-middle age range of teenaged years (approximately ages 15-17 years) is usually the most difficult time of the teenage years. The teen often sees himself/herself as "invincible." Risk-taking and experimentation tend to occur more frequently. These may include risks involving diabetes (e.g., "I don't need to wear a bracelet, I've got an ID card in my wallet," or "I'm not going to carry sugar—I can get something at my friend's house if I need it.") The need for experimentation may include new hair colors or styles, unusual clothing, perhaps ring piercing in an unusual place, or even a tattoo. The experimentation may also include diabetes-related behaviors such as eating high sugar foods, not doing blood sugars, or even missing shots. Regular (or more frequent) clinic visits and HbA_{1c} tests at this time may help to return the teen to reality. Parents need to let the teen know that they trust their child to act maturely. **Patience** on the part of the care providers and from the parents is a real virtue at this time.

THE PEERS

Peer relationships are very important to teenagers, often more so than relationships with parents. Early in adolescence, close friends are usually of the same sex. In later adolescence this often changes or is "added to" by members of the opposite sex. Being like their peers is very important; having diabetes and "being different" can be a problem. Some teenagers are comfortable doing blood tests or giving themselves injections in front of their friends. Others, particularly if acceptance of the diabetes has been a struggle, will absolutely refuse to let anyone other than the closest friend know that they have diabetes.

The willingness or refusal to wear an ID necklace or bracelet may reflect the teen's own acceptance of diabetes.

Much of a teen's identity (see section above) relates to conforming with their peer group. Peer groups can be important in helping the teen make decisions about the use of drugs, alcohol, or tobacco. If the peer group rejects or accepts these, the teen with diabetes will probably do likewise. Because smoking and chewing tobacco age the blood vessels and lead to a greater likelihood of diabetic kidney disease and later of heart attacks, tobacco use is particularly harmful to the individual with diabetes. As in all people, chewing tobacco can lead to dental problems and cancer of the mouth. Similarly, smoking cigarettes is associated with an increased likelihood of lung cancer and heart attacks. Alcohol consumption can result in delayed severe insulin reactions. (This is discussed in more detail at the end of Chapter 10, Normal Nutrition.) Drugs that alter awareness of time have their greatest effects on diabetes by interfering with consistency in eating and insulin injections.

Participation in a support group for teenagers with diabetes can be a help. A support group can be both a social and a discussion group. It may help the teenagers share their feelings with others who also have diabetes. They soon realize that others have many of the same feelings that they do, and that they are quite normal in spite of having diabetes!

Research has shown that the teen with diabetes who involves his/her peers by sharing knowledge about diabetes is more likely to achieve better sugar control. We encourage teens to bring a friend to the clinic visit to continue to learn how they can support their friend with diabetes.

SEXUALITY

Teenagers with diabetes run the same risk as non-diabetic teens of contracting diseases such as AIDS, herpes, chlamydia, and other sexually transmitted diseases. Pregnancy in adolescent girls with diabetes has added risks compared to non-diabetics. If a woman with diabetes is in excellent sugar control **PRIOR** to becoming pregnant, there will not be an increased risk for miscarriages or birth defects in the baby. However, if she is in poor sugar control, particularly in the early part of pregnancy, the baby will be at increased risk for birth defects. Thus, pregnancy must be carefully planned in women with diabetes, and should be undertaken only after the HbA$_{1c}$ has been in the "excellent" range for several months. This is an excellent time to use an insulin pump. The mother does not risk any worsening of kidney damage during the pregnancy (in contrast to the Hollywood production of "Steel Magnolias.") However, eye (retinal) changes do sometimes worsen during pregnancy and it is important to see the eye doctor more frequently at this time. It is generally wise for a woman with diabetes to consult with a doctor who specializes in diabetic pregnancies before and during her planned pregnancy.

Research has shown that there is no increased risk for teenage girls with diabetes to use birth control pills compared to non-diabetic teenage girls using birth control pills. The only sure way to absolutely prevent a sexually transmitted disease or pregnancy is to abstain from sex. If the teen chooses to have sex, a condom should always be used (even if other methods are already being used). The use of condoms can help prevent sexually transmitted diseases and AIDS, although they do not guarantee absolute protection. **If a male or female believes they cannot cause or become pregnant due to diabetes, they are absolutely wrong. People with diabetes can cause a pregnancy or become pregnant just like anyone else.** The stress of the teen years may be heightened by conflicts about emerging sexuality.

CONSISTENCY (EXERCISE, EATING, EMOTIONS, AND LIFESTYLE)

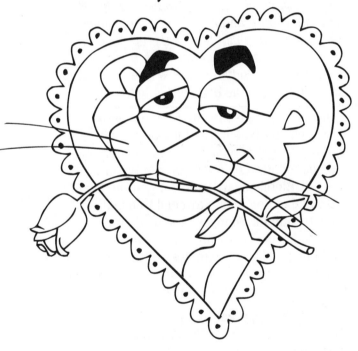

The word CONSISTENCY is in capital letters throughout Chapter 11, "Food Management and Diabetes." If everything could be the same every day, blood glucose control would be much easier. Unfortunately, there is no such thing as consistency in many teenagers' lives. Bedtime may be at 10:00 p.m. on school nights, but then at midnight or later on Friday and Saturday nights. Many teens like to sleep late on weekends. We suggest an absolute limit of 9:00 a.m. as the time when the insulin must be taken with at least a glass of juice. The teenager can then go back to sleep for an hour. If the teen sleeps later than 9:00 a.m. without juice or food intake, the insulin taken the previous evening may lead to hypoglycemia. Likewise, taking the insulin later than usual results in overlap with the evening insulin and a greater likelihood of low blood sugar. Once again, supportive adults must be available to make this plan work.

Tom is in his last year of high school and was recently diagnosed with diabetes. He feels confident that he can give his own injections and test his blood sugar. His greatest concern is that he enjoys sleeping in on weekends and that he no longer will be able to do this.

PLAN: *Tom's parents are very willing to help Tom with this problem. His Dad, the early riser in the family, agrees to draw-up Tom's insulin no later than 9:00 a.m. on weekends and to take the insulin and a glass of orange juice to Tom in bed. Tom can then wake up, take his shot, drink the juice and go back to sleep for another hour. Dad also agrees to wake Tom up at 10:00 a.m. so he can eat his breakfast.*

Consistent exercise is often a problem. Seasonal sports, such as football or soccer, call for heavy exercise for a few months, but may be followed by weeks or months of little activity. Blood sugars will vary and the insulin dose and eating plan may need frequent adjustments for changes in activity level. It is good to have a "back-up" activity such as walking, jogging, or aerobics so that there is some exercise every day. Daily exercise is also very effective in controlling weight.

It should be apparent that the saying **"DIABETES IS A COMPROMISE"** fits particularly well with the teenage years. Consistency in areas that would benefit diabetes control sometimes needs to be compromised in helping a teenager to develop normally.

OTHER CHALLENGES

Rapid mood swings are more common during adolescence. Mood swings may change the blood adrenaline level, affecting blood sugars. Adrenaline (epinephrine) causes the blood sugar to rise. In general, normal adolescent mood changes should not affect overall glucose control significantly. However, adolescence is frequently an age when other conditions may emerge; mood disorders (like clinical depression) and anxiety disorders are common, though they are often unrecognized conditions. If your teenager shows unusual changes that are concerning to you, please talk with your health care team. Such changes include: frequent irritability or anger; a drop in grades or school performance; loss of interest in activities that were previously enjoyable; suspected substance abuse; changes in sleep habits (unable to go to sleep or sleeping all the time); loss of appetite; and "hanging out" with a different group of friends or dropping friends all together. These may be symptomatic of an underlying mood disorder.

Teenagers' eating habits may be affected by their emotions. Teenagers are notorious for rather unusual eating habits and this poses a challenge for teens with diabetes who might not want to see themselves as "different." In addition, some teenagers develop mild to severe eating disorders (anorexia = not eating; bulimia = bingeing on food and self-induced vomiting and/or use of laxatives). Parents should be suspicious of eating disorders if their teen overeats, doesn't exercise and still doesn't gain weight. Weight loss without dieting or heavy exercise should also alert the parents to possible missed injections. More parental supervision and possibly professional help is then necessary.

Stress is a normal part of life (e.g., arguments with friends, worrying about grades, or concern about making a team). Learning to deal with stress is an important part of adolescence.

SUMMARY

The teen years are stressful for everyone. However, they can be the happiest years of an individual's life. The teen with diabetes has extra stresses, but with a supportive family, these can be managed. Diabetes is a partnership between the parents and the teenager. It is often important for parents to be patient and to remember that they, too, were once an adolescent. Parents must find ways to stay involved in the diabetes management, but not to be overbearing. Diabetes is a **"disease of compromise,"** as parents, teens and care providers must often compromise as to the level of care agreed upon. Parents must be available to help and to be supportive, but still let the teenager gain independence. The good news is, they do grow up!

DEFINITIONS

Adolescence: The term given to the teenage years.

Adrenaline (epinephrine): The stress hormone made in the adrenal gland in the abdomen. It causes blood sugars to rise.

AIDS: Acquired Immune Deficiency Syndrome. This is a serious condition acquired by sexual contact with an infected person or by sharing needles with an infected person. If a mother has AIDS, during pregnancy she can also pass it on to her baby.

Estrogen: Female hormone made in the ovary (located in the abdomen) that causes female body changes.

Growth hormone: A hormone (like insulin) made in the pituitary gland at the base of the brain that is important for growth. It blocks the insulin activity.

Peers: One's group of friends.

Self-consciousness (body image): Concern about how oneself appears to others.

Sexually transmitted diseases (STDs): Diseases contracted through sexual contact, such as herpes, chlamydia, gonorrhea (clap), or syphilis.

Testosterone: A male hormone made in the testes that causes male body changes.

QUESTIONS (Q) AND ANSWERS (A) FROM NEWSNOTES

Q. My son is going to college this fall and has asked if you will write a letter requesting that he has a private room in the dormitory because of his diabetes. Is this a good idea?

A. I have been asked this question many times and have generally replied, "No." First, this is using the diabetes as an excuse when, in reality, the usual reason for wanting the private room has nothing to do with the diabetes. People of all ages should be discouraged from "using" their diabetes.

A second reason for saying "No" is that a roommate can be a very important asset. If a person has a bad reaction and is in a room alone, it may not be discovered as quickly. Likewise, if a person has the flu, the roommate may be the best person to fetch a bowl of soup from the cafeteria across the street, etc.

Finally, if the person is shy about giving shots or doing blood sugars in the presence of another person, it is time to get over that shyness. It is all part of the adjustment to life with diabetes.

Q. Are birth control pills okay to use for a college-aged student with diabetes? Is there an increased risk for cancer if they are used? What are the main side effects?

A. Initial research reported from our Center and published in the *Journal of the American Medical Association* in 1994 (271:1099) did not show any bad effects on the eyes or kidneys of women with diabetes who used oral contraceptives for a mean of 3.4 years (range: 1.0-7.0 years).

Remember that it is important to plan pregnancies very carefully when a woman has diabetes. If a pregnancy occurs when the HbA_{1c} is low (near the non-diabetic normal), the fetus has little or no increase in risk for birth defects from the mother's diabetes. However, if the HbA_{1c} is high, the baby has a high risk for birth defects (abnormalities of the spinal cord, heart, lips and palate, and other organs). It is during the first 1-3 months of pregnancy when the vital organs are forming that excellent sugar control is critical to the fetus. Often, women do not even realize they are pregnant during this most crucial time. Therefore, the pill may be very important in allowing careful planning for a married couple who wants to plan the pregnancy around a time of excellent sugar control.

It must be remembered that much of the early research on the pill was done in the 1960s and 1970s when high-dose estrogen and progestin tablets were in use. The current pill has 1/3-1/4 the dose of the earlier pill. Also, women who smoked cigarettes were included in the early studies and it is now realized that smoking was a greater risk for some of the side effects being studied (e.g., blood clots) than was the pill. There is even evidence now to suggest that pill users may have a 20% reduction in risk for heart attacks.

In relation to cancer risk, the Food and Drug Administration (FDA) ruled that after evaluating 29 studies, they found no increased risk for breast cancer among pill users. In fact, epidemiological studies have shown the pill to help prevent ovarian and uterine cancer.

The main reasons women give for discontinuing the pill are acne, weight gain, no menses (amenorrhea), and breakthrough bleeding. In the clinic, we like to follow blood pressure, just to make sure it remains steady.

Q. Is it true that growth is reduced by poor sugar control?

A. Research published from our Center in 1995 (*Diabetic Medicine*, Vol. 12, 129-133) was one of the first studies to use longitudinal HbA_{1c} values to show that optimal growth is not reached if longitudinal HbA_{1c} values are not in a good range. In addition to the growth rate of the person with diabetes, the final adult height was compared to that of siblings, as well as the expected adult height based on the parents' heights. All were reduced in people with increased HbA_{1c} values. In contrast, growth was not altered in people who kept their HbA_{1c} values in a good range.

Q. Our teenage son has had a mildly elevated HbA_{1c} value (9%) over the past year. His physician and his mother and I have warned him about kidney failure and vision problems, but it doesn't seem to do any good. He currently receives Humalog and NPH insulin before breakfast and dinner. What would you suggest?

A. First, it has long been known that scare tactics do not work with teenagers. This is particularly true in the mid-teen period (15-17 years) when they are "invincible," which may in itself lead to risky behavior. If you want your son to change, you and his health care providers might start with "planting seeds." It might be suggested that a third shot each day, perhaps of Humalog using the insulin pen, would help at lunch or the afternoon snack. It is also sometimes helpful to switch the evening long-acting insulin (e.g., NPH) to bedtime and to just use the Humalog at dinner. At first, he may resist. Continue to offer education, but without the scare tactics. Eventually, he may be willing to try the third shot. Then praise him and offer support. Hopefully, this will help him to continue the positive action he has taken. It helps if he is able to feel a benefit (feeling better, less frequent voiding, etc.). However, he may not feel different. If growth picks up with the lower HbA_{1c} value, point this out to him. The lower HbA_{1c} value should also be a plus and give him positive feedback for this. Hopefully, the sum total will be such that he will want to continue with the new behavior (the third shot). This model for making change has many potential applications, both in diabetes-related change and in other areas.

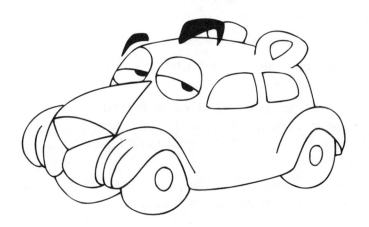

Chapter 19

OUTPATIENT MANAGEMENT, EDUCATION, SUPPORT GROUPS, AND STANDARDS OF CARE

Key ideas of this chapter:

* Use outpatient management methods to treat diabetes.

* Be aware of the minimum standards of care for diabetes treatment.

OUTPATIENT MANAGEMENT

The majority of new-onset treatment is now done in an outpatient setting when the Health Maintenance Organizations (HMOs) are cooperative in funding outpatient care. The primary reason is that it is less traumatic for the child and family. It usually also saves the HMO money compared to the cost of hospital treatment (if they are smart enough to realize this). Similarly, it is now relatively rare to hospitalize people with known type 1 diabetes in the U.S. to "assess how they are doing." Many of our patients who have had diabetes for over 20 years have never had a diabetes-related hospitalization in their entire lives. Good education, regular clinic visits (every 3 months), good communication with the diabetes health care providers, and fulfilling the diabetes standards of care all help to keep the person with diabetes healthy.

TELEPHONE MANAGEMENT

People with diabetes should have checkups with the health team approximately every three months. This is the recommendation of the ADA Standards of Care included at the back of this chapter. These visits allow for the HbA_{1c} to be done (Chapter 13), which reflects the number of high blood sugars for the past three months. Insulin adjustments can then be recommended. In between checkups, much of diabetes management can be dealt with over the telephone or by using a fax or e-mail message system. Some glucose meters now even have fax or e-mail capabilities if extra equipment is purchased from the company. The diabetes care provider should be called prior to the next regularly scheduled injection when a severe hypoglycemic reaction has occurred or if more than two mild reactions occurred within a short time. He/she should also be called anytime the urine ketones are moderate or large.

FAX MESSAGES

Most families now have access to a fax machine. The two blood sugar record sheets in Chapter 6 hold either one week or two weeks of blood sugar records and are an ideal size to send through the fax machine. We ask that records be faxed anytime the family feels things are out of control. If over half of blood sugar values at any time of day are above the upper level for age (see Chapter 6), and the family is uncertain what changes need to be made, it is wise to fax in the values and let one of the healthcare providers make suggestions. It is also wise to fax in blood sugars and insulin dosages if there are more than two values below 60 mg/dl (3.25 mmol/L) in one week. We prefer faxes to phone calls to report blood sugar values, as the fax saves time and confusion in trying to write down values over the phone. It has been our experience that if the parents do not have access to a fax machine, most schools (and especially the school nurse) will provide a way to fax in the blood sugars. It is only when records are kept that trends can be detected. Nothing is more frustrating to a health care provider than to have weeks of high values brought to the clinic with no attempts to make changes or to get help. The blood sugar testing is then a complete waste. If families wish to fax their data, they should remember to:

1. Include the insulin dosages

2. Record the time of any symptomatic low blood sugars (even if it was not possible to do a blood sugar test) and include any relevant information relating to why lows occurred

3. Include the sender's fax and phone number and when that person can best be reached

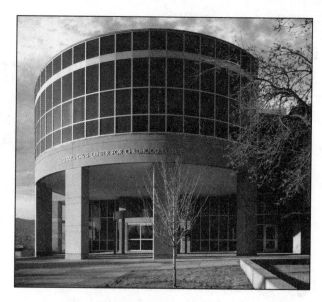

The Barbara Davis Center for Childhood Diabetes

CLINIC VISITS

In addition to reviewing blood sugars and the number of lows and having the HbA_{1c} test done, the visits every three months are important to follow growth, changes in insulin dosage, and to check for other problems. Education is continued and the family is taught new ideas. In the clinic, the family may see the following people:

Clinic Nurse, Medical Assistant, or Volunteer: weighs and measures the child, checks blood pressure, and helps with the blood sugar, hemoglobin A_{1c}, urine ketone and protein tests. Blood glucose meters are "downloaded."

Diabetes Nurse Educator: continues the diabetes education and reviews diabetes management.

Doctor, Child Health Associate, or Pediatric Nurse Practitioner: checks to see how the child is doing; may change insulin dosage and also do a physical examination; coordinates the recommendations of all team members.

Dietitian: reviews food intake and makes suggestions for changes. The dietitian provides nutrition education and information about snacks and other food needs.

Social Worker or Psychologist: can help with personal, family, school, or other problems.

When a family with a child or adolescent previously cared for elsewhere attends our Clinic for the first visit, it usually takes a half to a whole day. Later visits will be shorter. The family should bring snacks to the appointment.

Blood sugar records and meters must **ALWAYS** be brought along to the clinic visit. Occasionally, the nurse may wish to check the accuracy of your home meter with a more accurate meter that is kept in the clinic. All meters that we recommend have memories to store the last 100 to 250 blood sugar values and the ability to download the data upon arrival in the clinic. It is important to analyze this data at the time of the clinic visit. The nurse may also wish to review the method for cleaning the meter or to check the control standard with you. It is also helpful to bring this educational book so that it can be used to review knowledge about diabetes.

EDUCATION, SUPPORT, AND WORKING GROUPS

Some families gain extra support from meeting with other families who also have children with diabetes. This may happen at the time of the clinic visits, at special group meetings, or at special events, such as, sports picnics or Halloween parties.

Special education courses are important for families who do not live near a specialized diabetes clinic. These courses are important for children who were diagnosed at a young age and have reached teenage years because they are able to understand material they could not understand earlier. Courses dealing strictly with type 1 diabetes should be attended, as the problems of adult-onset (type 2) diabetes can be very different.

A special course, **"Transition to Work and College Bound Workshop,"** is offered as people become independent from their parents. A boost in knowledge at this time can be helpful in preventing later problems.

A one-day **"Grandparent's Workshop"** is offered at our Center, as well as regularly at several other centers throughout the U.S. It is important that children with diabetes have the same relationships with grandparents as do other children (see Chapter 23). This likely involves staying with the grandparents, which requires them to have basic knowledge about giving shots, checking blood sugars, and treating hypoglycemia. The grandparents may feel more confident in caring for their grandchild with diabetes as a result of such a course.

STANDARDS OF MEDICAL CARE

Standards of medical care for people with type 1 diabetes (and type 2—not included here) have been published by the American Diabetes Association (*Diabetes Care* 12:365, 1989; *Diabetes Care* 17:616, 1994 and more recently, *Diabetes Care* 21, Supplement 1:523, 1998). The standards are both for care providers and for people with diabetes, and should allow people with diabetes to:

1. Assess the quality of medical care they receive

2. Develop expectations for their role in the medical treatment

3. Compare their treatment outcomes to standard goals

The patient and/or family must assume some of the responsibility for meeting the standards of care outlined below. For example, if the family member with diabetes has reached puberty and has had diabetes for at least three years, annual eye and kidney evaluations are needed. The family must set up the eye evaluation with an ophthalmologist covered by their HMO. Similarly, they need to help the family member do two timed overnight urine collections for the important microalbumin test for the kidneys (directions at end of Chapter 21). Some of the American Diabetes Association's recommended standards of care with a few modifications are outlined below.

1. Insulin-treated patients should have regular clinic visits, including an HbA_{1c} or similar test, at least every three months.

2. All patients with type 1 diabetes must be taught a method of **blood glucose testing.**

3. A comprehensive physical examination, including sexual maturation in adolescents, should be performed annually. Parts of the physical exam

affected by diabetes (e.g., height, weight, blood pressure, eyes, thyroid, liver size, deep tendon reflexes, injection sites, feet, etc.) should be checked every three months.

🐾 Patients ≥10 years of age with type 1 diabetes should have a dilated eye examination by an eye doctor within 3-5 years after the onset of diabetes. Screening for diabetic eye disease is NOT necessary before 10 years of age.

🐾 Laboratory tests for determination of microalbuminuria should be done annually in postpubertal patients who have had diabetes for at least three years.

🐾 The occurrence of severe hypoglycemic episodes (episodes requiring the help of others [when not usually required], seizures, or loss of consciousness) are serious and require the help of a diabetes specialist in preventing further episodes.

🐾 The stress of illness frequently aggravates glycemic control and necessitates more frequent monitoring of **blood glucose and urine ketones** by the family. Medical help must be constantly available when moderate or large urine ketones are detected.

🐾 A lipid profile, including cholesterol, triglyceride, LDL and HDL should be performed at least every five years.

🐾 Hypertension and borderline elevations in blood pressure contribute to the development and progression of the chronic complications of diabetes. Elevations in blood pressure must be treated aggressively to achieve and maintain blood pressure in the normal range.

FOR PEOPLE WITH DIABETIC COMPLICATIONS

🐾 Established diabetic retinopathy and its complications require care by an ophthalmologist experienced in the management of people with diabetes.

🐾 The patient with abnormal kidney function (proteinuria or elevated serum creatinine) requires heightened attention, control of other risk factors (e.g., hypertension and smoking), and consultation with a specialist in diabetic renal disease.

🐾 Patients with cardiovascular risk factors should be carefully monitored. Evidence of cardiovascular disease (such as angina, decreased pulses, and ECG abnormalities) requires efforts aimed at correction of contributing risk factors (e.g., obesity, smoking, hypertension, sedentary lifestyle, hyperlipidemia, and poorly regulated diabetes), in addition to specific treatment of the cardiovascular problem.

DEFINITIONS

ADA: American Diabetes Association.

Child Health Associate: A doctor's assistant who is trained to care for children.

Standards of Care: Recommendations made by an ADA panel for the minimum levels of care for people with type 1 diabetes as included and modified in this chapter.

QUESTIONS (Q) AND ANSWERS (A) FROM NEWSNOTES

Q. Why are regular clinic appointments necessary and how often should these be scheduled?

A. It is our belief that clinic appointments should be scheduled approximately every three months. This is also the recommended interval for children in the ADA "Standards of Medical Care." The reasons for this are primarily preventive since this is where the emphasis in health care now lies. In the early 1900s the emphasis on health care was in the treatment of acute problems. This has now switched to a more preventive based health care, particularly relating to chronic diseases.

For people with diabetes, the visits every three months allow to continue education and to increase motivation for doing day-to-day monitoring of the diabetes. It is the experience of our Clinic and of other large diabetes clinics in the U.S. that if regular visits do not occur, diabetes monitoring and knowledge become lax.

In addition, it is very important to check the eyes and perform the remainder of the physical examination at regular intervals. We have seen a case where an eye specialist actually photographed the back of the eye and found normal eye photographs; four months later diffuse eye hemorrhages were present. The earlier such eye problems are detected and treated, the greater the chance for saving vision. In addition, with children, growth should be occurring. Many physicians believe that good diabetes control is one of the best means of assuring good growth. We feel that every three months is a good interval for checking the gain in height and weight. Other parts of the physical exam, such as the thyroid size, liver size, and the injection sites are also important to check at regular intervals. The liver can be enlarged if someone is receiving too much insulin (extra sugar is stored) or not enough insulin (extra fat is stored).

In summary, the best management occurs with the family and team working together. Although every three months seems to be an average best time to return to the clinic, there are obviously some situations where more frequent visits are important.

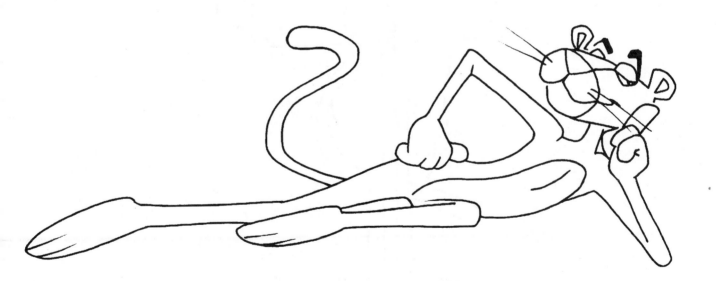

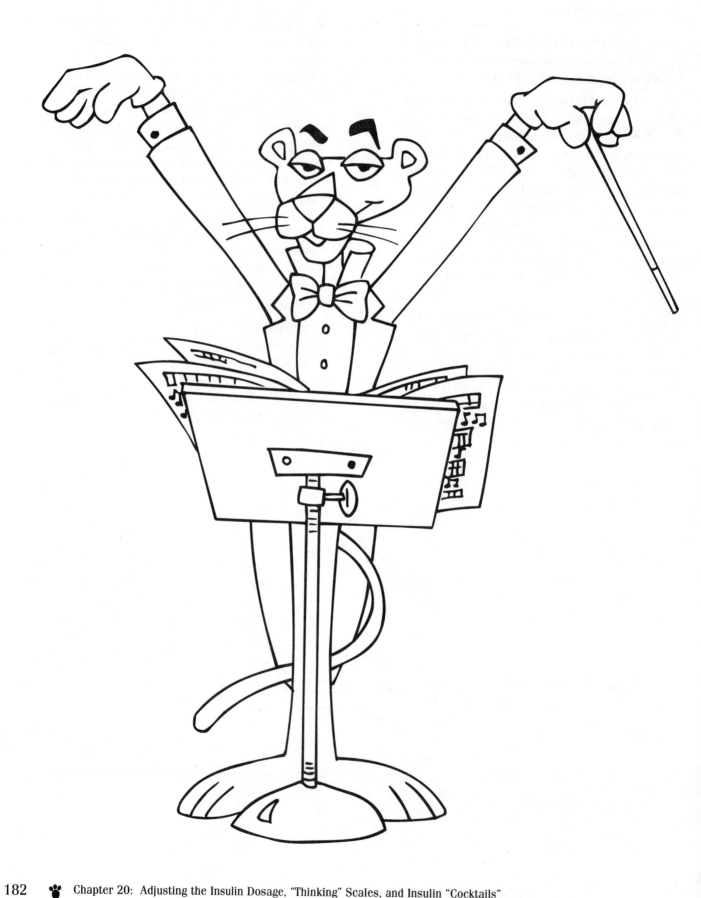

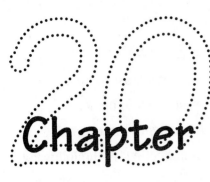

Chapter

20

ADJUSTING THE INSULIN DOSAGE, "THINKING" SCALES*, AND INSULIN "COCKTAILS"

(This chapter is not for newly-diagnosed families.)

Key ideas of this chapter:

* Understand when and how to increase or decrease the dosage of insulin.

* Appreciate "thinking" scales.

BLOOD SUGAR LEVEL GOALS (suggested ranges)

As noted in Chapter 6 on blood sugar testing, it is our general aim to keep preschool children's blood sugars between 80 and 200 mg/dl (4.5-11.1 mmol/L), 5 to 11-year-olds between 70 and 180 mg/dl (3.9-10.0 mmol/L), and 12-year-olds and older between 70 and 150 mg/dl (3.9-8.3 mmol/L) when no food has been eaten for at least two hours. A person who has difficulty recognizing low blood sugars or who has severe insulin reactions is usually asked to keep the blood sugar at a slightly higher level. Families and the diabetes care provider should discuss the desired range, and this range should be written down for future reference. It is important to remember that this is a target goal and that generally **if at least 50% of the sugar values are in the target range, the HbA$_{1c}$ level will also be in the target range.** Not all values will be in the target range, except possibly during the "honeymoon" period shortly after diagnosis.

After 6-12 months of dealing with diabetes, many families and older teens begin making some of their own insulin adjustments. This should be discussed with the diabetes care provider at a clinic visit, and if the decision is mutually agreeable, guidelines for insulin adjustments should be discussed.

ADJUSTING THE INSULIN DOSAGE

The first step is to understand the times of action of the insulin. Refer to the figures in Chapter 7 and Table 1 in this chapter, to review the times of action of various insulins.

*The term "sliding" scale is sometimes used and refers to basing an insulin dose just on a given blood sugar value and not as a result of thinking.

Table 1

THE FOUR TIME PERIODS OF INSULIN ACTIVITY FOR PEOPLE RECEIVING TWO SHOTS PER DAY

Period 1:	a.m.	Humalog and/or Regular	Works primarily from breakfast to lunch
Period 2:	a.m.	NPH or Lente	Works primarily from lunch to dinner
Period 3:	p.m.	Humalog and/or Regular	Works primarily from dinner to bedtime
Period 4:	p.m.	NPH or Ultralente	Works primarily from bedtime to the following morning

Changes in insulin dosage are best considered under two separate categories:

A) reducing the dose and B) increasing the dose.

Reducing the Insulin Dose
(TO PREVENT LOW BLOOD SUGARS)

Responding to trends in the blood sugar levels

If blood sugars below the suggested ranges are noted two or more days in a row at the same time of day, the insulin working at that time of day should be reduced (see Table 1). If all blood sugars in a day suddenly are running below the desired lower limit, the insulin dose should be reduced with the next injection. Even one value below 60 mg/dl (3.3 mmol/L), which is the level of true hypoglycemia, or below 70 mg/dl (3.9 mmol/L) in a preschooler, should cause one to consider lowering the insulin dose working at that time. We do not know why blood sugars will suddenly be low for a day or longer in a person who has been stable previously, but this does happen. Most often this is due to increased physical activity, eating less food, or opening new bottles of insulin.

How much the insulin is reduced depends on the age and size of the person and the dose being given. Sometimes all that is needed is to omit or reduce the short-acting (Regular or Humalog) insulin for a few days, particularly if the lows are in the morning or the evening. If the low values occur before dinner, the morning NPH or Lente insulin can be reduced by one or two units. If the reactions are in the early morning hours, the evening Ultralente, Lente or NPH can be reduced by one or two units. **Once again, think about what time of the day the reactions are occurring and**
which insulin is having its main action at that time of day, and reduce the insulin that is working at that time by one or two units. If the values are still low the next day, reduce the insulin again. It may be helpful to fill out Table 2 at the clinic visit as a guideline for insulin adjustments. Sometimes the values are high the day after the insulin dose is reduced. This is because the insulin-balancing hormones may require a day or two to adjust. It is important to be patient when a dose is reduced, and **DO NOT GO BACK UP ON THE DOSE** just because blood sugars are a bit higher. Wait a few days to let the balancing hormones re-adjust before deciding to go back up on the dose. Remember that even though we suggest waiting a few days to make further changes if the blood sugar is high, this is NOT necessary if it is low. **It is OK to make a further reduction the next day if values are still low.**

Thinking ahead to prevent lows (reactions)

Although discussed in more detail in Chapters 5 and 11, we would again remind families to **"think ahead" to prevent reactions.** This often involves reducing the insulin dosage during days of high excitement and activity or when eating less. When children stay overnight at a friend's house (or have a friend spend the night) there is often an increase in activity and less sleep. Thus, more energy is expended, and it is wise to reduce the p.m. insulin dose slightly. School trips and field days, family picnics, and playing with cousins, long hikes or bike trips, spending the night at a friend's, vacations to places like Disneyland® or the beach, or deciding to begin a diet can all lead to low blood sugars. Similarly, when school is out and the weather is nice, children will play outside after dinner and the evening Humalog and/or Regular insulins almost always have to be reduced.

Temporary omission of the Humalog or Regular insulin (but not of the long-lasting insulin) or appropriate reductions in dosage of insulins acting at the time of activity or excitement can help to prevent problems. If there are questions about reducing the insulin dosage, call the diabetes care provider during office phone hours (save home calls and pager calls for emergencies). **Remember that it is generally best to err on the safe side.** Alterations in the insulin dose for sick-day and surgery management are discussed in Chapter 15, Sick-Day and Surgery Management.

Responding to severe insulin reactions

If a severe insulin reaction occurs, we like all families to call us before giving the next scheduled insulin shot. The stores of balancing hormones (e.g., adrenaline) are reduced with a severe reaction and there is a greater risk for more reactions. Thus, the insulin dose should be reduced temporarily. We can also discuss what needs to be done to prevent similar severe reactions from occurring again. Sometimes it is helpful to schedule a clinic appointment to do this.

Increasing the Insulin Dose
(TO TREAT HIGH BLOOD SUGARS)

Understanding why more insulin is required

If the blood sugars have been above the desired range for three or four days in a row, and there is not an obvious illness or stress that will soon go away, the insulin dose should be increased. There are many reasons why people need more insulin. When children grow, their insulin needs generally increase by one unit for every two pounds gained. When growth hormone levels increase, insulin activity is blocked and the insulin dosage generally needs to be increased. Some people need more insulin because their own pancreas gradually makes less insulin. In the winter, many people exercise less and their insulin needs increase. If the blood sugars are above the desired range, or if HbA_{1c} values are high (reflecting blood sugars over the past three months), it is usually necessary to increase the insulin dose. Illness sometimes creates a temporary need

for more insulin (especially if ketones are present). This is discussed in Chapter 15, Sick-Day and Surgery Management.

Resistance to increasing the insulin dose

Some people resist increasing the insulin dose. When blood sugars have been running high, the person's body becomes accustomed to higher levels and may feel uncomfortable at lower blood sugar levels. It may be unpleasant for a short period to aim for the lower values, but this feeling gradually disappears. Also, the most frequent fear of people with diabetes (and their family members) is of low blood sugars. This is particularly true if severe reactions have occurred. Thus, people may resist (sometimes subconsciously) increasing the dose and lowering the blood sugars. Working with a counselor may help to remove this fear.

Knowing which insulin dose to increase

It is essential to know the times of action of the insulins and the desired ranges for the blood sugars. The four time periods of insulin activity shown in Table 1 are obviously the same when increasing the dose. Thus, when the blood sugars are above the desired range for 3-7 days with no obvious cause, insulin is increased in this manner:

- If the sugars are high before lunch, increase the morning Regular and/or Humalog insulin

- If the sugars are high before dinner, increase the morning NPH and/or Lente

- If the sugars are high before the bedtime snack, increase the dinner Regular and/or Humalog insulin

- If the sugars are high before breakfast, increase the dinner (or bedtime) NPH, Lente, and/or Ultralente insulin

The increases are usually by a half unit for a preschooler or by a unit for an older child. The blood sugars will tend to run lower on the first day of increased insulin, but may then increase again as the balancing hormones adjust. Extra snacks on the first day of an increased dose are often wise. We often suggest a slice of pizza at bedtime on the first night of increasing the insulin working during the night.

If the blood sugars are still above the desired range after 3-7 days, repeat the increase again. **Continue this program until at least half of the blood sugars at the time of day being worked on are in the desired range.** A general rule is to increase the dosage slowly. It may be helpful to fill out Table 2 at a clinic visit as a guideline for insulin adjustments. Remember, if you are not sure whether to make further increases in the insulin dose, fax the blood sugars and call to discuss changes with your diabetes care provider. Faxing in the blood sugar values allows the diabetes care provider time to review and think about recommendations and saves the need to be copying values over the phone. Try to do the reporting during office phone hours and save home calls and pager calls for emergencies.

ADJUSTING YOUR (OR YOUR CHILD'S) INSULIN DOSE

Date _____

1. The desired range for your blood sugar is _____.

2. If morning blood sugars are above _____ for three or more days in a row (with no illness or obvious cause), increase the evening Ultralente, Lente, or NPH by _____ unit(s) and wait 3-7 days to see if the values come down. If not, keep repeating this process until the blood sugars are in the desired range, waiting 3-7 days between each increase.

3. If morning blood sugars are below _____, decrease the evening Ultralente, Lente, or NPH by _____ unit(s). If the value is still low the next morning, make another similar reduction and repeat this process until the value is in the desired range.

4. If the blood sugar is above _____ at lunch for three or more days in a row, increase the morning Regular and/or Humalog insulin by _____ unit(s). Be consistent in the morning snack (if used). Wait 3-7 days and if the values have not come down to the desired range, make a similar increase. Continue this process until values are in the desired range.

5. If the blood sugar is below _____ at lunch, reduce the a.m. Regular or Humalog by _____ unit(s). If the value is still low the next day, make a similar reduction and repeat this process until the value is in the desired range.

6. If the blood sugar is above _____ at dinner for three or more days in a row (with no food eaten in the previous two hours, no illness and no obvious cause), increase the morning NPH or Lente by _____ unit(s). If the values are not down in 3-7 days, repeat this process at similar intervals until the blood sugars are in the desired range.

7. If the blood sugars are below _____ at dinner, decrease the morning NPH or Lente by _____ unit(s). If the value is still low the next evening, make another similar reduction and repeat this process until the value is in the desired range.

8. At bedtime, the desired range for blood sugars is _____ (usually a bit higher than at other times of the day). If the value is above _____ for three or more days in a row, increase the dose of dinner Humalog or Regular by _____ unit(s). If the value is still high after 3-7 days, repeat the process as needed until the values are in the desired range.

9. If the value is below _____ at bedtime, reduce the dinner Humalog or Regular by _____ unit(s). If the value is still low the next evening, make another similar reduction and repeat this process until the value is in the desired range.

10. Remember, if you need help, call the diabetes care provider (preferably during office hours). If you are ready to start making insulin changes yourself, ask your diabetes care provider if he/she will help you fill out this table. Work on it together!

POSSIBLE "THINKING" SCALE DOSAGES OF REGULAR (R) OR HUMALOG (H) INSULIN (IN UNITS) DEPENDING ON BLOOD SUGAR LEVELS AND SENSITIVITY TO INSULIN. EXERCISE AND FOOD INTAKE MUST ALSO BE CONSIDERED.

Child under four years old

Sensitive

mg/dl	mmol/L	
<200	<11.1	= OR/H
201-300	11.2-16.6	= 1R/H
>300	>16.6	= 2R/H

Less sensitive

mg/dl	mmol/L	
<100	<5.5	= OR
100-150	5.5-8.3	= .5R/H
151-200	8.4-11.1	= 1R/H
201-250	11.2-13.9	= 1.5R/H
251-300	14.0-16.6	= 2R/H
301-350	16.7-19.4	= 2.5R/H
>350	>19.4	= 3R/H

Child 4-10 years old

Sensitive

mg/dl	mmol/L	
<100	<5.5	= OR/H
100-200	5.5-11.1	= 1R/H
201-300	11.2-16.6	= 2R/H
>300	>16.6	= 3R/H

Less sensitive

mg/dl	mmol/L	
<70	<3.9	= OR/H
70-150	3.9-8.3	= 1R/H
151-200	8.4-11.1	= 2R/H
201-250	11.2-13.9	= 3R/H
>250	>13.9	= 4R/H

Child 11-14 years old

Sensitive

mg/dl	mmol/L	
<70	<3.9	= OR/H
70-150	3.9-8.3	= 1R/H
151-200	8.4-11.1	= 2R/H
>200	>11.1	= 3R/H

Less sensitive

mg/dl	mmol/L	
<70	<3.9	= OR/H
70-150	3.9-8.3	= 2R/H
151-250	8.4-13.9	= 4R/H
>250	>13.9	= 6R/H

Above 14 years old

Sensitive

mg/dl	mmol/L	
<70	<3.9	= OR/H
70-150	3.9-8.3	= 3R/H
151-250	8.4-13.9	= 4R/H
>250	>13.9	= 5R/H

Less sensitive

mg/dl	mmol/L	
<70	<3.9	= 1R/H
70-150	3.9-8.3	= 4R/H
151-250	8.4-13.9	= 6R/H
>250	>13.9	= 8R/H

Table 3

"THINKING" SCALES (AND REPLACING THE TERM "SLIDING" SCALES)

It is important to emphasize that "sliding" scales are really "thinking scales. They give the person or family ranges of Humalog and/or Regular insulin to "think about." **The blood sugar level SHOULD NEVER be the only factor considered. Food intake and both recent and expected exercise also need to be considered with every shot.** An example would be a five-year-old going out to play with friends after dinner in the summer. Even if the blood sugar was 200 mg/dl (11.1 mmol/L) before dinner, it would be wise to reduce (or omit) the evening dose of Humalog or Regular insulin. This would also apply if Mom (or Dad) were making tuna noodle casserole for dinner, and they knew that the five-year-old disliked tuna noodle casserole. **Sliding scales require careful thinking prior to giving each insulin shot, and it is better to call them "thinking" scales.** Sample thinking scales for different aged children, based on whether they are still quite sensitive to Regular or Humalog insulin or not as sensitive, are shown in Table 3. **These are examples only and may not be correct for your child.** We would not recommend using any of them unless you first discuss them with your diabetes care provider.

Many families adjust Humalog and/or Regular (not NPH or Lente) insulin dosages with every injection by using a thinking scale in which the amount of Humalog or Regular insulin given is based on the blood sugar level, the expected food intake, and both recent and expected exercise. The amount of insulin is usually preset by the family and the diabetes care provider working together. The insulin scale can be written down in Table 4. Thinking scales are particularly helpful when parents alternate giving injections and desire a pattern that both can follow. **The amount of Humalog or Regular insulin given is based on the blood sugar level, the expected food intake, and both recent and expected exercise.** If the blood sugar is low, the amount is decreased. In contrast, the dose is increased for higher blood sugars, if less exercise is expected, or if a large meal is to be eaten. Smaller children obviously have lower dosages than larger children. Children in the first year after diagnosis (who make more of their own insulin) are usually more sensitive to Regular and Humalog insulin and will have lower dosages.

One advantage of thinking scales is that the blood sugar level must always be measured if the scale is to be used. Sometimes the family and diabetes care provider will decide on a dose of insulin to give in case a blood sugar test is not done. A disadvantage of the thinking scales is that often one scale must be used for the morning and a different scale for the evening. As indicated in Table 4, it may even be necessary to use one scale for an active day, and a different scale for a quiet day.

SUGGESTED "THINKING" SCALE FOR REGULAR OR HUMALOG INSULIN DOSAGE

Blood Sugar Level	Morning Regular or Humalog		Afternoon Regular or Humalog	
	If active (or if not eating much)	If not active (or if eating much)	If active (or if not eating much)	If not active (or if eating much)
_____ =	_____	_____	_____	_____
_____ =	_____	_____	_____	_____
_____ =	_____	_____	_____	_____
_____ =	_____	_____	_____	_____
_____ =	_____	_____	_____	_____
_____ =	_____	_____	_____	_____

Note: *This table does not apply to sick-day management (see Chapter 15). Call your diabetes care provider AFTER CHECKING THE BLOOD SUGAR AND THE URINE KETONES if you have questions. Scales may also be used for Humalog or Regular insulin dosages given at other times during the day. Copy this table as often as you wish.*

It is important to remember that thinking scales are not "written in stone." A scale that works fine for a few months may have to be altered if the blood sugars are not in the desired range. Always bring the scale along to clinic visits so the dose can be reviewed with the diabetes care provider. Also, write down the dose of insulin given in each shot on the blood sugar record sheet (see Chapter 6). This makes it possible for you and the diabetes care provider to more easily review dosages and how the scales being used are working.

INSULIN "COCKTAILS"

This is a term applied to mixtures of three or more insulins in the same syringe—often of Humalog and Regular insulins and of a long-acting insulin (NPH, Lente, or Ultralente). As noted in Chapter 7, it is fine to mix the Humalog and the Regular insulins, and either can be drawn into the syringe first. Both should be in the syringe prior to drawing the long-acting insulin into the syringe. It should be remembered that the NPH insulin delays the activity of Humalog slightly (but not of Regular), Lente and Ultralente delay the action of Regular insulin slightly (but not of Humalog). The advantage of using a mixture of Humalog and Regular is that there is an immediate effect from the Humalog (especially good when eating right after the shot or if the blood sugar is high) and a later effect from the Regular (often important for school children in the morning to cover lunch—as Humalog activity is mostly gone after four hours).

The adjustments in the insulin cocktails can be somewhat tricky. For example, if the blood sugar level is on the low side, if not much is going to be eaten (e.g., a teenager rushing to school in the a.m.), or if there is to be heavy exercise in the hour after the meal, a lower dose of Humalog and more Regular insulin should be used. In contrast, if the blood sugar level is high, if there is to be exercise in three or four hours (but not in 1-2 hours), or if a big meal is to be eaten, a higher dose of Humalog and a lower dose of Regular might be used. **This really does require "thinking"** and remember that two heads are better than one—particularly early in the morning. An example of an "insulin cocktail" for a 15-year-old boy receiving 6-8 units of short-acting insulin is shown below. Note that when the blood sugar is low (less than 60 mg/dl [3.25 mmol/L] for some, or less than 100 mg/dl [5.5 mmol/L] for others), it might be better to wait to give the shot after the meal if Humalog is to be given.

Units of Humalog (H) and of Regular (R) Insulins

Blood Sugar		Not eating much or exercising in next hour		Eating now and not exercising in next hour	
mg/dl	mmol/L	H	R	H	R
<100	<5.5	0	6	2*	2
100-200	5.5-11.1	2	4	4	4
>200	>11.1	4	4	6	2

*Might best be given after eating

Sometimes the insulin cocktail is judged more on the blood sugar level such as the example below. However, we still encourage families to try to think about food intake and exercise as well (as in the example above).

Units of Humalog (H) and of Regular (R) Insulins

Blood Sugar		H	R		Total
mg/dl	mmol/L				
<100	<5.5	0	4	=	4
100-200	5.5-11.1	2	4	=	6
200-300	11.1-16.6	4	4	=	8
>300	>16.6	6	4	=	10

In this example, more Humalog is added primarily to reduce higher blood sugar levels.

The mixing of three or more insulins (an insulin "cocktail") can also refer to the mixing of a short-acting insulin with two long-acting insulins in the same syringe. For example, a child who receives Humalog and NPH insulins in the morning, and whose parent arrives home late (so that supper will be delayed), may need to add Ultralente (a longer-acting insulin) to the morning NPH insulin. Similarly, when puberty comes and growth hormone levels are high from 4-9 a.m. (the "Dawn phenomenon"), a child who was previously well controlled on Humalog and Ultralente insulin at dinner may now do better with adding a bit of NPH insulin to the evening Humalog and Ultralente insulins.

The current **"extreme cocktail"** is one in which four insulins are mixed in the same syringe. This might be Humalog, Regular, NPH and Ultralente insulins. Obviously, keeping the dosages and insulins accurate is essential and, once again, "two heads are better than one."

SUMMARY

In summary, it is important for families to consistently look at blood sugar levels and to make needed insulin adjustments to obtain or maintain optimal diabetes control. **Keeping a blood sugar and insulin dose log (record) will allow the family to see patterns to make the insulin adjustments.** It is most frustrating when high blood sugars are obtained week after week and no adjustments are made. If a family is uncertain whether changes in insulin need to be made, fax the blood sugar values and insulin dosages to the diabetes care provider to get help.

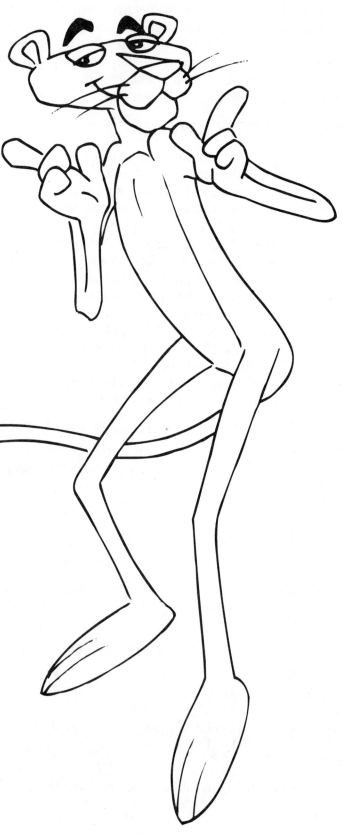

QUESTIONS (Q) AND ANSWERS (A) FROM NEWSNOTES

Q. What is meant by "sliding" scales for insulin adjustments and who should use them?

A. "Sliding" scales generally refer to giving different dosages of Humalog or Regular insulin depending on the level of blood sugar. They should not be used for the long-acting insulins (usually NPH, Ultralente, or Lente). We prefer the term **"thinking" scale** to emphasize that the blood sugar level, food intake, and exercise must all be considered before each insulin dose is chosen. The diabetes care provider should discuss the "thinking" scale for the dose of Humalog (H) or Regular (R) insulin individually for each person. Some people are still making their own insulin and will need less Humalog or Regular insulin, particularly at younger ages. Thus, a four-year-old diagnosed at age three might do fine with a thinking scale of:

Blood Sugar		Dose of Humalog (H) or Regular (R) Insulin
mg/dl	**mmol/L**	
<100	<5.5	= 0H/R
100-200	5.5-11.1	= 1H/R
201-300	11.2-16	= 2H/R
>300	>16.6	= 3H/R

However, a 16-year-old who developed diabetes at age three might have an entirely different scale:

Blood Sugar		Dose of Humalog (H) or Regular (R) Insulin
mg/dl	**mmol/L**	
<70	<3.9	= 2H/R
70-150	3.9-8.3	= 4H/R
151-200	8.4-11.1	= 6H/R
>200	>11.1	= 8H/R

Some people even need a different scale for their morning compared to their evening dosage of Humalog or Regular insulin. It should always be remembered that the scale may have to be reduced if heavy exercise has just been done or is about to be done. There is no good substitute for thinking and reasoning! If you do at least three blood sugar tests per day and want to try a thinking scale, you should discuss this with your diabetes care provider.

Q. Do the needs for insulin change with the seasons?

A. The short answer is "yes." To illustrate this, think of summer camp.

Nearly every person going to camp has their routine dose of insulin substantially reduced because of all the extra activity. To a lesser degree this happens in spring—over a week or two the snow suddenly disappears, the sunshine appears and children are out playing, bicycling, etc. With the increased activity, low blood sugars are more likely. Snacks may have to be adjusted and/or insulin doses may need to be lowered.

In contrast, the opposite happens with going back to school in the fall, especially for those going to new schools. This may be a time of extra stress as well as reduced activity. Activity is decreased with the evening homework. Blood sugars may go up and insulin doses may need to be raised.

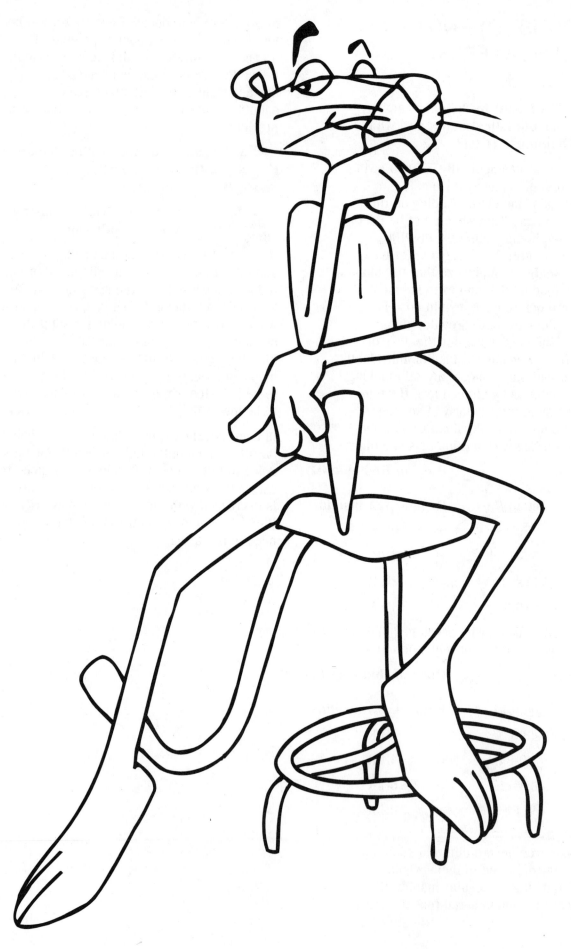

❦ Chapter 21: Long-term Complications of Diabetes

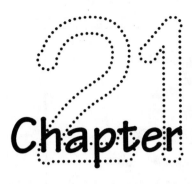

Chapter 21

LONG-TERM COMPLICATIONS OF DIABETES

(Do not read until psychologically ready.)

Key ideas of this chapter:

❧ Introduce some of the complications that can occur in people with diabetes.

❧ Recognize some of the things that help reduce the risk for diabetes complications.

❧ Be aware of the importance of urine microalbumin tests and of eye exams.

In addition to the acute complications of diabetes—insulin reactions and acidosis—there are also problems known as "long-term" complications. Many families may prefer to read this chapter when they are ready to deal with the subject. Also, teenagers may be able to understand the material better than pre-teenagers. Many new and difficult words are used in this chapter. They are introduced (and defined in the back) so that if your diabetes care provider uses them you will have a place to find out what they mean. For the most part, the long-term complications occur in people who have had diabetes and high blood sugar levels for many years. The three most common parts of the body to be involved are the eyes, the kidneys, and the nerves.

THE DCCT

The Diabetes Control and Complications Trial (DCCT) has been mentioned previously in this book. The results of this study became available in 1993 and proved without question that **the eye, kidney, and nerve problems of diabetes were decreased in people ages 13-39 years whose blood sugars were kept closer to normal.** Although blood sugar control is one important factor in relation to these three complications, **IT IS NOT THE ONLY FACTOR**. As will be discussed in this chapter, data from our Center and others has shown that blood pressure is also important in relation to both the eye and the kidney complications. Smoking cigarettes also adds to the risk for the kidneys. Increased blood clotting is also a likely risk factor and there are other factors that are still unknown.

Most of the long-term complications do not occur in young children. The years of greatest risk for complications seem to start after puberty. Research has shown that in people with diabetes, the small blood vessels show no changes before puberty, whether good sugar control was present or not. After puberty, the blood vessels usually remain normal in people with good sugar control, but changes may appear in people with poor sugar control. Around the time of puberty, levels of growth hormone, sex hormones, and other hormones increase greatly. The risk of complications after puberty may increase because of the changes in hormone levels, because of poor sugar control caused by the changes in hormone levels, or possibly due to both.

We do not know how the high blood sugar levels cause the complications. It is possible that sugar attaches to proteins in the blood vessels or other parts of the body when the blood sugar levels are very high. We know this happens with the protein (hemoglobin) in the red blood cells (to form hemoglobin A_{1c} or HbA_{1c}, see Chapter 13). We also know that sugar attaches to the skin proteins in people who have curvatures of several fingers (see "finger curvatures" in this chapter). Once the sugar attaches to any body protein, the protein may not work as well as when sugar is not attached.

Even though the actual complications are not usually seen until puberty, it is important to work for good sugar control in the pre-puberty years. There are some side effects of poor sugar control that can occur at any time (see Chapter 13 on Diabetes and Blood Sugar Control). Also, the habits for the future are formed when the person is young.

We have divided complications into two groups: complications related at least in part to blood sugar control and complications not related to blood sugar control.

COMPLICATIONS RELATED AT LEAST IN PART TO BLOOD SUGAR CONTROL

 Eye Problems

Cataracts

Cataracts are small thickenings in the lens (which is located at the front of the eye; see picture). The damage to the lens is believed to be caused by sorbitol, a compound made in the

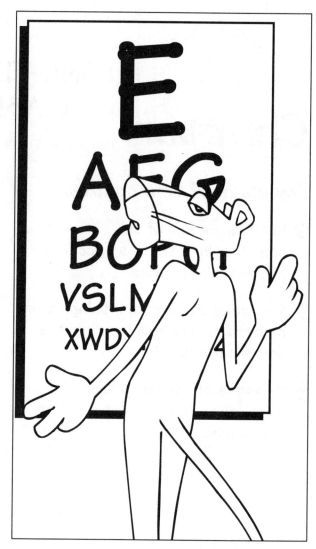

lens from glucose. Sorbitol damage occurs when blood glucose (sugar) levels have been very high in the body for a long time. Sorbitol in foods is changed by the body (liver) and does not cause this damage. Damage to the lens can happen at any age. It can even be present at the onset of diabetes if sugar levels have been high for a long time before insulin is started. Cataracts may show some improvement with good sugar control. These lens changes are not the same as the more severe retinal complications in the back of the eye that are discussed. The eye doctor (ophthalmologist) will do a detailed exam for cataracts in the yearly eye exam. If cataracts interfere with vision, they can be removed surgically by the eye doctor.

Retinal Changes or Retinopathy

The word retinopathy refers to changes of the retina, which is the layers of tissue at the back of the eye. This part of the eye has many small blood vessels similar to those found in the kidney. Research in children and teenagers with diabetes has shown that the changes in the small blood vessels, such as those found in the eyes and kidneys, occur mainly after puberty. These changes depend on various factors. One is the duration of diabetes after puberty. Another is the degree of blood sugar control. The DCCT showed that in people without eye changes from diabetes, lower blood sugars delayed development of retinopathy by 76%. The DCCT also showed that intensive therapy slowed the progression of retinopathy by 54% and reduced the incidence of severe retinopathy by 47% in people with known early eye changes from diabetes. Similarly, increased blood pressure results in a greater risk for retinal changes. Smoking also makes these changes progress more rapidly. However, we do not understand all of the causes of the eye changes of diabetes. There is a small group of people for whom the presence or absence of eye changes show no relation to sugar control.

Retina (back of eye)

Lens

Early detection of eye changes is very important and is one clear argument for having diabetes check-ups every three months. The diabetes care provider doing the physical exam should be able to detect eye changes and make appropriate referrals to an eye doctor (ophthalmologist) who specializes in diabetic changes (retinal specialist). The ADA does not suggest seeing an eye doctor for diabetic reasons before age 10 years. Thereafter, if there are no diabetic eye changes, or if the changes are minor, yearly visits to the diabetes eye specialist are adequate. Minor eye changes include a ballooning of the small retinal blood vessels; these changes are reversible and are called "**microaneurysms.**" Some people can have these minor changes for many years and not develop more severe eye disease. Careful blood sugar control is particularly important when any changes are detected. If more severe eye changes occur, then more frequent visits to the diabetes eye specialist are needed.

The more severe eye disease usually involves formation of new retinal blood vessels (proliferation) which are then at a greater risk for breaking (hemorrhaging). These more severe changes are referred to as "**pre-proliferative**" and "**proliferative**" retinopathy. Laser treatment, using a very bright light, was begun in the 1970s as a way to save vision in people with diabetes who have severe eye changes. Laser treatment destroys the fragile (proliferative) new blood vessels and has been very effective in preventing loss of vision. The most important factor is to have close follow-up once the more severe changes appear. Then, laser treatment can be done at the proper time to prevent loss of vision. The biggest danger is a hemorrhage that could damage the retina or send blood into the vitreous fluid between the lens and retina (vitreous hemorrhage) or cause the retina to separate from the other layers in the back of the eye (retinal detachment).

Studies are now in progress to determine if antioxidants or other medicines might help to prevent or to slow diabetic retinopathy.

Kidney Disease or Diabetic Nephropathy

Kidney disease is one of the most feared of the complications of diabetes and is spoken of as "nephropathy." As with the eye disease discussed above, kidney disease generally happens after puberty and is more likely to be present in people who have had diabetes for a long time. It is also more likely in people with poor sugar control or elevated blood pressure, ad in those who smoke or chew tobacco. It occurs in about one in three people with type 1 (insulin-dependent) diabetes, and in about one in four people with type 2 (adult onset) diabetes.

The kidneys normally filter wastes and water from our blood to make urine (Chapter 2). When blood sugar levels are high, sugar is excreted in the urine, pressures are higher in the kidney filtering system (the glomerulus), and changes in the small blood vessels of the kidney can occur. This increased pressure causes damage to the filtering system so that some proteins start leaking through the filter and appear in the urine. Eventually the signs of kidney disease may include:

- i. increased blood pressure
- ii. ankle swelling, also known as edema (due to fluid collection)
- iii. excessive urine protein spillage
- iv. elevation of the waste materials in the blood (increased blood creatinine and urea nitrogen or BUN)

The Microalbumin Test

Fortunately, a test is now available to detect diabetic kidney involvement at an early stage when it might still be reversible. This is called the **microalbumin test** and is usually done on a timed overnight or on a 24-hour urine sample. The test should be done after having diabetes for five years or at the time of puberty (11-13 years), whichever comes first. It should then be done once yearly so that the interval is not missed when the early damage is still reversible.

The method for collecting the overnight sample is included at the end of this chapter. IF THERE IS INCREASED MICROALBUMIN (ABOVE 20 MICROGRAMS [ug] PER MINUTE), IT IS NOW ACCEPTED THAT THERE IS A 95% RISK FOR DEVELOPING NEPHROPATHY AND KIDNEY FAILURE (if nothing is done). A "borderline microalbumin level" for timed overnight urine collections is a value between 7.6 ug/minute and 20 ug/minute. This "borderline" range represents a time period when good sugar and/or blood pressure control

will help to lower the value, or to keep it from going higher. Medications are not usually given for a "borderline" level, as it may still be possible to return the value to normal by lowering the HbA_{1c}. If the urine microalbumin value is between 20 and 200 ug/minute, it is called **"microalbuminuria"** and may still be reversible with good sugar and blood pressure control and medications. Smoking cigarettes and chewing tobacco lead to a greater likelihood of kidney damage and must be avoided by people with diabetes. A decrease in protein intake is recommended (to lessen the load on the kidneys) for anyone who has microalbumin levels above 20 ug/minute, but particularly for those who have levels above 300 ug/minute (**nephropathy** or **macroalbuminuria**).

The DCCT showed that improved glucose control reduced the occurrence of microalbuminuria by 39% and of gross kidney damage (nephropathy or albuminuria) by 54%. It must once again be remembered, though, that glucose control is NOT the only cause of diabetic kidney damage.

The 1980s and the 1990s have brought significant advances in the prevention, detection, and treatment of diabetic kidney damage. However, as recommended in the ADA Standards of Care listed at the end of Chapter 19, it is up to the family and the physician to make sure that the urine tests to detect kidney changes are done at the recommended times. If not, the "window" during which changes may be reversible could be missed. If the microalbumin levels are high on the overnight or 24-hour urine test, medicines may be effective in reversing or slowing the kidney involvement. The usual medicine that is tried first is an ACE-inhibitor (angiotensin-converting enzyme). This medication prevents formation of angiotensin II, which is a very potent constrictor of blood vessels. The result is less pressure build-up in the kidneys. There are several varieties of ACE-inhibitors, all of which are probably effective if given in adequate dosage. Thus, early kidney damage is detectable and methods to reverse or slow down kidney damage are available. This has now resulted in a decline in the cases of renal failure from diabetes.

Neuropathy

Diabetic neuropathy, or "damage to the nerves," is a condition seen after puberty, usually in people who have had very high sugar levels. Neuropathy is a complex condition that we still do not completely understand. The DCCT found that the incidence of people complaining of neuropathy was 60% less in the group with the lower blood sugar levels. As with cataracts, neuropathy is believed to be related, at least in part, to increased sorbitol levels deposited in the nerves. The sorbitol is made from sugar. There is also a decrease in another compound (myo-inositol) which is important for the nerves. For some reason, neuropathy seldom occurs unless diabetes has been present for at least 10 years. The neuropathy usually makes itself known with numbness, tingling, and sharp pains in the lower legs or feet. It can also affect other inner parts of the body. For example, neuropathy may change the rate at which food moves through the intestines. This is referred to medically by a big word, **gastroparesis**. Much research is being done to find new and better medications for the treatment of neuropathy.

Joint Contractures

Some children with diabetes cannot touch the knuckles of the second joint in their fifth fingers when their hands are in a "praying" position. At times, the joints of the other fingers or other joints in the body can also be involved. When other joints or fingers other than just the fifth finger are involved, there has usually been a period of very high sugar levels and sugar has attached to the proteins in the skin over the joints. No pain or other problems are usually related to these changes. Some doctors believe the curvatures of the fifth fingers may be partly inherited. Parents and siblings of people with diabetes often have curvatures of the fifth fingers, even though they don't have diabetes. It is not yet known if the more severe curvatures will disappear as blood sugar control improves.

Birth Defects

This complication is primarily important to a woman who might get pregnant. If her diabetes is not well controlled, a pregnant woman with diabetes is more likely to have a baby with one or more birth problems or defects. The first few months of pregnancy are the most important in preventing defects. A woman should not stop using birth control or decide to get pregnant until her diabetes is well controlled. IT IS VERY IMPORTANT TO TALK TO YOUR DIABETES PHYSICIAN BEFORE GETTING PREGNANT. Insulin pumps and intensive diabetes management must be considered **PRIOR TO THE PREGNANCY**.

If the HbA_{1C}, blood pressure, ad kidney tests are normal or low prior to the pregnancy, the likelihood of kidney deterioration during pregnancy is minimized. Diabetic retinal changes do sometimes worsen during pregnancy and it is wise to be followed more closely by one's retinal specialist during this time.

COMPLICATIONS NOT PRIMARILY RELATED TO SUGAR CONTROL

Macrovascular (large blood vessel) Problems

The "large" blood vessels are in contrast to the very small (sometimes microscopic) blood vessels in our eyes and kidneys. They include the coronary blood vessels that provide blood (and thus nutrition and oxygen) to our heart. When a coronary blood vessel is blocked, a "heart attack" can result.

People with diabetes have an increased likelihood of heart attacks. Heart attacks have many causes, but high risk factors include **increased blood pressure**, a **family history** of relatives who had heart attacks before age 50, **smoking**, **elevated LDL** (low-density lipoprotein) cholesterol, **reduced HDL** (high-density lipoprotein) cholesterol (the "good" cholesterol), and **elevated total blood cholesterol** levels. Until a few years ago, diets that contained 40% of calories from fat were routinely recommended for people with diabetes and this may have added to the high blood fat levels. Most dietitians now recommend that no more than 30% of calories be from fat sources. Heredity and poor sugar control also can be causes of high cholesterol levels. It will be many years before we know if the reduced fat intake and better sugar control lower the likelihood of heart attacks in people with diabetes. Blood cholesterol levels, which are influenced by heredity and blood sugar control, should be checked each year. Medications that block our body's cholesterol synthesis (the "statins") are now available for people who have very high cholesterol levels. The blood pressure should be checked at regular clinic visits. Increases in blood pressure should be treated early. Finally, people with diabetes should not smoke!

🐾 Foot Problems

Foot problems due to poor or decreased blood flow and neuropathy do not occur in children. Some families who are educated by diabetes care providers who care mainly for adults with diabetes will be told that children must "wash their feet daily" or "never go barefoot." Although it is nice to have clean feet for clinic visits, these precautions are NOT necessary for children. They are usually a problem of older adults and may be related to the blood fat levels and poor circulation or to neuropathy. There is recent research suggesting that regular exercise may help to maintain normal foot circulation in later life (see Chapter 12). It is important for diabetes care providers to do careful examinations of feet in post pubertal patients. It is also important for the patient to know to call the doctor if a foot lesion does not heal well or if there is any sign of an infection (redness, warmth, or pus) or ulcer.

Ingrown toenails (an infection) occur with similar frequency in children with or without diabetes. However, they are more of a problem in people with diabetes, as infections cause high sugar levels. The high sugar levels, in turn, support the infection. The ingrown toenails are usually caused by toenails that are cut too short at the corners. The toenails should be cut straight across and the length should be even with the end of the toe. Good prevention is much easier than treatment, and use of a straight nail clipper helps. (By the way, this is true for everybody!)

🐾 Thyroid Disorders

Some thyroid enlargement occurs in about half of people with type 1 diabetes, although only about one in 20 ever needs treatment. The reason for this is believed to be a similar "self-allergy" (autoimmune) type of reaction that causes both diabetes and the related thyroid enlargement. As discussed in Chapter 3, people who get diabetes often have an antibody (allergic reaction) in their blood against their pancreas (specifically, the islet cells in the pancreas). Likewise, people with diabetes who get thyroid problems usually have an antibody (allergic reaction) in their blood against the thyroid gland. Thyroid antibody tests can be done, but are usually not done as they are expensive and are often not paid for by insurance. It is important for the diabetes care provider to always check the size of the thyroid gland at the time of clinic visits. If the thyroid is not functioning normally, body growth may be slowed. Also, the person may feel tired all the time. If the gland is enlarged, specialized blood tests should be done (**particularly a TSH test**, as this is almost always the first test to become abnormal). If the thyroid tests are abnormal, a thyroid tablet can then be taken once daily. Thyroid problems are not serious unless unrecognized or untreated. The treatment is excellent, easy, inexpensive, and involves taking pills (not shots). Sometimes the tablets can be discontinued (under a doctor's supervision) when the person is finished growing. Thyroid problems are common even in people who do not have diabetes (about one in 50 adults).

🐾 Adrenal Disorders

Autoimmunity (self-allergy) against the adrenal gland can occur just as with the pancreas (type 1 diabetes) and the thyroid gland. It is quite rare (about one in 500 people with type 1 diabetes), but it is important to diagnose and treat, as it can result in death if untreated. President Kennedy is an example of a famous person who had autoimmune adrenal insufficiency. The most common early sign for someone with diabetes may be an increased frequency of severe low blood sugars. Episodes of feeling weak or faint (with normal blood sugars—but sometimes low blood pressure) can occur. The two electrolytes in the blood, sodium (Na+) and potassium (K+), may be low and high, respectively. Later, increased pigmentation over the back of the hands (or knuckles or elbows) may occur. Initial screening may be for an antibody against the adrenal gland. Eventually, cortisol (cortisone) blood levels must be obtained. The treatment (as with thyroid disease) is with tablets. Treatment includes training the person (or family) to increase the tablets during periods of stress (as with an infection or with surgery).

Celiac Disease

Celiac disease (Sprue, Gluten-enteropathy) is carried on one of the DR types (DR3) that is also related to being at high risk for type 1 diabetes (see Chapter 3). Thus, although celiac disease and diabetes are separate and different diseases, it is not uncommon for the two to occur in the same person. Approximately one in 20 people with diabetes also has celiac disease. As other family members who do not have diabetes may also have the DR3 genetic type, they are also more likely to have celiac disease (even though they do not have diabetes).

Celiac disease is an allergy to the wheat protein, gluten, and can be diagnosed using a blood antibody test (transglutaminase and/or anti-endomysial antibodies). At present, an intestinal biopsy is usually also done to confirm the diagnosis. Some people with celiac disease have symptoms, whereas others may not have any symptoms at all. Symptoms may include abdominal pain, gas, diarrhea and, in children, decreased height or weight gain. The symptoms, the abnormal blood tests, and the intestinal biopsy changes all return to normal within a few months after treatment is begun.

The treatment involves removing all wheat, rye, and barley products from the diet. Rice, corn, oat products, and all foods, except those containing gluten, can still be eaten. It is important to work with a dietitian to learn which foods have the wheat protein, gluten, in them. Adults who have no symptoms may not wish to restrict all gluten from their diet. The main argument for doing so is that in a few case reports of adults dying with a cancer (lymphoma) of the intestine, celiac disease has been found present (and a possible causative factor). There is much that we still do not know about this disease.

 Skin Problems

Yellow fatty deposits (**necrobiosis**) can collect in the skin over the front of the lower legs. No one knows what causes these fat deposits.

A rare condition called **dermatitis herpetiformis** is also related to a sensitivity to the wheat protein, gluten (see celiac disease). It is characterized by blisters on the elbows, buttocks, and knees. Like celiac disease, it responds to a gluten-free diet.

Sexual Function

Some males with diabetes have problems with penile erections. The cause of this problem is unknown. The medicine Viagra® may be helpful to some men with diabetes who have this problem. There is no evidence that women with diabetes have problems with sexuality related to diabetes.

SUMMARY

In summary, much is still unknown about the long-term complications of diabetes. However, recent research suggests that good sugar control, normal blood pressure, and not smoking can help prevent some of these complications.

DEFINITIONS

Adrenal gland: A hormone-producing gland located above each kidney which has the function of making cortisone, salt-retaining hormones and other hormones.

Autoimmunity (self-allergy): As defined in Chapter 3, this involves forming an allergic reaction against ones own tissues. This happens in type 1 diabetes and can happen in thyroid disorders and, more rarely, with the adrenal gland.

Blood pressure: The blood pressure consists of a higher (systolic) pressure that reflects the pumping or working pressure of the heart and a lower (diastolic) pressure which reflects the resting pressure of the heart between beats. It is important to have the blood pressure checked regularly.

Blood Urea Nitrogen (BUN): A material in the blood normally cleared by the kidneys. It is elevated in advanced kidney disease as well as with dehydration.

Cataract: A density (clouding) in the lens that may cause spots or blurred, or reduced vision.

Celiac disease (Sprue, Gluten-enteropathy): An allergy to the wheat protein, gluten.

Creatinine: A material in the blood normally cleared by the kidneys. The test to measure its clearance from the blood is called a creatinine clearance test.

DCCT: Diabetes Control and Complications Trial. A very large trial of people ages 13-39 years old which showed that lower HbA_{1c} values resulted in a lower risk for diabetic eye, kidney, and nerve problems. It ended in June, 1993.

Edema: Collection of fluid (swelling) under the skin.

Filter: To separate out or remove. The kidneys filter wastes from our blood.

Gastroparesis: Neuropathy involving the stomach and/or intestine.

Glomerulus: Small groups of blood vessels in the kidneys that filter the blood to remove wastes and water to make urine.

Hemorrhage: The breaking of a blood vessel. In the eye, this can occur in the retinal layer or, in more advanced cases, in the fluid (vitreous) in front of the retina (vitreous hemorrhage).

Laser treatment: Using a very bright beam of light to destroy the new (proliferative) blood vessels in the retina which are at high risk for hemorrhaging and causing a loss of vision.

Lens (see picture of eye): The oval structure in the front of the eye that changes shape to allow the eye to focus on near or distant objects.

Microalbumin: A test that can measure small amounts of a protein (albumin) in the urine to detect kidney damage from diabetes at a stage in which it might still be reversible.

Microaneurysm: A small dilatation of a blood vessel, which is a minor change caused by diabetes that can be reversible.

Myo-inositol: A compound which is reduced in nerves when sorbitol levels are elevated (in neuropathy).

Necrobiosis: The name for yellow fatty deposits that can occur over the lower legs in people with diabetes.

Nephropathy: A generic name for kidney disease. It is usually used to indicate a more advanced stage of kidney involvement.

Neuropathy: A disease of the nerves. This is believed to happen in people with diabetes due to accumulation of sorbitol (formed from blood glucose), or possibly due to deficiency of another metabolite, myo-inositol.

Ophthalmologist: The name for a doctor (MD) who specializes in eye diseases. The ophthalmologist may further specialize in the retinal layer in the back of the eye which is affected by diabetes. The doctor is then called a "retinal specialist."

Optometrist: A person who is primarily trained to check for the need for glasses. An optometrist is not an MD (although they are still important care providers).

Podiatrist: A person who is specially trained in the care of the feet. They are not MDs (although they are still important care providers).

Pre-proliferative or proliferative retinopathy: Terms for more advanced stages of eye involvement from diabetes (when a diabetes eye specialist needs to be seen more frequently).

Puberty: The time in a teen's life when adult sexual changes start to occur.

Retina: The layers of small blood vessels and nerves in the back of the eye that are very important for vision.

Retinal detachment: Separation of the retinal layer in the back of the eye from other layers in the eye.

Retinopathy: Changes in the retinal (small blood vessel) layer in the back of the eye from diabetes. These are more apt to occur after puberty in people who have had diabetes for a long time and who have been in poor sugar control.

Sorbitol: A compound derived from glucose which collects in the lens and nerves when blood sugars are high and is believed to cause cataracts and neuropathy.

Thyroid: A hormone-producing gland in the lower front of the neck on each side of the windpipe (trachea). The hormone is called thyroid hormone.

Vitreous fluid: The fluid between the lens and the retina. When retinal blood vessels break, they can bleed into the vitreous fluid (vitreous hemorrhage).

QUESTIONS (Q) AND ANSWERS (A) FROM NEWSNOTES

Q. What is the best way to screen for early microvascular (small vessel) disease of the kidneys and the eyes in people with diabetes and when should it be done?

A. The microalbumin urine test is the best way to currently diagnose early kidney involvement in people with diabetes. The test is done by measuring the microalbumin in a timed overnight or 24-hour urine. It is very important to repeat the two overnight (or 24-hour) urine collections every year. If a person has begun pubertal changes (usually ages 11-13 years) and has had diabetes for at least three years, we recommend doing the two overnight urine collections for microalbumin and having an eye exam by an ophthalmologist once yearly. Directions for the urine collections are in the back of Chapter 21.

Q. Why is it necessary to reduce my protein intake as I lose protein in my urine? Shouldn't I eat more protein?

A. The protein (albumin, microalbumin) loss in the urine is most likely due to kidney damage from diabetes. This is a result of HbA_{1c} levels being too high, the blood pressure being too high, or as a result of smoking cigarettes. There are probably other causes as well that we do not yet understand. When someone gets kidney damage from any cause (diabetes, hypertension, nephritis, lupus, etc.), it generally helps to slow down the process by eating less protein. The protein seems to be an extra load for the kidney to handle, and reducing the protein will make less

work for the damaged kidneys. It is wise to meet with the dietitian at this stage to discuss what the correct amount of protein should be.

Q. What level of glucose control is necessary to prevent the eye and kidney complications of diabetes?

A. Our longitudinal study reported in the *Journal of the American Medical Association* in 1989 correlated glycohemoglobin (hemoglobin A_1) values with complications and showed that blood sugar control (HbA_1 levels) were definitely related to the eye and kidney complications. No person who had kept their HbA_1 (reflecting frequency of high blood sugars over the previous three months) below 9% by the affinity column method (normal to 8.0 %) or below 6.8% for the DCA 2000 method (normal to 6.2%) had evidence of eye or kidney changes. Likewise, no person who had kept their HbA_1 below 9.8% for the column method (7.4% for the DCA 2000 method) had kidney changes, and only two of 23 had serious eye changes. This is in contrast to people who had a mean HbA_1 above 12.3% for the column method, or above 9.3% for the DCA 2000 method, where 41% of people had more severe eye changes and 28% had evidence of kidney damage.

The extra effort to stay in good blood sugar control may indeed save much work in later life in dealing with the eye and kidney complications of diabetes.

Q. Is cigarette smoking bad for someone with diabetes?

A. Yes. It is linked to lung cancer, high blood pressure, and heart attacks in ALL people and is thus a poor choice for everyone.

In addition, data from our Center has shown that smoking results in about a three-fold greater likelihood of diabetic kidney complications. Smoking also causes diabetic eye disease to progress more rapidly. The mechanism by which smoking does this is unknown, but as people who chew tobacco seem to have the same consequences, it may be from the absorption of nicotine into the body.

Glycohemoglobin (HbA_{1c}) levels are often high in smokers with diabetes. Therefore, these effects had to be removed before a conclusion about smoking could be reached. Smoking results in higher HbA_{1c} levels by increasing levels of other hormones, such as adrenaline, which raise the blood sugar. The heart rate and blood pressure also increase and this may be related to the increased eye and kidney problems.

Q. Dr. Chase, our son has been chewing tobacco. Is this really bad? Should we be bothered by it or just be glad he is not smoking cigarettes?

A. The use of "smokeless" tobacco is increasing greatly in teenagers and should be actively discouraged. One study of Denver high school students (mean age = 16 years) showed that more than 10% used smokeless tobacco.

The tobacco contains dangerous components that could be cancer-causing. In addition to the increased risk for cancer of the mouth, the nicotine is absorbed from the tobacco and can cause any of the following: stimulation, increased muscle tone and aggression, increase in heart rate and blood pressure, dizziness, nausea, and shakiness of the extremities. **The latter three symptoms may be confused with the symptoms of low blood sugar.** Reduced taste is common and increased use of salt (and sugar) often occurs. Dentists note that users typically have discolored teeth, receding gums, periodontal destruction, and excessive wear of the teeth due to abrasives in the tobacco. Withdrawal symptoms of irritability and decreased cognitive functions are frequently found between doses.

Fortunately, the Comprehensive Smokeless Tobacco Health Education Act, which bans radio and TV advertisements, was signed into law during the Reagan Administration. As a result, famous sports and movie stars are no longer seen promoting chewing tobacco on TV. Needless to say, it is well worthwhile for responsible people (including parents) to take a strong stand against chewing (or smoking) tobacco!

Q. Do children with diabetes have to take special care of their feet?

A. Much is written about diabetes and foot care, and this was one of the initial stimuli to write this educational book. All of the books available at the time talked about washing the feet daily and taking special care of the feet. Although it is nice to have clean feet (especially when coming for clinic check-ups), children with diabetes do not have any more problems with their feet than do other children. Foot problems for people with diabetes occur in older age, particularly in relation to two problems:

i. Neuropathy: People in poor glucose control accumulate sorbitol in their nerve fibers and develop neuropathy and a loss of normal feeling. It may then not be possible to feel hot or cold normally, thus the need to be careful when getting into hot bath water, etc.

ii. Atherosclerosis: If blood vessels age and the walls thicken, less blood flow will go to the feet. This happens only in later years—and one precaution we take in the clinic is the yearly check of blood cholesterol levels. High cholesterol levels, high blood pressure, ad smoking are all believed to hasten the aging of blood vessels.

One problem with the feet which is no more common in children with diabetes than in other children, but which is more difficult to cure in children with diabetes, is INGROWN TOENAILS. These usually occur because toenails (especially the large nails) are cut too short and the surrounding skin then grows over the nail. The nail then grows into the skin and an infection is set up. The infection can cause high sugars—and the high sugars can help the infection grow. The result is often a chronic problem cured only by removal of the toenail. A better solution is PREVENTION. Cut the toenails straight across, preferably with a straight toenail clipper and not a rounded fingernail clipper. The length should be out to the end of the toe. Ingrown toenails are rare when nails are properly cut!

Q. Are thyroid problems more common in children with diabetes, and if so, why?

A. Yes, thyroid problems are more common in children with diabetes. They are caused by an "autoimmune" or allergic-type reaction that is very similar to the allergic-type reaction that is believed to be important in causing diabetes. Thus, most people with new-onset diabetes have islet cell antibodies (an allergic reaction against the islet cells that make the insulin) at the time of diagnosis of type 1 (but not type 2) diabetes. Likewise, the people with diabetes who develop thyroid problems have an antibody in their blood against the thyroid gland. Both the pancreas and the thyroid are endocrine glands that make the hormones insulin and thyroid hormone, respectively. Thus, the two glands have much in common. Some physicians recommend thyroid blood tests yearly in children with diabetes. The practice in our Clinic is to do the tests if the thyroid gland is large or if there is a special indication, such as a fall-off in height. Fortunately, when low thyroid function is detected, it can be treated with a tablet. Also, the pills can sometimes be discontinued after a few years. Thus, most people handle the problem easily.

Q. How common is kidney disease in association with diabetes, and can it be prevented?

A. Kidney problems occur in up to 30% of people with type 1 diabetes, usually when the person reaches their 30s or 40s. There are things that we can do now to help reduce the likelihood of kidney problems. These include:

❧ Good sugar control

There is evidence to suggest that the kidney problems may result from the increased sugar load the kidney constantly has to handle. Gradually, the tissue starts to thicken due to increased pressure resulting from this increased sugar load. The closer to normal the blood sugars are kept, the less likely the kidney has to handle an excessive load. Thus, good sugar control may be the most important parameter in preventing kidney disease.

❧ Blood pressure

It is important to have the blood pressure monitored at regular intervals to make sure the systolic and the diastolic pressures are not above the 90th percentile for age. If blood pressure elevations are found, early treatment is important in preventing kidney disease. It is also advisable to avoid adding extra salt to foods, which can increase blood pressure in some people.

❧ Prompt treatment of urinary tract infections

It is important to treat infections that might get to the kidneys and cause damage. Problems with infections are more common in women than in men. It is important to repeat urine cultures after the antibiotic treatment to make sure the infection has really gone away.

❧ Dietary protein

There is evidence that a high protein diet adds to the material that must be filtered by the kidneys and the likelihood of kidney problems from diabetes. Most Americans eat much more protein than is needed and it would be wise to reduce the quantity of protein. This can be discussed with the dietitian at the time of clinic visits.

❧ Avoid medicines that list kidney damage as a possible side effect

When your physician chooses a medicine (e.g., an antibiotic to treat an infection), make sure that he/she is aware you have diabetes and that he/she is using a medicine that does not have possible side effects of damaging the kidneys. There is often an alternative medicine which may be used that does not have this potential side effect.

❧ Smoking

Data from our Clinic has clearly shown that smoking adds to the likelihood of diabetic kidney damage. Smoking must be avoided in people who have diabetes.

❦ Regular check-ups

Protein is evaluated in the urine with every three-month check-up at the clinic because it may indicate kidney problems. Having the microalbumin tests done yearly is the best way to detect early problems.

❦ Preventive medicines

Recent studies have shown that at least one type of blood pressure medicine (an ACE-inhibitor) also has an effect of reducing kidney filtration pressure. Eventually, it may be possible to give medications to specifically prevent kidney problems from diabetes.

Q. Are contact lenses OK for a person with diabetes to use?

A. Yes, people with diabetes can wear contact lenses, but there are some extra precautions. The contact lens fits over the superficial layer of the eye called the cornea. The cornea needs a constant supply of oxygen and tears to keep it healthy. Thus, the contact lens must fit properly so that the cornea is not injured and the tears are able to continue to flow. A qualified (experienced) eye doctor should fit the lenses—probably in a contact lens clinic.

It is even more important for people with diabetes to follow the instructions for care and cleaning of the contact lenses than it is for other people. The corneas of people with diabetes are sometimes less sensitive to pain or irritation, so people may be less apt to tell when their contacts are causing problems. Infections may also not clear as quickly if they do occur. Thus, use the solutions and disinfectants exactly as your eye doctor recommends. Don't get lazy in cleaning or try to cut corners. Don't leave the contacts in any longer than recommended. Don't mix cleaning solutions. Finally, it is probably better not to get the extended wear lenses.

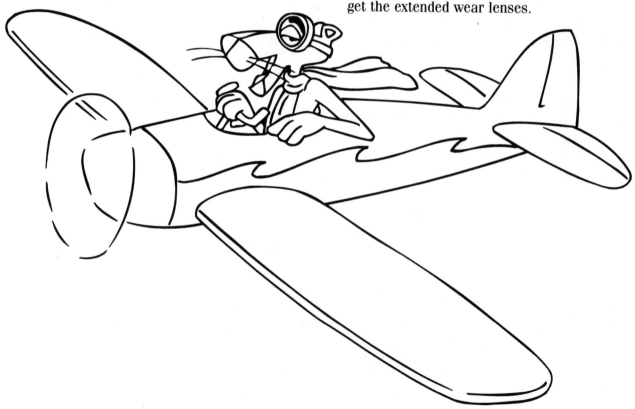

MICROALBUMINS

Doctor: _____   Your Name: _____

A. INSTRUCTIONS FOR DOING THE OVERNIGHT URINE COLLECTIONS

COLLECTION #1   DATE: _____

1. Empty your bladder at bedtime and discard this sample.
                                           TIME: _____

2. Save **EVERY DROP** of urine during the night.

3. Save **EVERY DROP** of the first morning sample. **ALL** urine from collection #1 should be placed in the same container.
                                           TIME: _____

4. Measure the volume of the urine sample.   TOTAL VOLUME: _____

COLLECTION #2   DATE: _____

1. Empty your bladder at bedtime and discard this sample.
                                           TIME: _____

2. Save **EVERY DROP** of urine during the night.

3. Save **EVERY DROP** of the first morning sample. **ALL** urine from collection #2 should be placed in the same container.
                                           TIME: _____

4. Measure the volume of the urine sample.   TOTAL VOLUME: _____

B. IMPORTANT TIDBITS ABOUT YOUR COLLECTIONS

1. **Label each container with your name and #1 or #2**.

2. You may use any **CLEAN** container you have at home that will not leak to collect the sample. We do not provide containers.

3. Store urine aliquots in fridge until your visit (samples are good for one week if kept **cold**).

4. **DO NOT** mix collections #1 and #2 together in the same container.

5. **DO NOT** drink caffeinated or alcoholic beverages or use tobacco after 10 p.m. the evening of the collections.

6. **DO NOT** exercise strenuously for the four hours prior to bedtime.

7. **DO NOT** collect specimens during a menstrual period.

8. Failure to follow directions exactly may cause incorrect results.

9. If you have any questions, please call your health care provider.

C. DIRECTIONS FOR MEASURING THE VOLUME

1. Have a measuring cup or (better) a cylinder—preferably marked in cc (mL). One cup is 240cc. Urine is sterile and it is ok to use cooking measuring cups (just wash prior to next use for cooking).

2. Measure the total cc of each overnight sample and put the amounts in the blanks for step 4 for collections #1 and #2.

3. Put a sample of each urine collection in a clean tube. Any clean red top tube from a doctor's office, clinic, or hospital lab will work. Label which sample (#1 or #2) it is, put your name on the tube, and put the tube in a cup in the refrigerator until you get to your clinic. Bring this sheet with the times and total volumes with you.

SCHOOL DIABETES MANAGEMENT CHECKLIST FOR PARENTS:

_____ Discuss specific care of your child with the teachers, school nurse, and other staff who will be involved.

_____ Complete the individualized school health care plan with the help of school staff and your diabetes care staff (see two examples in this chapter).

_____ Make sure your child understands the details of who will help him/her with testing, shots, and treatment of high or low blood sugars at school.

_____ Keep current phone numbers where you can be reached.

_____ Collect equipment for school:

meter, strips, and finger-poker

lancets

logbook or a copy of testing record page included in this chapter

insulin, insulin syringes, insulin pens and needles, and extra pump supplies

Ketostix

_____ Food and drinks: (parents need to check intermittently to make sure supplies are not used up):

4-6 oz juice cans or boxes

glucose tablets, instant glucose, or cake decorating gel

crackers (± peanut butter and/or cheese)

quarters to buy sugar pop if needed

fruit-roll ups, dried fruit, raisins or other snacks

box with the child's name to store these food and drink items

The School and Diabetes

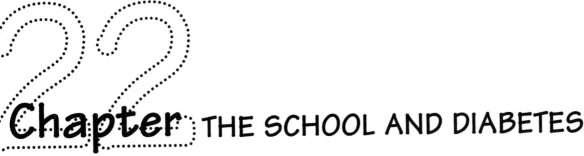

Chapter 22 THE SCHOOL AND DIABETES

Key ideas of this chapter:

- Help parents feel secure about the handling of their child's diabetes while the child is at school.

- Assist parents in providing the essential diabetes supplies and information for the people at their child's school.

The first and main job of parents in relation to school is to educate those who will be working with the child at school about diabetes. Parents want to feel that their child is in safe hands while at school (often the place where the majority of the child's waking hours are spent). Parents also want to make sure their child is not treated differently because of having diabetes. The next few pages are meant to be cut out or copied (permission is granted to copy as often as wished) for the school. It is wise for the parent to phone the school nurse, teacher, or principal to discuss the best way to get all of the necessary people informed. This is usually best to do in the week before classes start. Some parents in our area will buy or borrow a copy of one of the videos (see next page) on diabetes and the school and take it to show the nurse, teachers, and others likely to be involved with their child. It can be a good take-off place for the discussion of the most likely emergency to occur at school, hypoglycemia. It is essential that the family educate the teachers, school nurse, bus driver, gym teacher, lunchroom workers, and others involved with their child at school. Sometimes the school nurse or the teacher will help educate other staff people. It is also important that when a substitute teacher is at school, the substitute knows that a child in the classroom has diabetes, and that the time is taken to read this summary. **It is important NOT to leave it up to the child to inform and educate the school.** They may be self-conscious or embarrassed and not get the job done.

A second job of parents is to keep an adequate supply of instant glucose, small cans of juice, peanut butter or cheese and crackers, and/or graham crackers in a container in the teacher's, principal's, or nurse's drawer. The child's name and a set of instructions (with phone numbers written in) should be taped to the container. It is also wise to include a can of sugar pop (or some quarters so the school can purchase this).

A third job might be to leave a finger-poker and an extra meter (with appropriate strips) or some Chemstrips bG in the classroom, office or nursing station in case a blood sugar test has to be done at school (e.g., for a low blood sugar reaction or for a sick-day). Often children carry their own meter in their backpacks. Many children now routinely do a test every day before lunch, whereas others do a test only if feeling low. Phone numbers where the parents can be reached should be recorded on the form that follows and a copy left with the meter.

There is a special anxiety about a young child starting preschool. The young child may not yet be able to recognize low blood sugars and may not be mature enough to help remember snacks (see Chapter 17, Responsibilities of Children at Different Ages). In addition, the child might not have been away from the care of the parents for any significant period of time prior to starting preschool. Separation may be more difficult for the parents and may also be more difficult for the child. And yet, preschool may be important for the child in learning social and other skills. Thus, it is important to allow participation just as one would if the child did not have diabetes. The information at the end of this chapter may be given to the preschool teacher just as it is to regular school teachers.

Schools in many states now require a School Health Plan. We have included two possible plans in this chapter. The first (I) is one page and concise. It would be appropriate for all children and schools. The second (II) is longer with a more detailed educational element, and might also be filled out for some schools. The parents and school personnel can decide which is needed. You have our permission to copy the forms as often as you wish. There is also a generic school letter at the end of this chapter which may be of help in introducing your child's diabetes to the school. Also note that there is a letter for sports coaches at the end of Chapter 12. Either of these letters may be copied as often as desired.

Two videos parents often take to show the school personnel are:

1) "The Care of Children With Diabetes in Child Care and School Settings." (This comes as two tapes, with the skills part sold separately for $198.00 or both tapes for $279.00.) The address is:

Managed Designs, Inc.
P.O. Box 3067
Lawrence, KS 66046
Phone: 785-842-9088
Fax: 785-842-6881

2) "Living With Diabetes: Tips for Teachers," is a 19-minute video tape available from Maxishare for $59.00 plus $5.00 for shipping and handling. Their address is:

Maxishare
P.O. Box 2041
Milwaukee, WI 53201
Phone: 1-800-444-7747
Fax: 414-266-3443

A customer service representative for Maxishare can be contacted at 414-266-3428. Hospitals can pay for this video with purchase orders, and individuals can pre-pay with a check or credit card. Some diabetes clinics have copies of this video which they can sell at a reduced rate. Also, some clinics have copies of these videos which can be loaned to parents to take to their school.

School Health Plan: I

SCHOOL: _____ **GRADE:** _____

STUDENT: _____ **ADDRESS:** _____ **DOB:** _____

PHYSICIAN/PHONE: _____

MEDICATIONS: Insulin,_____

PARENT'S PHONES: Home: _____ Mom's work: _____ Dad's work: _____

HEALTH CONCERN: INSULIN-DEPENDENT DIABETES DATE OF DIAGNOSIS _____

1) **ROUTINE MANAGEMENT:** 1) Morning snack: (time: _____) snacks to be kept in the classroom and in the clinic; 2) tests blood sugar daily (time: prior to lunch or anytime there are symptoms of low blood sugar). Exercise should be delayed or avoided if the blood sugar level is lower than 60 mg/dl (3.25 mmol/L).

2) **LOW BLOOD SUGAR OR HYPOGLYCEMIA:** Can be a result of receiving too much insulin, skipping a meal or snack, or an unusual amount of exercise. Hypoglycemia can happen quickly and must be corrected immediately.
   THE SYMPTOMS ARE:
   1) shakiness   3) "feels hungry"   5) looks dazed   7) confused   9)_____
   2) "feels low"   4) very tired   6) sweaty   8) pale or flushed face 10)_____

INTERVENTION: A blood sugar should be done, ideally in the classroom so that energy is not spent going elsewhere. If it is necessary to go elsewhere, **someone must accompany the student.**

The target range of blood sugar is 70-180 mg/dl (3.9-10.0 mmol/L)
If blood sugar is **60-70** mg/dl (3.25 mmol/L-3.9 mmol/L):
   1) Give four ounces (one small can) of juice **OR** 2-3 oz of sugar pop
   2) Follow with snack (crackers) in 5-10 minutes
   3) Symptoms should subside in 10-15 minutes
If blood sugar is **below 60** mg/dl (3.25 mmol/L):
   1) Give four ounces juice and one glucose tablet, or 2-3 oz sugar pop
   2) Follow in 10-15 minutes with a snack of crackers or dried fruit, etc.
   3) Symptoms should subside in 10-15 minutes
   4) Do not allow adult supervision to leave
   5) Re-test blood sugar in 15-30 minutes
   6) Let parents know
If unable to take the juice:
   1) Administer 1/2-3/4 tube of glucose gel or 2-4 tsp cake decorating gel
   2) Place between cheek and gum and massage the outside of cheek with head elevated
   3) Follow this treatment in 10 minutes with a small snack if symptoms have subsided
   4) Call parents

IF ANY OF THE FOLLOWING OCCUR, PLEASE CALL 911 AND THE PARENTS; if RN in school, give 0.5cc (0.5 mg) glucagon subcutaneous or intramuscular:
   1) Loss of consciousness
   2) Seizure
If to be taken to the hospital, preferred hospital: _____

3) **HIGH BLOOD SUGAR:** Especially with stress or illness, the blood sugar may be high and extra insulin may be needed. Instructions for insulin supplements are: _____
(to be given by: child ___, parent ___, school RN ___, school staff ___). A child should be supervised. (If the blood sugar is above 300 mg/dl [16.65 mmol/L], urine ketones should also be checked and the parent may wish to leave foil-wrapped ketostix at school _____ or to be called to come and do the test _____.) If ketones are present, drinking extra fluids is also helpful. Extra bathroom privileges will be needed.
                    Physician's signature (for insulin): _____

4) **FIELD DAYS OR TRIPS:**   1) Notify parents ahead of time so insulin dose can be reduced
                               2) Extra snacks, glucose monitoring kit, and glucose gel should be taken
                               3) Copy of Health Plan with emergency numbers should be carried by staff

----

As parent/guardian of the above named student, I give my permission for use of this plan in my child's school and for the school to contact the above named physician if necessary to complete the Health Care Plan.

_____ date   _____ date
School Nurse   Parent

_____ date   _____ date
Clinic Aide   Physician

_____ date   _____ date
Principal   Reviewed

INSULIN-DEPENDENT DIABETES
HEALTH CARE PLAN: II

DATE: _____

SCHOOL: _____ **GRADE:** _____

STUDENT: _____ **BIRTHDATE:** _____

HOME ADDRESS: _____

PARENT/GUARDIAN: _____

PARENT'S PHONE: Home:_____ Mom's work: _____ Dad's work: _____

EMERGENCY CONTACT (NAME, NUMBER AND RELATIONSHIP):

_____

MEDICATION: Insulin,_____

ALLERGIES: _____

HEIGHT: _____ **WEIGHT:** _____

EMERGENCY MEDICAL INFORMATION

PHYSICIAN AND PHONE: _____

HOSPITAL PREFERENCE: _____

❧ I. GENERAL INFORMATION FOR SCHOOL PERSONNEL

Diabetes is not contagious. Type 1 diabetes is caused by the pancreas not producing enough insulin. The result is too much sugar in the blood. Treatment consists of daily shots of insulin, blood sugar tests, food management, and exercise. It is an entirely different condition from adult-onset diabetes, in which shots may not be required. The priority for a child with diabetes is to lead a normal life. Children with diabetes can participate in all school activities, including sports. They should not and do not want to be singled out. They should be treated in the same way as others. Although performance may be impaired during and after low blood sugars, schoolwork and grades should not be affected by diabetes.

❧ II. FOODS AND SNACKS

In general, large amounts of high-sugar foods are avoided. The child with diabetes may need snacks in the morning and/or afternoon as these are often the times when insulin has its greatest effect and blood sugars are lowest. In general, the morning snack should be around 10:30 or 11:00 a.m., depending on the child. If not too disruptive to the class, most children do best just eating their snack at their desk. By doing this they will not miss as much school time. Others may prefer to eat their snack in the nurse's or school office. If gym class is in the last hour of the morning or afternoon (the parents should find out before the first day of school), a snack is usually needed before gym. If other children question why the child with diabetes is having a snack, the teacher should explain that it is because he/she has diabetes. It is usually then well-accepted.

TIME SNACK USUALLY EATEN: _____ A.M.

EXAMPLES: _____

AND/OR _____ P.M.

EXAMPLES: _____

III. BLOOD SUGAR TESTING

There may be times that blood sugar testing needs to be done at school. This may be at a set time (e.g., before lunch) or it may be when a low blood sugar is suspected. A form is included at the end of this chapter to use to keep records of blood sugars at school. This might be copied weekly or at some regular interval to send home to the parents. Children have their own testing equipment. This should be kept in their backpack or an extra set should be in their desk, the nurse's or the principal's office. When possible we prefer that the student be allowed to test their blood sugar at their desk. School personnel may need to be taught how to do blood sugar testing to help younger children.

IV. LOW BLOOD SUGAR ("Insulin Reaction" or "Hypoglycemia")

This is the only emergency likely to occur at school.

A. Onset: SUDDEN and, if not treated promptly, can be an emergency.

B. Signs: Variable, but may be **any** of the following:

- Hungry
- Eyes appear glassy, dilated, or "big" pupils
- Personality changes such as crying or stubbornness
- Inattention, drowsiness, or sleepiness at unusual times
- If not treated, loss of consciousness and/or seizure

- Pale, sweating, shaking
- Pale or flushed face
- Headaches
- Weak, irritable, or confused
- Speech and coordination changes

C. Student's usual symptoms are: _____

_____

D. Most likely time to occur is before lunch or after gym class.

E. Causes: Too much insulin, extra exercise, a missed snack, or less food at a meal than is usually eaten. Field days or trips with extra exercise and excitement may result in reactions. The parents should be aware of all field days or trips so that the insulin dose can be reduced and/or extra snacks provided.

F. Treatment:

1) Mild Reaction

Symptoms: Hunger, shaking, personality changes, drowsiness, headache, paleness, confusion, or sweating.

Blood sugar: If equipment is available to do a blood sugar test, this is ideal to do even if juice has been taken. We prefer this to be done by the student (if old enough) in the classroom so that extra energy is not spent going elsewhere. However, we realize that for some schools this is not possible (note G). It takes 10 minutes for the blood sugar to rise after the juice has been given. Doing the blood sugar tests will help to tell if the blood sugar was truly low and how low (70-120 mg/dl or 3.9-6.7 mmol/L is normal for a person without diabetes) or if the symptoms were just due to a rapid fall in blood sugar.

Treatment: two or three sugar packets, cubes or tablets (can dissolve in warm water), or
one small can (4-6 oz or 1/2 cup) of juice, or
instant glucose, or
any sugar-containing food or drink

Liquids are absorbed in the stomach more rapidly than are solid foods. However, INSULIN REACTIONS TREATED WITH LIQUIDS INITIALLY SHOULD BE FOLLOWED IN 10 MINUTES WITH MORE SUBSTANTIAL FOOD (e.g., cheese and crackers or 1/2 sandwich, etc.).

2) Moderate Reaction

Symptoms: Combative behavior, disorientation, lethargy.

Blood sugar: Do the same as in a Mild Reaction (see above).

Treatment: Instant glucose immediately, then give sugar or juice. After the person is feeling better (10 minutes), give solid food as above.

3) Severe Reaction

Symptoms: Seizure or unconsciousness

Treatment: **CALL 911 IMMEDIATELY**

Give glucagon (0.5cc) subcutaneously or intramuscularly if nurse is available to administer

G. IF YOU SEND THE CHILD TO THE OFFICE, HAVE SOMEONE ACCOMPANY HIM/HER. The child may become confused and not make it to the office, if he/she is alone.

H. If you suspect that the child is having a low blood sugar reaction and it is not possible to do a blood sugar, do not hesitate to give the child something sweet to drink (such as juice or sugar pop).

I. In general, it is helpful if the school will notify the parents whenever an insulin reaction occurs at school. This will allow for adjustment of the insulin dose the next day so that hopefully further reactions can be prevented. Children often forget to tell their parents that they had an insulin reaction.

❧ V. HIGH BLOOD SUGAR

People with diabetes may have high blood sugars and spill extra sugar into the urine on some occasions. These occasions include periods of stress, illness, overeating, and/or lack of exercise. High sugars are generally NOT an emergency (unless accompanied by vomiting). When the blood sugar is above 300 mg/dl (16.65 mmol/L), the urine ketones also need to be checked (a urine dipstick). When the sugar is high, the child will have to drink more and urinate more frequently. **It is essential to make bathroom privileges readily available.** If the teacher notes that the child is going to the bathroom frequently over a period of several days, the parent should be notified. The diabetes care provider can then adjust the insulin dose.

The student may also occasionally need to check the urine ketones at school. This may be because ketones were present earlier at home, because the blood sugar is above 300 mg/dl (16.65 mmol/L), or because the child is not feeling well. The parents should be notified if moderate or large urine ketones are present as extra insulin will be needed.

Extra insulin possibly needed at school by our child:

For blood sugar above: _____ give: _____

To be given by: child _____, parent _____, school RN _____, school staff _____

(If insulin is given by the child, it should be supervised.)

Physician's signature: _____

❧ VI. CLASS PARTIES

If the class is having a special snack, the child with diabetes should also be given a snack. Please notify the parents ahead of time so that they can decide whether the child may eat the same snack as the other students or they may want to provide an alternate food. Preferred types of snacks are: fruit (fresh or dried), trail mix, pretzels, diet soda, sorbitol candy, sugarless gum, etc.

Suggested treats for school parties: _____

_____

If an alternate snack is not available, the student should be given the same snack as the other children.

❧ VII. BUS TRAVEL

Please allow _____ to take some food with him/her on the bus. It would also be helpful if the teacher checks with the bus driver to see what arrangements parents can make for allowing snacks on the way to or from school. At times, bus rides take longer than usual due to bad weather or stalls, and the child needs to have **a snack available and permission from the bus driver to eat it if necessary.**

❧ VIII. SUBSTITUTE TEACHERS

Place a copy of this information sheet in either the substitute teacher's folder or mark the attendance register so that a substitute would know:

1) there is a child with diabetes in the class; 2) when he/she usually eats a snack; and 3) symptoms and treatment of an insulin reaction.

IX. GYM (PHYSICAL EDUCATION) TEACHERS AND COACHES

It is particularly important for the gym teacher or coach to also have a copy of this information. Low blood sugars may occur during exercise, and a source of instant sugar should be nearby. Often a snack is recommended before gym and the child may be delayed in getting started. Exercise is even more important for children with diabetes than for other children. They should not be excluded from gym or sports activities.

X. AFTER SCHOOL DETENTION

Children with diabetes should not be singled out or treated differently from the rest of the class. However, if required to remain after school (at noon or in the afternoon) for a longer time than usual, an extra snack should be given. Most parents will have packets of cheese and crackers, peanut butter and crackers, or some such snack for the teacher to keep in the drawer. This is a common time of the day for the morning or afternoon insulins to be peaking. If a snack is not taken, an insulin reaction is likely to occur.

OTHER SPECIFIC INSTRUCTIONS

_____

_____

_____

TO THE PARENT/GUARDIAN: If your child experiences a change in health condition (such as a change in medication or a hospitalization), contact the School Nurse so that this Health Care Plan can be revised.

I give permission for the staff at _____ to carry out this Health Care Plan for _____ effective until revised.

PARENT/GUARDIAN: _____ **DATE:** _____

SCHOOL NURSE: _____ **DATE:** _____

CLINIC AIDE: _____ **DATE:** _____

ADMINISTRATOR: _____ **DATE:** _____

PHYSICIAN: _____ **DATE:** _____

DATE REVIEWED/REVISED: _____

BLOOD SUGAR RECORD SHEET

Student:_____ Date of Doctor's Order: _____
School Year: _____ School: _____ Grade: ____ Teacher: _____
Medication: Insulin, _____ Dosage: _____
Special Instructions: _____
Initials and Signatures of persons giving medication

_____ _____
_____ _____
_____ _____

Abbreviations:
A= Absent   NS= No show
C= Comment on back
PN= Parent Notified   FT= Field trip

Please note time and result of each blood sugar

Aug./Sept.
M	T	W	Th	F

Oct.
M	T	W	Th	F

Nov.
M	T	W	Th	F

Dec.
M	T	W	Th	F

Jan.
M	T	W	Th	F

Feb.
M	T	W	Th	F

March
M	T	W	Th	F

April
M	T	W	Th	F

May/June
M	T	W	Th	F

QUESTIONS (Q) AND ANSWERS (A) FROM NEWSNOTES

Q. **With school starting, what special precautions should we take for our child with diabetes?**

A. It is wise for the parents to go in and meet with the child's school teacher and school nurse (if there is one). This is particularly true if the child is attending a new school, but it is also true if the child just has a new teacher. If there is no school nurse, sometimes an individual in the principal's office or elsewhere is defined as a "clinic aide" and it would be wise to talk with this person. It is important for the teacher to be aware of the diabetes in case reactions or other problems occur in the classroom. Many of the parents have taken a video on the topic of school and diabetes to show to school personnel.

It is also frequently necessary to emphasize the importance of consistency in the time of eating snacks and lunch. Extra snacks and sources of sugar should be taken to school and left in the classroom and/or office. It is important to point out to the teacher that on some occasions, such as with a cold, the sugars may be higher and the child may have to leave the classroom more frequently to go to the bathroom. It is also important to remind the teacher that a child having a reaction should not be sent to the nurse's office without someone else going along. The child having a reaction could faint, get confused, or lost on the way. If the child must leave the classroom, the teacher must always send a second person along to accompany them.

Our educational book has two school health plans describing the symptoms of low blood sugar (and what to do) for school teachers. It is important that school teachers, bus drivers, lunchroom personnel, playground supervisors, and P.E. instructors be aware of these symptoms. They should be aware that the administration of food or sugar is essential for the child having a reaction, and that if there is ever a question, sugar should be given. The child should then rest until the sugar is back up to a normal range.

Finally, it is important to advise your child's teacher to let any substitute teachers know of the diabetes by putting a note on the attendance record or lesson plan to please look at the child's school health plan. The substitute teacher must know the symptoms of a reaction, the steps to take if the child has a reaction, and the snack schedule. Often the child's teacher will be well-trained and cooperative concerning the diabetes, only to have a substitute teacher there on a day of problems.

Q. **My son recently had a cold and small ketones when he woke up. He felt good enough to go to school and wanted to go. Was I wrong in letting him do this?**

A. As long as he felt well enough and wanted to go, I think it was good that you let him do so. At least he wanted to go and must like school! You might have sent one of the large plastic drinking cups with a straw so that he would remember to drink fluids to help wash away the ketones. Probably a special note to the teacher explaining the situation and the possible need for extra bathroom privileges would be wise. Finally, it would be important for a parent (or the child, if old enough) or the school nurse to make sure the urine ketones were checked again at lunchtime to make sure they went away and did not increase to the moderate or large level. Children with moderate or large urine ketones are usually better off staying at home until the ketones have gone down.

Date: _____

Attention: Principal
Attention: School Nurse

Dear Principal and School Nurse,

_____ is a _____ year-old child with type 1 diabetes who will be attending school at _____ this year. In order for _____ to maximize his/her learning potential in the classroom, it is important that staff be aware of the need for properly timed snacks and meals to keep his/her blood sugars as stable as possible. Low blood sugars are an emergency and must be treated by the school staff promptly and correctly. Some education on this topic is important.

Children with type 1 diabetes usually test their blood sugars 3-4 times per day by poking a finger and placing the blood on a strip in a meter that gives a number. The blood sugar tests are often done at school prior to lunch, and must be done if the child is having a possible low blood sugar. These children also must get at least two injections of insulin each day, usually before breakfast and dinner. Some children require insulin before lunch to prevent high blood sugars.

Children with diabetes can participate in all activities without restrictions, but may need extra snacks to prevent low blood sugars before or during P.E. or other activities. Please refer to the school health care plan for details.

Children with type 1 diabetes may not feel well if they have high blood sugars, which require increased water intake and access to restroom facilities without embarrassing restrictions. Please refer to the school health care plan for details.

There is a school video available through Maxishare (1-800-444-7747) to educate your staff. The video is titled "Living With Diabetes: Tips for Teachers." The video is approximately 19 minutes long. If you would like to purchase this video for your staff, please contact Maxishare directly for pricing. It is also possible for the parents to borrow (or purchase) a copy to bring to the school to share with the school staff. Please let them know if you would like them to do this and the preferred date and time.

If you or your staff have any questions, you may contact one of our nursing staff at

_____.

Sincerely,

_____, MD   _____, RN
Physician   Nursing Case Manager

_____   Parent's phone # _____
Parent

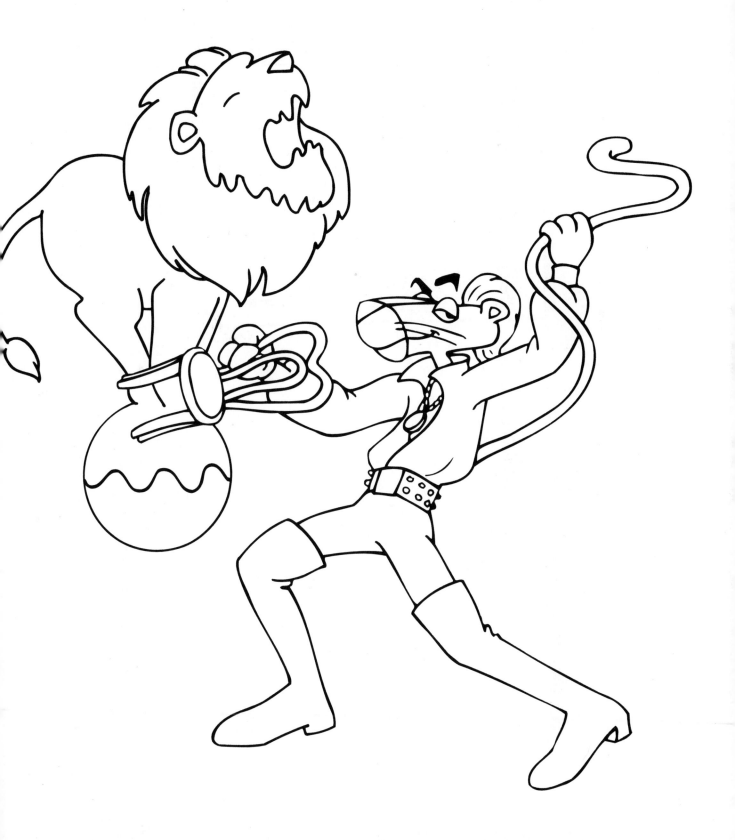

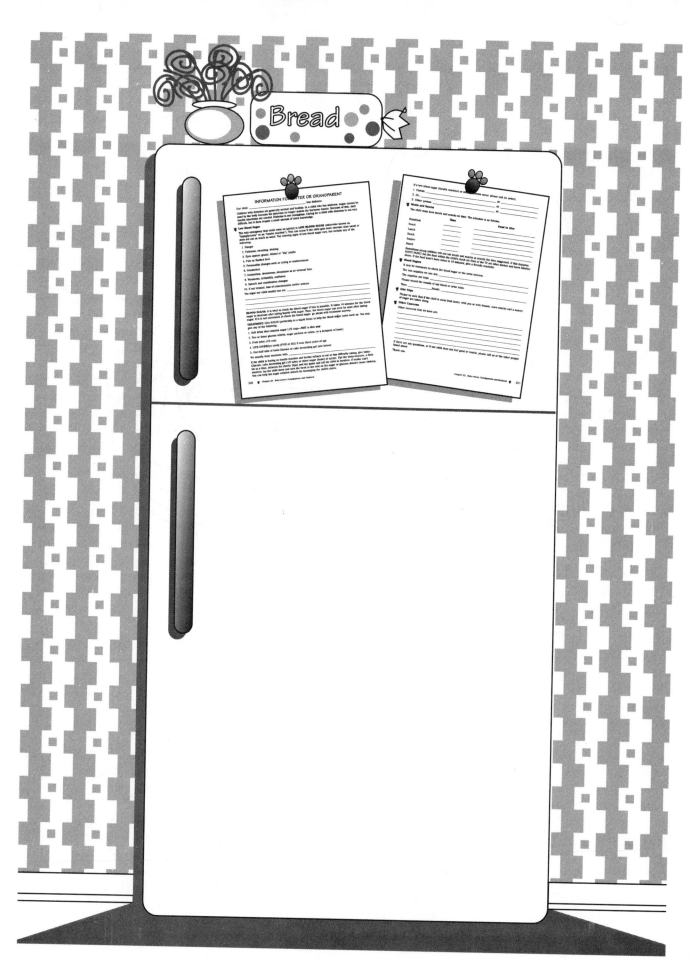

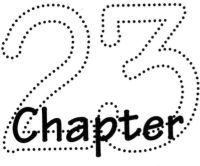

Chapter 23
BABY-SITTERS, GRANDPARENTS AND DIABETES

Key ideas of this chapter:

🐾 Assist parents in providing the essential diabetes supplies and information for the baby-sitter or grandparents.

🐾 Feel secure about the handling of their child's diabetes when the child is with the baby-sitter or with grandparents.

Cut out these pages and/or make copies of them to have available for baby-sitters or grandparents. The time required to instruct a sitter or grandparent will depend on how long he/she will be with your child. A person helping for a few hours will generally do fine after you teach him/her the basics in this handout. A person staying with a child for a longer time, or day-sitting for many weeks, will require more time to learn to give shots and to gain other knowledge. You are welcome to bring the sitter or grandparent along to diabetes clinic visits. In some cities, baby-sitting courses are offered to teach people diabetes-related skills.

Our center has offered a one-day course several times each year for grandparents of children with diabetes. It is important for grandparents to have a normal relationship with their grandchildren. This includes having the children for a day or, when parents are away, caring for them for a longer period. This requires having some knowledge and skills in many areas of diabetes management. Certainly recognizing low blood sugars and knowing how to treat them is essential. Checking blood sugars and, if the child is going to spend more than the day, knowing how to draw and give insulin also becomes essential. Grandparents do not usually need to know how to manage illness or how to adjust insulin doses for other reasons. They should be in contact with the parents or health care team if the child is ill or has high blood sugars for other reasons. Grandparents who take the time to learn about diabetes are showing love and support for their children and their grandchildren.

INFORMATION FOR SITTER OR GRANDPARENT

Our child, _____, has diabetes.

Children with diabetes are generally normal and healthy. In a child who has diabetes, sugar cannot be used by the body because the pancreas no longer makes the hormone insulin. Because of this, daily insulin injections are needed. Diabetes is not contagious. Caring for a child with diabetes is not very difficult, but it does require a small amount of extra knowledge.

Low Blood Sugar

The only emergency that could come on quickly is **LOW BLOOD SUGAR** (otherwise known as "hypoglycemia" or an "insulin reaction"). This can occur if the child gets more exercise than usual or does not eat as much as usual. The warning signs of low blood sugar vary, but include any of the following:

1. Hunger

2. Paleness, sweating, shaking

3. Eyes appear glassy, dilated or "big" pupils

4. Pale or flushed face

5. Personality changes such as crying or stubbornness

6. Headaches

7. Inattention, drowsiness, sleepiness at an unusual time

8. Weakness, irritability, confusion

9. Speech and coordination changes

10. If not treated, loss of consciousness and/or seizure

The signs our child usually has are: _____

_____

_____

_____

BLOOD SUGAR: It is ideal to check the blood sugar if this is possible. It takes 10 minutes for the blood sugar to increase after taking liquids with sugar. Thus, the blood sugar can even be done after taking sugar. If it is not convenient to check the blood sugar, go ahead with treatment anyway.

TREATMENT: Give SUGAR (preferably in a liquid form) to help the blood sugar come back up. You may give any of the following:

1. Soft drink that contains sugar (1/2 cup)—**NOT a diet pop**

2. Two or three glucose tablets, sugar packets or cubes, or a teaspoon of honey

3. Fruit juice (1/2 cup)

4. LIFE SAVERS(r) candy (FIVE or SIX) if over three years of age

5. One-half tube of Insta-Glucose or cake decorating gel (see below)

We usually treat reactions with: _____

If the child is having an insulin reaction and he/she refuses to eat or has difficulty eating, give Insta-Glucose, cake decorating gel (1/2 tube) or other sugar (honey or syrup). Put the Insta-Glucose, a little bit at a time, between the cheeks (lips) and the gums and tell the child to swallow. If he/she can't swallow, lay the child down and turn the head to the side so the sugar or glucose doesn't cause choking. You can help the sugar solution absorb by massaging the child's cheek.

If a low blood sugar (insulin reaction) or other problems occur, please call (in order):

1. Parent: _____ at: _____

2. Dr.: _____ at: _____

3. Other person: _____ at: _____

Meals and Snacks

The child must have meals and snacks on time. The schedule is as follows:

	Time	Food to Give
Breakfast	_____	_____
Snack	_____	_____
Lunch	_____	_____
Snack	_____	_____
Supper	_____	_____
Snack	_____	_____

Sometimes young children will not eat meals and snacks at exactly the time suggested. If this happens, DON'T PANIC! Set the food within the child's reach (in front of the TV set often works) and leave him/her alone. If the food hasn't been eaten in 10 minutes, give a friendly reminder.

Blood Sugars

It may be necessary to check the blood sugar or the urine ketones.

The test supplies we use are: _____

The supplies are kept: _____

Please record the results of any blood or urine tests.

Time: _____ Result: _____

Side Trips

Please be sure that if the child is away from home, with you or with friends, extra snacks and a source of sugar are taken along.

Other Concerns

Other concerns that we have are:

_____

_____

_____

_____

_____

_____

If there are any questions, or if our child does not feel good or vomits, please call us or the other people listed above.

Thank you.

QUESTIONS (Q) AND ANSWERS (A) FROM NEWSNOTES

Q. What is the Grandparents' Workshop and why does the Center have this?

A. The Center has the Grandparents' Workshop (usually 2-4 times per year based on need) so that grandparents can have grandchildren and grandchildren can have grandparents! Both are very important to each other! I recently had a family tell me that when their five-year-old was diagnosed with diabetes, one set of grandparents jumped in and learned about diabetes including how to check blood sugars, give insulin shots and the whole "ball of wax." The other set of grandparents were scared of the diabetes and never learned any of the needed diabetes skills. Needless to say, the first set of grandparents gained a grandchild while the second set lost a grandchild (and the grandchild lost the opportunity for a close relationship with the second set of grandparents). For most grandparents, attending the one-day workshop, and possibly reading the Center's educational book or coloring book, results in enough skills to be able to have the child spend a night or a week with the grandparents like any other grandchild. Perhaps even more importantly, attending the workshop helps alleviate the fears of diabetes, particularly involving hypoglycemia. This is important and the child does not then feel different or punished because of having diabetes (particularly if siblings get to stay at the grandparents). It is also a chance for the child (and parents) to break inter-dependencies. Finally, all parents need a break and an occasional vacation without the children. Grandparents are not only often the best possible option, but they are also often the only option. The chance to get to know one's grandparents better, and to have memories of staying with them, is something that is valued for many years to come.

Chapter 24 VACATIONS AND CAMP

Key ideas of this chapter:

* Assist the family in planning for diabetes management for a vacation or for a camp away from home.

* Support the family in allowing the child with diabetes to develop independence skills apart from the family.

* Encourage having fun.

VACATIONS

Diabetes should not interfere with vacations, which are a normal part of life. Some extra "planning ahead" should help prevent problems related to the diabetes. It is often wise to plan a clinic visit in the week or two prior to leaving on vacation. Possible changes in insulin dosage can then be discussed. If more activity is likely, the insulin dose should be reduced. If traveling overseas, it may be necessary to reduce the dose for a shortened day, or to take extra insulin for a lengthened day. Insulin pumps can be reset for the new time zones prior to arrival. Some diabetes care providers also reduce the insulin dose when people travel east by airplane with a loss of three hours, particularly between coasts. It is not necessary to alter the insulin dosage for the changes in time when traveling across the United States by car. Sick-day management can also be reviewed with your diabetes care provider at that visit. Always remember to take strips for checking urine ketones (preferably foil-wrapped or a fresh bottle). If traveling to an area where the risk for diarrhea is high, a plan should be outlined for prevention and treatment. Kaopectate® (sugar-free) and Imodium AD® tablets may be wise to take along. You may wish to take this book along to quickly review the chapter on sick-day management in case it is needed.

There have been no problems with taking insulin or other diabetes supplies (including meters and insulin pumps) through airport security (x-ray) devices. Do remember to take extra batteries for meters and insulin pumps.

Eating times and amounts of food are often altered on vacations. Meals are rarely served at expected times on airplanes. Extra snacks such as pre-packaged cheese or peanut butter crackers must be available for emergencies. A source of sugar should be carried. Food served in a restaurant or in a relative's home may contain more or less calories than are usually eaten. The importance of consistently eating on time is often not appreciated by other people. Foods that increase the blood sugar greatly may be more available and hard to resist when on vacation.

Exercise may be quite different on vacation than at home. If traveling in a car, it is wise to plan to stop in time to get some exercise each day. A few extra units of Humalog and/or Regular insulin may have to be taken to make up for the lack of exercise during travel times. Some vacations may include days of much more activity than usual, and the insulin dose might best be reduced on those days.

Blood sugar monitoring will allow you to know how your diabetes is being affected by the vacation. If the values are consistently high, a bit more insulin may be needed. If they are low, the insulin dose may need to be decreased. Doing the tests and making appropriate changes will help prevent problems. Some specifics to remember are:

🐾 Pack enough **insulin** and supplies to last the whole time you are away (generally twice the amount you think you'll need). Take extra batteries for meters and pumps. Supplies may not be available at your vacation area.

🐾 Make a **check list** ahead of time of things to take. Double check this list at the last minute. If using an insulin pump, take long-acting insulin and syringes in case it malfunctions and you need to return to shots.

🐾 If you are traveling in a hot car, keep **glucagon, insulin, and blood sugar strips** in an ice chest or thermos bottle **with ice**. They spoil if they get above 90° or if they freeze. Bring the strips to room temperature before using. If you travel by plane, keep all of your supplies in your carry-on luggage (or if traveling with someone, put 1/2 of the supplies in their carry-on in case one is lost). Supplies may freeze in the plane's luggage compartment and be ruined!

🐾 **ALWAYS** carry a form of **sugar** with you to treat reactions.

🐾 Have adequate **snacks** available in case meals are not served on time.

🐾 Always wear a diabetes **identification tag**.

🐾 Get the name of a **doctor** in your vacation area so that you can call him/her if necessary. Take your own doctor's phone number, too. He/she knows your case best, and it may be reassuring to make a long distance phone call when help is needed.

🐾 Visit your doctor **two weeks** before you leave so that you can work out any problems before the last minute. Remember to take his/her list of suggestions with you.

🐾 If you expect to be **more active** on the vacation (hiking, camping, skiing, etc.), you may need to decrease the insulin dose. Discuss this with your doctor or nurse.

🐾 For international travel, remember to check far enough ahead of time to see if you need special immunizations. The state health departments usually can help provide this information.

🐾 If international travel is planned, it is wise to carry a letter from the physician explaining why insulin syringes and other supplies are being transported through customs. It is wise to check to see if your health insurance covers you in other countries, or if you need supplemental insurance.

🐾 The most important advice is to **HAVE FUN!**

CAMP

Children with diabetes are very dependent on their parents for blood sugar tests and injections, proper nutrition, and help with preventing and treating potentially dangerous low blood sugars, in addition to their other needs. Likewise, the diabetes management for their child can become one of the main functions in life for a parent. Thus, it is not unexpected that children with diabetes may become overly dependent on their parents, and that taking care of their child may become a major part of life for the parent. Diabetes camp often offers the first chance to alter these relationships. Most diabetes camps have doctors and nurses at the camp so that the parents can feel their children will be safe. The food is monitored so that high-sugar desserts will not be a constant temptation. Adequate snacks are routinely provided. It is often a major help for children to meet other friends who take shots and do tests just like they do. Children who are old enough and who do not give their own shots or do their own blood sugar levels may try doing these tasks at camp. It is also a chance for a child to realize that he/she is not the only person in the world who has diabetes. The children also realize that with proper planning, they can do the same hiking, overnights, and other activities that other children do. Older teens with diabetes may serve as junior counselors and find that they must take good care of themselves in order to set a good example for younger campers.

It is important for parents not to be upset if they receive the "typical" camp letter from their child asking the parents to come and get them immediately. This type of letter is not unusual and should not cause concern. Most campers are having a wonderful time. If you are overly concerned, call the camp coordinator for reassurance. Whatever you do, don't upset the child by trying to call them at camp, and don't suddenly appear at camp ready to take the child home.

Most diabetes camps also have some educational programs. These may be "rap-sessions," problem-solving sessions, or skills demonstrations. The major goal of the camp, however, should be to have fun and to make new friends. It is not unusual for pen pals to develop and who can't wait until the next summer at camp when they can meet again.

Scholarship programs are offered at most diabetes camps. If finances are a problem, a request for financial help should be made. Sometimes children can earn part of their own expenses.

After having tried diabetes camp, the child may decide to try other camps. When this happens, the parents will need to discuss insulin dosage and other changes with their diabetes care provider a few weeks before camp. They will then need to relay this information to the camp nurse. Telephone numbers for emergencies and methods to handle low blood sugars and illnesses should also be discussed with the camp nurse. He/she may wish to phone or fax blood sugar results to the family, or to the child's diabetes care provider after the first few days of camp. Attending a diabetes camp or another camp is often the first step toward independence for the child with diabetes. Encouraging camp attendance can result in a healthy parent-child relationship.

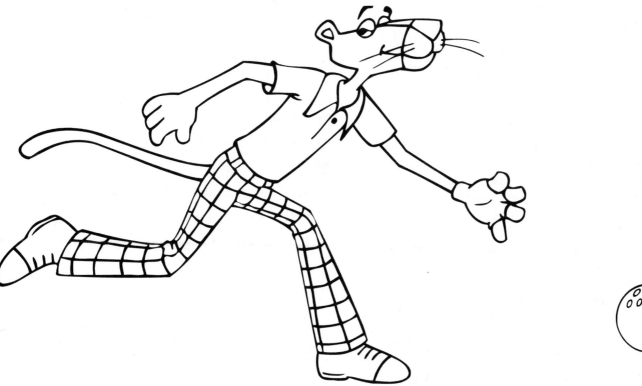

¡QUESTIONS (Q) AND ANSWERS (A) FROM NEWSNOTES

Q. Should my child go to diabetes camp?

A. We are often asked this question. The lower age limit for the Colorado camp is eight years, although not all eight-year-olds are mature enough to be away from home. Some camps (Texas) take children at even younger ages. This question was directed to me specifically as it relates to a 10-year-old and I replied without hesitation, "Yes, your child should go to camp."

Camp offers many benefits: fun (our major emphasis!) and getting to know and live in a cabin with other children the same age who also have diabetes. It is a great help for children to learn that they are not the only persons their age in the world with diabetes—that 10 others in the cabin also have to take shots and do blood sugars. Camp is often the first chance to break the inter-dependencies (child on parents and parents on child) which usually develop when diabetes is diagnosed at a young age. It is often a good time for parents to also get a vacation!

Q. Our family is going on a two-week vacation this summer. Are there any special concerns regarding our son's insulin?

A. The method of travel and the type of vacation are important. If you are traveling by plane, make sure the insulin is carried with you and not in the luggage. Freezing or pressure changes in the baggage compartments may change the insulin. It is also wise to have two vials of each insulin in case one is broken. Many foreign countries do not have U-100 insulins. Do not forget that meals on airplanes are never served on time, so extra snacks are essential. If time changes during travel to foreign countries are known, it is wise to call and discuss these with your nurse or physician so that the insulin can be adjusted accordingly.

Long trips in cars frequently result in excess sugar spillage and frequency of urination. Stopping for regular exercise at two-hour intervals, eating less, or taking extra Humalog and/or Regular insulin may all help. If the car is likely to be hot, remember that insulin does lose activity at temperatures above 90°. Insulin, glucagon, and blood sugar strips must always be kept in the thermos or cooler with ice. The strips should be brought to room temperature before use.

Do not forget to take your ketostix (preferably foil-wrapped) and a card with your doctor's phone numbers. It is often wiser to call your physician long-distance when you have questions than to get advice from someone who may be unfamiliar with your child.

Routines are often broken during vacations. Sleeping late or eating snacks or meals late can result in insulin reactions. Be aware of the likelihood of inconsistencies and try to prevent problems. Thinking ahead can help prevent problems and result in more fun!

Q. We are going to the East Coast on vacation this summer. Will we need to adjust the times for giving shots?

A. No, a change of one or two hours does not generally make a difference; simply adjust to their time zone.

This is not the case when traveling to Europe, the Far East, or Hawaii. When greater time changes are to occur, call your diabetes care provider with:

- The time of leaving home and/or the U.S.
- The number of hours you will be traveling
- The time of planned arrival (a.m. or p.m.)
- The same calculations for the return trip
- Scheduled meals on planes

Your diabetes care provider can then help you with the insulin adjustments.

A special note: If you are taking syringes and needles through customs, it is also generally wise to have a letter from your physician stating that you have diabetes. Examples of possible letters are shown in the Table.

EXAMPLES OF TRAVEL LETTERS

The first letter (Example 1) is a generic letter to allow diabetes supplies to be taken through customs. Example 2 and the pump card are, as suggested by MiniMed, for people who use insulin pumps. As faxed signatures are now legal, a family could fax a letter to their physician to be signed and then have it faxed back.

Travel Letter Example 1

To Whom It May Concern:

Please allow _____ to carry medical supplies in order to manage his/her diabetes.

_____ must take insulin shots daily to control his/her blood sugar. It will be necessary for him/her to carry supplies to monitor blood sugar levels as well as extra food. It is important to guard against low blood sugars and we advise enough food to last one day or more.

Sincerely,

(Doctor's signature, stamp and phone number)

Travel Letter Example 2

To Whom It May Concern:

_____ is a patient in this office being treated for insulin-dependent diabetes mellitus. He/she is currently using an insulin pump and does blood sugar monitoring by finger poke. Hypoglycemic reactions (low blood sugars) are always a possibility and require treatment with glucose (sugar) tablets or other sugar-containing drinks or foods. Therefore, it is essential that he/she have in his/her possession at all times insulin, insulin syringes, and the equipment to test his/her blood sugar levels. It is also essential that he/she wear the insulin pump at all times, as it is continuously supplying the medication, insulin, which is required for the patient's survival.

If you have any questions, please contact this office.

Sincerely,

(Doctor's signature, stamp and phone number)

Insulin Pump

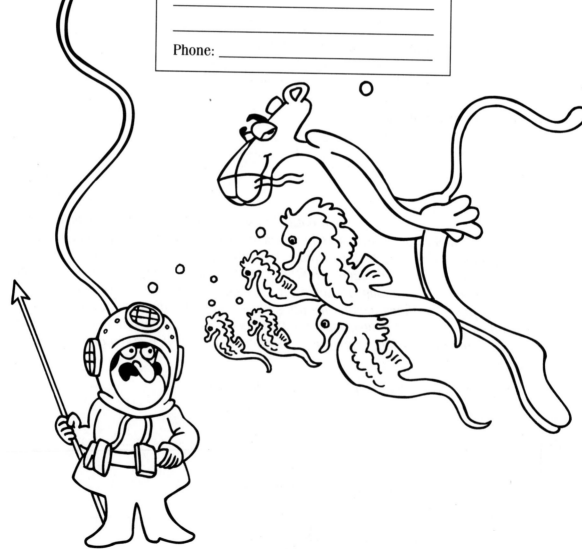

INSULIN PUMP

INSULIN PUMP

Identification Card For:

_____

ATTENTION: *A medical device containing metal is being worn by the bearer of this card. This device cannot be removed. "This person has insulin-dependent diabetes mellitus and is wearing an insulin pump which delivers insulin continuously into the subcutaneous tissue to control diabetes."*

DO NOT REMOVE THIS PUMP

Physician's Signature: _____

Physician's Name: _____

Address: _____

_____

_____

Phone: _____

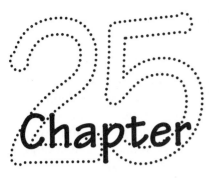

Chapter 25 INSULIN PUMPS

(This chapter is not for newly diagnosed families.)

Key ideas of this chapter:

- Provide an overview on the use of an insulin pump.

- Appreciate some of the advantages and disadvantages of using an insulin pump.

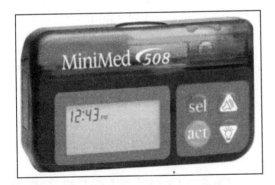

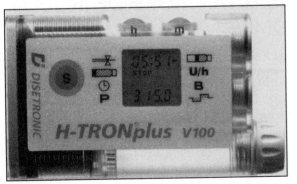

This chapter is not meant to teach everything that one needs to know about insulin pumps. There are entire books (see end of chapter) written about pump therapy, and this chapter is only meant to provide an overview. An insulin pump is a microcomputer (the size of a pager) that constantly infuses insulin. When an insulin pump is used, insulin is first put into a special syringe, which is then placed within the pump case. A small plastic tube within a needle is put under the skin (the needle is then withdrawn, leaving the plastic tube in place). Insulin is infused through the small plastic tube to an area under the skin (most commonly the abdomen). Tape is placed over the catheter to keep it in place for up to three days.

It is important to realize that the current insulin pumps do not know what the blood sugar level is and give 0.1 unit of insulin every few minutes (called the "basal" rate). Each time the person eats, buttons on the pump must be pushed to give an additional "bolus" insulin dose. There is not a "closed-loop" pump that measures blood sugars and turns off the basal insulin if the blood sugar is low or gives more insulin if the blood sugar is high. This will likely become possible at some time in the future.

Four visits are generally required to begin treatment with an insulin pump. A nurse educator, social worker, dietitian, and physician usually spend 4-6 hours with the patient and family in the two pre-pump visits, another 4-6 hours at the time of starting the pump and then another 3-4 hours at the first follow-up visit.

ADVANTAGES OF INSULIN PUMPS

1 Improved Glucose Control

The Diabetes Control and Complications Trial (DCCT), as discussed in Chapter 13, showed that improved glucose control lessened the likelihood of the eye, kidney, and nerve complications of type 1 diabetes. Glucose control is measured by doing a HbA_{1c} test (see Chapter 13) every three months. Most people who use pump therapy have some decrease in their HbA_{1c} values and thus some decrease in their risk for complications. People who are not able to obtain optimal glucose control on multiple daily injections of insulin may benefit from insulin pump therapy.

2 Insulin Delivery

One of the big advantages of using a pump is that the insulin is readily available; it is relatively easy to push a few buttons to take extra insulin (this could possibly also be an added risk for young children). The insulin pump is designed to deliver insulin in two ways:

i. A programmed basal rate (0.1 unit delivered every few minutes)
ii. A user-initiated bolus dose (a quick burst) of insulin with meals or with high blood sugars

This is similar to the insulin output by the normal human pancreas, with a constant (basal) output of insulin and boluses of insulin with meals. The pump has advantages over multiple daily shots in that the absorption of the insulin is more consistent and is thus very predictable. Only short-acting insulin is used in the pump (usually Humalog). Long-acting insulins (such as NPH or Lente), which vary in their absorption in the same person from day-to-day, are NOT used in a pump.

3 Decrease in Total Insulin Dose

The total daily insulin dose is usually decreased (by about 30%) when changing from multiple shots of insulin to an insulin pump due to more efficient delivery and use of insulin. Some people think the lower total insulin dose may be important in helping to prevent hardening of the arteries or elevated blood pressure, but this is not proven.

4 Reduction of Blood Sugars after Meals or Whenever High

With the quick-acting Humalog insulin, the high blood sugars after meals can now be reduced using boluses at mealtime without having to remember to give pump bolus doses 30-90 minutes before eating. In addition, extra doses of insulin are easy to take if a high blood sugar is found between meals. The Humalog insulin in the pump works just like when it is given in shots. It starts to work in 10 minutes, peaks in 30-40 minutes and is gone in four hours.

5 Flexibility and Freedom

For some people, using a pump has psychological advantages, where as for others, there are disadvantages (see next section). Being able to sleep late in the morning or to alter the time of meals or exercise represents an advantage for many pump users. Basal rates can easily be altered to meet special circumstances. Extra or increased boluses can be taken (e.g., when ill) without having to take extra shots. Many people express an increased sense of freedom and flexibility. The "Quick-Release" now found on the pump tubing makes it easy to remove the pump for showers or exercise. (One should not remain disconnected for more than two hours without checking the blood sugar.) The long plastic tube permits placement of the pump on the bed stand while sleeping at night. Several special holders are available for the pump. Miss America (1998), Nicole Johnson, wore her pump strapped to her leg during the evening gown competition (she disconnected it for the swim suit competition).

DISADVANTAGES OF INSULIN PUMPS

1 Psychological Factors

Wearing a pump, even though it is not much bigger than a pager, is difficult for some people. We have heard the comment that "Starting the insulin pump was like getting diabetes all over again. People who had not known that I had diabetes now asked me what the pump was." A considerable amount of learning about the pump is necessary, and it is not that much different from the amount required when diabetes was first diagnosed. There are other feelings expressed—such as "constantly being hooked to an instrument." (In contrast, as discussed earlier, some people like always having insulin with them.)

Expense

Pumps are expensive and some insurance companies may refuse to pay for them. Initial expenses include buying the pump (approximately $5,000), starting the pump ($1,500-$10,000, depending on whether the pump start is done as an outpatient or in the hospital) and yearly pump supplies (about $2,000). Although this may seem like a lot, the cost savings in the prevention of the eye, kidney, and nerve complications of diabetes more than offsets these expenses.

Hypoglycemia

Severe low blood sugars were three times more common in pump users or in people taking three or more shots per day (all using Regular insulin) compared with people receiving one or two shots of insulin per day in the DCCT (see Chapter 13). The use of Humalog with more timely absorption, action, and disappearance has now made pumps safer in relation to hypoglycemia.

Weight Gain

People using insulin pumps (resulting in better glucose control) may gain weight as a result. The sugar is absorbed rather than going out in the urine. The weight gain can happen in any person who improves their sugar control. Working with a dietitian before and after starting the pump can help to prevent this from happening. It may be less of a problem with the pump in comparison to multiple injections because it is not necessary to eat to keep up with insulin previously injected.

Skin Infections

Infections can occur at the infusion sites— particularly if the infusion sets are left in for longer than three days. However, if proper cleaning techniques are followed, this is a minimal risk. If redness and pus are noted, the physician should be called to get a prescription for antibiotics.

Ketonuria or Ketoacidosis

When problems occur with insulin delivery,

there is no long-acting insulin in the body. Ketones will start to form in 4-6 hours (the duration of the last Humalog infused). There are now warnings on pumps to help indicate a plugged line or catheter, or the syringe being out of insulin. If more frequent urination or thirst are noted, people are taught to do an immediate blood sugar, urine ketone test, pump and site inspections (particularly to check for leaks, plugged line or catheter that may have come out). If sugar control has been good for a period of time, ketones will generally not form as rapidly and/or can be cleared more easily. In contrast, if glucose control has been poor, the ketones will develop more rapidly and build up more easily. In our experience, most pump users have times when their catheter comes out or plugs. Insulin and syringes must be kept available in case they are needed. Urine ketone strips (see Chapter 4) must always be readily available.

Insulin Availability

One must remember to routinely fill the insulin reservoir (syringe) in the pump so that the pump does not run out of insulin at an awkward time. Also, remember that insulin spoils if it freezes (unlikely next to the body) or reaches temperatures above 90°. One of our patients "cooked" her insulin by wearing her waterproof pump into a hot tub. Others have frozen insulin by exposing tubing while skiing.

Visits

Pre-pump Visits

Insulin pumps are not for everyone. The patient (not just other family members) must be ready for the insulin pump, want the pump, and be fully committed to using the pump; otherwise it will fail. Our greatest success has been with people 13 years of age and older. We usually have the patient and their family or a close friend meet with the physician, nurse, dietitian, and social worker in the first pre-pump visit. The basics of pump therapy and the advantages and disadvantages are discussed. We ask that four or five blood sugars be done per day, recorded, and faxed to us weekly (often for one-month). This gives us an idea of the commitment of the person and the family, as well as their reliability. If the person is not already counting carbohydrates, the dietitian will give instructions in this area. We usually ask that potential pump users be old enough to count carbohydrates and that they bring or send completed blood sugar and food records, as well as insulin doses, to the dietitian. They must also be able to reliably give bolus dosages, and must be old enough to be able to deal in tenths of units of insulin. We send a video on the pump and other information home with the family for review. In general, a person who finds it difficult to let others know that they have diabetes, who is considering the pump mainly because a parent or other person is pushing them to do so (and not because they want to), or who finds frequent blood sugar testing difficult will not do well on the pump. **It must be realized that insulin pump therapy is more work than other diabetes management regimens. If the person is not committed to doing the extra work, glucose control will not improve.**

In the second pre-pump visit we lend the person an insulin pump to use for one week. They use only sterile saline (salt water) in the pump, but can get used to wearing it to see if they like it, and to find out if they can deal with the every two- or three-day changes in infusion sets. It is important to practice using the pump and to become comfortable with how it works. We recommend that the instructional video be viewed at least two times to learn all the basic pump functions. If this introduction is successful, we then start the insurance process in tandem with the pump company to see if insurance coverage is possible. (Most families have already obtained some information about this, so they know if their insurance company will support pumps with proper communication.) Further instruction with the dietitian around carbohydrate counting usually is necessary. The social worker is also available to discuss concerns about starting the pump.

Starting the Insulin Pump
We encourage having a significant other(s) along with the person beginning pump therapy. The significant other(s) may help with future pump problems, may assist with blood sugar testing (particularly in the middle of the night), and must be available to help with possible hypoglycemia. Glucagon administration should be reviewed. The support of the significant other(s) adds to the likelihood of success with the pump. The physician sets initial basal and bolus insulin dosages (see below), the dietitian again reviews carbohydrate counting and the food records that were sent in, and the nurse educator usually does the technical training for the insulin pump. The social worker is available to discuss concerns or fears.

Post-pump Visits
The person (or family member) faxes blood sugar results daily for the first week, then weekly for several weeks, and then every 2-4 weeks. Good communication at this time is essential.

We usually have the initial post-pump clinic visit in the first 1-3 days after starting the pump. This visit is primarily so the nurse can observe a set change and be certain that good techniques are being used. After 1-4 weeks, another visit is scheduled to bring in a food record to discuss and determine the insulin-to-carbohydrate ratios with the dietitian. Other methods of preventing high blood sugars after meals (such as the square-wave bolus) are discussed. Sick-day management, site care and hypoglycemia are reviewed. If the Soft-Set® is primarily being used, the Silhouette Infusion Set® is demonstrated. The physical exam includes a careful eye check at this time (particularly if the blood sugar control is rapidly improving).

METHODS OF INSULIN DELIVERY BY PUMP

The pump delivers insulin in two ways: 1) a basal dosage that is programmed into the pump and remains the same day-after-day unless the user changes the rate, and 2) bolus dosages that are taken before meals or when a blood sugar is high, but which must be programmed in by the user at the time the dose is taken or it will not be given.

Basal Insulin Dosages
The basal rate reflects the units of insulin per hour that would be needed if a person were not eating meals. The basal rate is similar to the small amount of insulin released by the pancreas every few minutes to turn off sugar

production by the liver and to prevent fat breakdown. Usually the basal dose consists of 50-60% of the total daily pump insulin dose. The number one goal in the first week is to calculate and fine-tune the desired basal dosages. Most people reduce (by half) or omit their evening long-acting insulin the night prior to starting the pump and take a shot of Humalog insulin at breakfast prior to coming to the clinic. Others do not take any long-acting insulin the night before starting the pump, but take shots of Regular insulin at dinner, bedtime, and 2 a.m. There is then less insulin activity remaining as the pump dosages are begun the next morning. This should be discussed with the physician or nurse.

Some doctors start with approximately two-thirds of the estimated basal doses, and as the person's long-acting insulin wears off (1-2 days) and blood sugar levels are reported each day, the dosages are gradually increased. The number of basal dosages to be used varies between doctors. Some start with one or two basal rates and others with 8-12 basal dosages. Most teenagers and young adults need more insulin in the early morning hours to cover the body's normal increase in hormones (the "Dawn phenomenon"). All people are different, and the use of different basal doses allows for fine-tuning. Once the basal rates are set they tend to stay quite consistent, except with large changes in body weight, change of time zones, injuries, some medications (e.g., steroids), and temporary reductions for exercise.

Bolus Insulin Dosages

Approximately 40-50% of the daily pump insulin doses are given as boluses before meals or snacks. (Some people give the bolus at the end of the meal when they can better judge amounts eaten.) Everyone is different and boluses can be chosen to fit individual eating habits. However, **the first goal is to get the basal doses adjusted,** so we usually suggest keeping the carbohydrate intake relatively consistent and using a "Thinking Scale" for bolus doses. Table 1 gives an example of suggested boluses for a 15-year-old young man in our clinic, but will obviously vary for different people. Dosages for the initial basal and bolus insulin doses can be filled in for a given person in Table 2.

After collecting adequate information on carbohydrates eaten, insulin dosages, and resulting blood sugars (usually at least a week after the pump-start), an insulin-to-carbohydrate ratio can be set for each meal. (Some pump clinics prefer to start with insulin-carbohydrate ratios right from the beginning and not use set bolus dosages.) Ratios vary by the person and meal, but the most commonly used ratio seems to be one unit per 15 grams carbohydrate (CHO). Another example might be one unit of insulin per 15 grams CHO in the morning, one unit per 20 grams CHO at lunch, and one unit per 10 grams CHO at dinner. The dietitian is an important member of the pump team and will need to review and reinforce carbohydrate counting. They often make the recommendations for insulin; CHO ratios for

Examples of Bolus Insulin Dosages

	Blood Sugar Levels in mg/dl (mmol/L)			Approximate
	<100 (<5.5)	100-200 (5.5-11.1)	>200 (>11.1)	Carbs (gms)
Breakfast:				
Light*	3 units	4 units	5 units	30-60
Standard	4 units	6 units	8 units	60-90
Lunch:				
Light*	3 units	4 units	5 units	45-60
Standard	4 units	5 units	6 units	60-90
Dinner:				
Light*	4 units	6 units	8 units	45-75
Standard	6 units	8 units	10 units	75-105

Or planned exercise (if heavy exercise, reduce further)

INITIAL INSULIN PUMP INSTRUCTIONS

Table 2

A. Check Blood Sugars:

1. <u>ALWAYS</u> before breakfast, lunch, dinner, and bedtime
2. Two hours after breakfast, lunch, and/or dinner (pick two after meal checks the first week on the pump, one after meal check the second week on the pump and intermittently thereafter)
3. Between 1 a.m. and 6 a.m. (every night for one week and intermittently thereafter)

B. Your Initial Basal Rates:

Time Period	U/hr	Total (U/hr x hrs)
1. _____	_____	_____
2. _____	_____	_____
3. _____	_____	_____
4. _____	_____	_____
5. _____	_____	_____
6. _____	_____	_____
7. _____	_____	_____
8. _____	_____	_____
9. _____	_____	_____
10. _____	_____	_____

_____ = Total U's/24 hours

C. Initial Units Of Insulin For Your Boluses:

	Blood Sugar Level			Usual Carb Intake
For blood sugar:	<___mg/dl	____ to ____mg/dl	>____mg/dl	____(gm)
or	<___mmol/L	____ to ____mmol/L	>____mmol/L	____
Breakfast:				
Light*	____	____	____	____
Standard	____	____	____	____
Lunch:				
Light *	____	____	____	____
Standard	____	____	____	____
Dinner:				
Light *	____	____	____	____
Standard	____	____	____	____

*Also use lower dose if exercise is planned in next 1-2 hours

D. If Using Carbohydrate Ratios* (CHO):

Breakfast ratio is: one unit of insulin for each ____ gm of CHO
Lunch ratio is: one unit of insulin for each ____ gm of CHO
Dinner ratio is: one unit of insulin for each ____ gm of CHO
Snack ratio is: one unit of insulin for each ____ gm of CHO

E. If Doing Carbohydrate Ranges For Meals*:

Breakfast: Bolus ____ units of insulin and eat between ____ and ____ gm of CHO
Lunch: Bolus ____ units of insulin and eat between ____ and ____ gm of CHO
Dinner: Bolus ____ units of insulin and eat between ____ and ____ gm of CHO
Snacks: Bolus ____ units of insulin and eat between ____ and ____ gm of CHO

*For both of these methods, you will compensate for high blood sugars by adding ____ units of insulin for each ____ mg/dl (____ mmol/L) above ____. For example, with a blood sugar of 241 mg/dl (13.3 mmol/L), you would add two units to your bolus if adding one unit for each 50 mg/dl (2.75 mmol/L) over 150 mg/dl (8.3 mmol/L).

the different meals after reviewing food records, insulin dosages taken and blood sugars two hours after meals.

Supplemental Insulin Dosages

Extra (unscheduled) insulin boluses are important to use if the blood sugar level is high. These can be determined in one of several ways and, once again, it is best to try different methods and see what works. It is important to remember that larger dosages will be required if ketones are present. The health care team should be contacted if moderate or large ketones are found.

i.   Some people just take a dose that fits their body and insulin sensitivity based on the level of blood sugar. For example, one unit for every 50 mg/dl above 150 mg/dl might be used as a bolus to get the blood sugar back down. Thus, if the blood sugar level was 300 mg/dl, three units of insulin would be bolused. This calculation and a new bolus can be repeated after two hours if the blood sugar is still high and Humalog insulin is used. (For people using mmol/L for glucose, use one unit of insulin for every 2.7 mmol/L above 8.3 mmol/L. For a level of 16.6 mmol/L with a desire to reach 8.3 mmol/L, divide 2.7 into 8.3 (16.6 minus 8.3 = 8.3) and give three units of insulin.

ii. The "Rule of 1500" works for some people. This involves dividing the number of units of insulin usually taken in 24 hours (e.g., 70 units) into 1500, which equals 21. One then takes one unit of insulin for every 21 mg of glucose that one wishes to lower the blood sugar. For example, if the value is 255 mg/dl and one desires to lower the glucose to 150 mg/dl, one divides 105 by 21 and gets 5, which is the number of units of insulin to take. (For people using mmol/L for glucose, it is the "Rule of 83," using 83 rather than 1500. Seventy units divided into 83 gives 1.2. To lower the glucose 5.8 mmol/L [14.1-8.3 = 5.8], divide 5.8 by 1.2 and get 5 units of insulin.)

Table 3

DAILY RECORD FOR INSULIN PUMP MANAGEMENT

Day/Date	12MN	1AM	2AM	3AM	4AM	5AM	6AM	7AM	8AM	9AM	10AM	11AM	12 Noon	1PM	2PM	3PM	4PM	5PM	6PM	7PM	8PM	9PM	10PM	11PM	NOTES
BG																									
CARBS																									
BASAL																									
BOLUS																									
BG																									
CARBS																									
BASAL																									
BOLUS																									
BG																									
CARBS																									
BASAL																									
BOLUS																									
BG																									
CARBS																									
BASAL																									
BOLUS																									
BG																									
CARBS																									
BASAL																									
BOLUS																									
BG																									
CARBS																									
BASAL																									
BOLUS																									
BG																									
CARBS																									
BASAL																									
BOLUS																									

Phone Numbers:

(Family) Home _____

Work _____

Fax _____

Health Care Team:

Home _____

Work _____

Fax _____

Home _____

Work _____

Fax _____

This table may be copied as often as desired.

BLOOD SUGAR TESTING

More frequent blood sugar testing is required in the first week or two to help set the basal rates. At a minimum, tests should be done prior to each meal and the bedtime snack, two hours after eating one or two meals each day (to help with bolus doses), and once or twice during the night. This amounts to seven or eight tests per day—although this number may start to be reduced in the second week to five or six per day. It is obvious that parents or a significant other are extremely helpful at this time to help get all the testing done. The minimum eventually will be four tests daily with occasional checks during the night. The form we like for reporting (faxing) blood sugar results is shown in Table 3 and may be copied as often as desired.

HYPOGLYCEMIA

The three main causes of low blood sugars for people using an insulin pump are all related to human (and not pump) errors. They are:

Too few blood sugars

Some people go through periods when they do not do the extra required work of more frequent blood sugar checking necessary for intensive diabetes management. They may be having lows and not be aware this is happening. They may then have a severe hypoglycemic event.

Incorrect bolus dose

This may be because carbohydrate counting is not being done, or because the person calculated wrong. It can also happen when a bolus is taken and a meal is then interrupted.

Wrong adjustment for exercise

Some people fail to think ahead and make needed changes in insulin dosage for exercise. At other times it may be a new exercise or one that is more intense than usual, and they just did not realize how much it would lower their blood sugar. The answer is to test blood sugars before, during, and after exercise and to have extra drinks or food available.

Symptoms of Hypoglycemia

The symptoms and treatment of low blood sugar (hypoglycemia) are the same as those for people receiving insulin shots (Chapter 5). Some keys to avoiding lows are given in Table 4. Additional symptoms which should alert people/families to think of hypoglycemia during the nighttime are:

1. Inability to sleep or waking up "alert"
2. Waking up sweating
3. Waking up with a fast heart rate
4. Waking up with a headache
5. Waking up feeling "foggy-headed" or with memory loss
6. Unusually high blood sugar or with positive urine ketones (rebounding?)

IF ANY OF THESE DO OCCUR, DO A BLOOD SUGAR CHECK IMMEDIATELY. If low, treat appropriately and call the doctor or nurse the next day. Also think about what was different the previous day (extra exercise, bolus insulin, less food, etc.). This will allow planning ahead to prevent the low with a similar occurrence in the future. A summary of some key ideas for avoiding lows is given in Table 4.

Treatment

If hypoglycemia is suspected, the person with diabetes should be treated. If the blood sugar is below 60 mg/dl (3.25 mmol/L), we prefer 15 grams of "quick-acting" carbohydrate first (four ounces of juice or sugar pop or four glucose tablets). If it is still below 60 mg/dl (3.25 mmol/L) after 10 minutes, repeat this treatment. When it is above 60 mg/dl (3.25 mmol/L), give solid food.

If the glucose value is below 50 mg/dl (2.75 mmol/L), or if the person is "out of it" or unconscious, THE PUMP SHOULD BE PLACED ON "SUSPEND" for a period of 30 minutes. A parent or significant other must know how to do this, as the person with low blood sugar may be confused. It must be remembered that insulin already infused will not yet have peaked, so giving the sugar is essential. Instant Glucose (or cake decorating gel) and glucagon must be readily available, as must someone who knows how to give them (as with all people with diabetes).

Table 4

KEYS TO AVOIDING LOWS

1. Always do **AT LEAST** four blood sugars daily (and occasional checks during the night)

2. Count grams of carbohydrate to be eaten (or just eaten) accurately to give correct bolus

3. Test before, during, and after exercise

4. Be aware of symptoms of lows and treat promptly

5. Think ahead regarding variations in daily schedule that could cause low blood sugars

6. Subtract one unit of insulin if it is time to give a bolus dose and the blood sugar level is below 70 mg/dl (3.9 mmol/L)

HIGH BLOOD SUGARS

Some of the causes of high blood sugars for pump users are the same as for people taking their insulin by shots (e.g., extra food intake, lack of exercise, forgetting boluses, and illnesses). An additional cause in pump users is the pump not delivering insulin. The most common causes of this problem are an empty reservoir (insulin syringe) or a clogged infusion set. If there is still insulin in the syringe, changing the infusion set is usually a wise decision. In order to prevent running out of insulin, the syringe should be filled every 2-3 days as the set is changed. If more insulin has been used than usual (illness, driving in a car, etc.), bolus doses can be taken using a syringe. Table 5 summarizes some other possible pump problems. With leaks in the infusion set, a bead of insulin may be noted or the odor of insulin may be detected.

EXERCISE

There are several options for altering the insulin dose with exercise and experience is usually the best teacher to see which works. **Doing more frequent blood sugars to determine the effects of the exercise and the changes in insulin dosage is MOST helpful!** Many athletes find pumps are better than injections for dealing with exercise. It is generally not as necessary to eat and then perform on a full stomach.

1. If the exercise is mild to moderate (walking, golf, dancing, etc.), reducing the basal dosages by half during the exercise may be sufficient. Some people start the reduction 30 minutes before the exercise and continue it for 30 minutes after the exercise is over.

2. If it is intense exercise (jogging, football, basketball, etc.), most people just disconnect from the pump (some disconnect 30 minutes before the start of the exercise). There are then several options for insulin adjustments:

i. Some people do a blood sugar test and bolus after the exercise (particularly if the epinephrine out put with the exercise raises the blood sugar). Some people use a bolus of the entire amount missed while disconnected, while others use 1/2 of the amount missed AFTER the exercise.

ii. Some people estimate the amount of insulin to be missed while disconnected from the pump and take part of the dose before the exercise (particularly if the blood sugar is high) and the rest of the dose after the exercise.

In general, if the pump is to be disconnected for more than two hours, a blood sugar must be done. If the blood sugar is rising, it is easy to reconnect, take a small bolus, and again disconnect.

3. If it is to be an all day exercise (e.g., a long hike), it may work best to reduce the basal rates (perhaps by half) and to not give any bolus doses. People must determine what works best for them.

4. With exercise, it is important to remember to stay hydrated and to take extra snacks (see Chapter 12). Drinking water or Gatorade (or other sports drinks) works for some people. Snacks such as granola bars provide extra carbohydrates and calories. Make sure that coaches or others around at the time know that you have diabetes and wear an insulin pump.

POSSIBLE PUMP PROBLEMS

	Pump Alarm
1 Empty insulin reservoir (syringe)	Yes
2 Clogged infusion set	Yes
3 Leaky infusion set	No
4 Weak or dead battery	Yes
5 Pump malfunction	Yes

SCHOOL

If the person using the pump is in school, the school nurse should have some knowledge of the pump. You may wish to copy Table 6 (or this entire chapter) for the school nurse. (You have our permission to make copies as desired.)

SUMMARY

Insulin pumps have advantages and disadvantages. It is up to each person and family, working with their health care team, to decide if a pump would be good for a given person.

DEFINITIONS

Basal dose: A pre-set hourly rate of insulin as programmed into an insulin pump.

Bolus dose: An amount of insulin taken prior to a meal or when the blood sugar is high as entered at any time of the day by the person wearing the insulin pump.

Carbohydrate ratio (see Chapter 11): The number of units of insulin to be taken for a certain number of grams of carbohydrate eaten (e.g., one unit for 15 grams of carbohydrate).

Closed-loop pump: An insulin pump (not currently available) which would increase insulin infused for high blood sugars or decrease insulin infused for low blood sugars.

Insulin pump: A microcomputer with a syringe of insulin within the pager-sized device that can infuse a basal insulin dose at a pre-set hourly rate. Bolus insulin dosages can also be entered at any time by the person wearing the pump.

Additional Reading

1. *Pumping Insulin (Everything In A Book For Successful Use Of An Insulin Pump)*, Second Edition, by John Walsh, P.A., C.D.E. and Ruth Roberts, M.S. Torrey Pines Press, 1030 West Upas Street, San Diego, CA 92103-3821

2. *Teens Pumping It Up! Insulin Pump Therapy (Guide for Adolescents)*, by Elizabeth Boland, MSN, APRN, PNP, CDE. MiniMed Technologies, 12744 San Fernando Road, Sylmar, CA 91342, 1-800-933-3322

3. *The Insulin Pump Therapy Book. Insights from the Experts,* edited by Linda Fredrickson, MA, RN, CDE. MiniMed Technologies, 12744 San Fernando Road, Sylmar, CA 91342, 1-800-933-3322

4. *H-TRONplus® Advanced Insulin Pump Programming and Practices,* by Disetronic Medical System, Inc., 5201 East River Road, Ste. 312, Minneapolis, MN 55421-1014, 1-800-280-7801

Table 6

INSULIN PUMPS IN THE SCHOOL SETTING

_____ is a student in your school who has diabetes and is wearing an insulin pump. An insulin pump is a device which infuses a very small amount of fast-acting insulin every few minutes through a small catheter under the skin. The student then takes additional insulin through the pump for meals and for snacks. We would like to emphasize that problems and complications with insulin pumps are very seldom seen. For the most part, you will not be aware that the student is using the pump, although you may hear an occasional quiet beep when insulin is taken for a meal or a snack. The following information may assist you in helping the student wearing an insulin pump.

BLOOD SUGAR TESTING

When a student is on an insulin pump, more frequent blood sugar testing may be necessary. If the testing can be done easily in the classroom, that would be preferred, as the student will miss less classroom time. Testing can also be done in the office or clinic, if necessary.

LOW BLOOD SUGARS

If a student who is on an insulin pump experiences a low blood sugar reaction, the following guidelines should be followed:

*If the blood sugar is between 50-60 mg/dl (2.7-3.2 mmol/L), the student needs to take about 15 gms of liquid carbohydrate, which is equivalent to four ounces of juice or regular sugared pop, or four glucose tablets.

*If the blood sugar is less than 50 mg/dl (2.7 mmol/L), the student may treat as above, suspend the pump for 30 minutes, and once the sugar level is up, eat 15 gms of solid carbohydrate (e.g., cheese crackers, peanut butter crackers, or a granola bar).

*If the student is not able to cooperate with the treatment due to drowsiness, combativeness, or has slurred speech and is "out of it," squirt instant glucose or cake decorating gel between the cheek and the gum, and massage from the outside until the student can take oral fluids better. Then treat as above with 15 gms of liquid carbohydrate followed by a solid snack.

*If the student should experience a severe low blood sugar where the student is unconscious or is having a convulsion, 911 should be called and/or Glucagon may be given by appropriately trained staff. The pump should be placed on "suspend."

HIGH BLOOD SUGARS

High blood sugars over 250 mg/dl (13.9 mmol/L) may be an early indication that the pump is not infusing the insulin as it should or that the child is ill. When the student's blood sugar is this high, urine ketones should be checked. If the urine ketones are negative, the student can give an additional insulin dose through the insulin pump. The student should then re-check the blood sugar in one hour to be sure the blood sugar is coming down. If the blood sugar is still high and the ketones are small, moderate, or large, the student will need to give an insulin dose with a syringe and drink 16 oz of water per hour until the ketones disappear. The student will also have to change the infusion tubing for the insulin pump. The student should have a vial of fast-acting insulin and insulin syringes available in the clinic in case they need to give an additional injection.

EXERCISE

During times of vigorous exercise, the student may need to disconnect the pump. For this, the student needs to place the pump in a safe place where it will not be damaged. During prolonged exercise, many students reconnect the pump periodically and take insulin. Some students wear their pump during exercise and use a special case to protect it.

QUESTIONS?

If you have any questions, speak with the student and the student's family. They can be a tremendous resource for you. You may also wish to contact the health care providers for your student.

QUESTIONS (Q) AND ANSWERS (A) FROM NEWSNOTES

Q. At what age should children with diabetes be considered for insulin pump therapy?

A. This question is often asked. There is no "magic" age, although in general, teenagers tend to do better than pre-teens. Other factors which are also important are: **a.** the person must be faithful in doing at least four blood sugars daily; **b.** the desire of the patient, and not just the parents, to use a pump; **c.** the patient's maturity and ability to problem solve; **d.** the patient's ability to faithfully give the bolus dosages; **e.** the ability to use carbohydrate counting, and **f.** family support.

In addition, the pumps are expensive at $4,000-$5,000, and it is important to make sure the insurance company will support this expense. The Diabetes Control and Complications Trial (DCCT) showed that the reduction in cost of caring for diabetes complications in later years more than makes up for this cost. However, not all insurance companies are willing to invest in prevention.

Starting insulin pump therapy is time-consuming. We require an initial 3 to 7-day period of wearing the pump using saline (salt water). Then, if the person is still motivated, another day is spent in the clinic to begin insulin treatment. We do NOT hospitalize people. Daily phoning and faxing of 6-8 blood sugars per day follows in the first week.

Some people have said that starting the pump can be like getting diabetes all over again. Instead of taking shots in private, a pager-sized device is now constantly attached to the belt. This is removed during intensive exercise. People may ask questions such as, "What is that on your belt?"

An additional drawback of pumps is that if the plastic catheter accidentally pulls out and insulin is not being infused, high sugars and ketones may develop in 2-6 hours. This is because only Humalog insulin is used in the pump, and it is a short-acting insulin.

The rewards are also plentiful. The HbA_{1c} usually declines (average for our Center's patients = 7.4%). Using Humalog, the likelihood of severe low blood sugars is less than for three shots of insulin daily. Finally, blood sugars are "smoothed out" with more consistent absorption of the Humalog insulin, in contrast to long-acting insulins injected subcutaneously. It is common for people to comment, "I have more energy now," or "I just seem to feel better." Finally, people who lead inconsistent lifestyles can have more flexibility in what time they eat meals or even what time they arise in the morning. However, some degree of consistency still helps.

Although pumps are not for everyone, if it is something you want to know more about, ask your health care providers at the time of your clinic visit.

Q. My son is going on a trip without other family members. He uses an insulin pump. Could you remind us of supplies he should be taking along?

A. In case of pump malfunction, we generally recommend he take extra syringes and bottles of the long-acting insulin he was on prior to starting the pump. You should also look back in your records to send the dosages he was last on along with him. A summary of important items to include are:

1. Clinic phone number
2. Humalog (or Regular) insulin
3. Long-acting insulin
4. Insulin syringes
5. Extra pump batteries
6. Glucose meter/strips
7. Extra meter battery
8. Extra infusion sets
9. Extra pump syringe (reservoir)
10. Alcohol pads
11. Dressing, tape
12. Glucose tablets/instant glucose
13. Ketostix

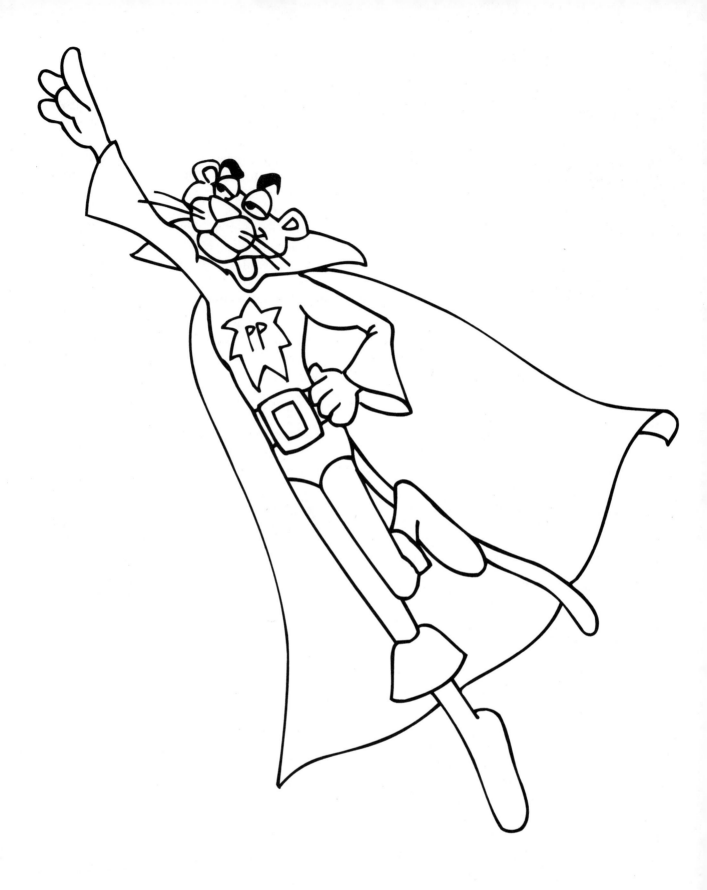

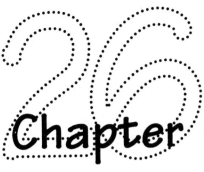

Chapter RESEARCH AND TYPE 1 DIABETES

Key ideas of this chapter:

🐾 Be aware of the research that is currently being done and, in some cases, how to participate.

🐾 Separate fact from fiction so that families do not have unrealistic hopes and expectations.

The four questions about research that are most frequently asked are listed below. Each of these topics will be briefly addressed.

I. When will non-invasive glucose monitoring (no finger pokes) be available?

II. When will there be a cure?

III. Can diabetes be prevented?

IV. Have there been clinical advances in the morbidity or mortality of diabetes?

Extraordinary developments have been realized in type 1 (insulin-dependent) diabetes research over the last decade, and the next decade is charged with much promise for the management of diabetes and, as important, its prevention.

NON- OR MINIMALLY INVASIVE GLUCOSE MONITORING

We were all misled for a number of years to think that it would be possible to put a finger in a hole of a box, shine a wavelength of light at the finger, and have a glucose level accurately determined. Most researchers now doubt that this will ever be possible as too many other substances (including water) overlap with the wavelength that represents the blood sugar.

Fortunately, two non- or minimally invasive alternatives are about to be (or have recently been) approved by the FDA that do measure glucose levels accurately. These are the GlucoWatch by the Cygnus Company and the Continuous Glucose Monitoring System (CGMS) by MiniMed, Inc. Both measure subcutaneous rather than blood glucose levels, but the glucose levels are very similar. The subcutaneous glucose levels are approximately 10 minutes behind the blood glucose levels, but this does not seem to be a major problem.

The **GlucoWatch** does not involve any pokes or blood draws, but has a pad on the back of the watch which draws extra-cellular fluid from under the skin by a small battery-powered current. (This initially results in some tingling or itching which is minor and soon passes.) A glucose level is determined three times per hour (every 20 minutes). If excessive sweating or heat are present, the determination is voided for that reading. The watch requires an initial three-hour equilibration time and a single finger-poke blood sugar for calibration. It is then ready to give three readings per hour for the next 12 hours. The glucose levels can be read on the watch and it has a memory to print out the values. An alarm can be set to warn about low or high sugar values.

The only negatives are that the watch leaves a mark under the pad and/or irritation from the adhesive material around the outer edges of the watch in some people. These areas of irritation gradually disappear over 1-2 weeks. It is likely that a major use of the watch will be to monitor glucose levels in people suspected of having lows during the night or for those who have had seizures during the night. Perhaps it will be worn on nights when children have had heavy daytime exercise. Most families will probably not have the child wear the watch every night unless methods are found to prevent the areas of irritation.

The **Continuous Glucose Monitoring System (CGMS)** by MiniMed, Inc. was the first such device to be approved by the FDA. Unfortunately, in order to get it on the market, the initial device:

> i. does not have an alarm system to warn of low or high glucose levels;

> ii. does not display the glucose levels but must be taken into the doctor's office to have the values downloaded.

The company will gradually make improvements and collect information to hopefully persuade the FDA to allow these two deficiencies to be changed. The monitor will read glucose levels 288 times in 24 hours (every five minutes). A plastic cannula is inserted under the skin which, as with the insulin pump cannula, can stay in place for up to three days. A sample tracing is shown in the figure. The system will be particularly useful as people change from standard diabetes management to intensive management (e.g., an insulin pump). Because the CGM system is capable of determining such frequent sugar measurements, it will likely be the precursor, along with the MiniMed insulin pump, of the "closed-loop" pump, the **"bionic pancreas."** The CGM system will be hooked up to the pump in such a way that it will turn off or increase insulin output as the glucose levels indicate. It is now predicted that this will be possible within 5-10 years. This will revolutionize the treatment of type 1 diabetes.

A CURE: PANCREAS OR ISLET TRANSPLANTATION

Banting and Best received the Nobel prize for their discovery of insulin in 1921. It was originally believed that a "cure" for diabetes had been found in January, 1922, when the first person with diabetes was treated with insulin. As the disease had been known for approximately 4,000 years, and people with the more severe form (now called type 1) lived only about one year, this represented a great advance. Insulin was not a "cure," but was a life-saving treatment. Several decades later, people began to understand the long-term complications of diabetes. A cure continues to be hoped and prayed for, and the following continue to show promise:

Pancreas Transplantation

Surgeons can now cure type 1 diabetes by doing a whole (or partial) pancreas transplant. The immunosuppression medications that must be taken to prevent the body from rejecting the foreign tissue are the same as those that must be used to prevent rejection of any transplanted organ (e.g., kidney, liver, heart). The medicines have improved, but they still have dangerous side effects (e.g., infections, low white blood cell counts, and possibly types of cancer). However, if it is necessary to have a kidney transplant due to kidney failure from diabetes (so that one has to be on the medicines anyway), a pancreas transplant should now also be done.

Figure: Example of CGMS

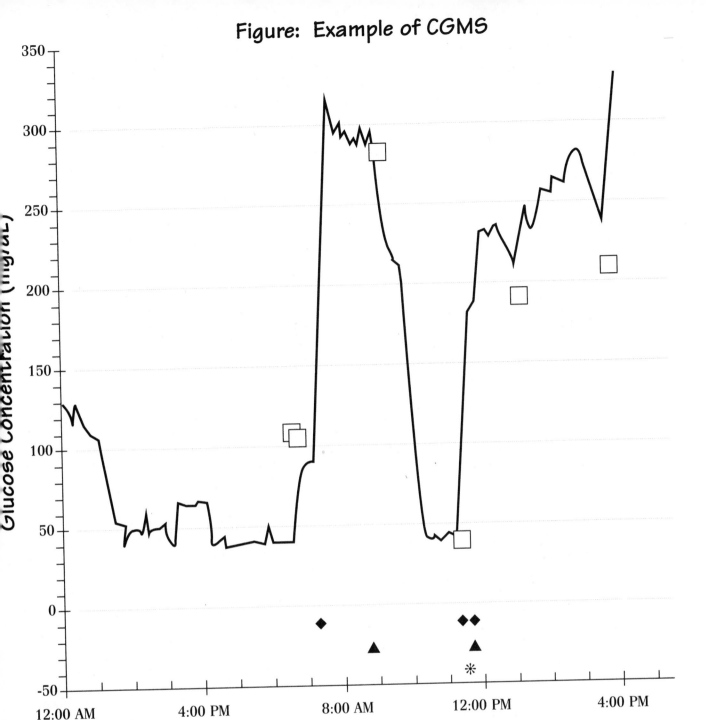

A tracing of glucose levels using the Continuous Glucose Monitoring System (CGMS) by Minimed, Inc., versus finger stick glucose readings (squares). This tracing is from a boy who receives insulin pump therapy. His hemoglobin A_{1c} was 8.5%, which is above our acceptable level (<8.0%). It can be seen that the morning blood sugar level of 105 mg/dl looked excellent (see open square = meter value). However, the sensor graph, giving readings every five minutes, showed low glucose values (around 50 mg/dl) from 1a.m.-6a.m. There were also low values just prior to lunch (also detected by meter—see open square). It also became apparent from the CGMS tracings that the boy was sometimes forgetting to bolus with his meals. The basal dosages were decreased during the night and late morning as a result of two tracings showing similar patterns. Later CGMS graphs (not shown) confirmed that the periods of hypoglycemia were resolved. Adult supervision was enlisted to help resolve the missed meal boluses. (The diamonds represent bolus insulin administration and the triangles represent food intake [as entered by the patient].)

Islet Transplantation

The islets, where insulin is made (see Chapter 2), make up less than 1/100 of the total volume of the pancreas. Methods have improved to harvest the islets from a pancreas, although many are destroyed in the process. It may take islets from as many as five pancreases in order to get enough islets to cure one person. Also, the same immunosuppression medications must be used as with whole pancreas transplants as discussed above. Even with the potent immunosuppression medications, there are only one or two "cured" patients reported in the medical literature who have been able to remain off insulin for five years or longer.

Although there would never be enough human pancreases to get enough islets to cure everyone with type 1 diabetes, several other options are possible. One such option would be the possibility of cloning a new pancreas or new islet cells. This is not possible at this time. However, some scientists are working on putting the genetic information into cells for insulin production. This is complex and requires the cells to be able to turn off and turn on insulin production safely and reliably. Although not possible at this time, this research offers hope for the future.

Other researchers are trying to find out if islets from other animals, such as pigs, could be transplanted into humans. (Pork insulin worked satisfactorily in humans for approximately 60 years.) The transplanted islets could probably be partially protected from attacking white blood cells by encapsulating them with an alginate material, although it is likely that immunosuppression therapy would still be necessary. As the FDA is now placing very strict guidelines on transplanting animal tissue into humans, this area of research is moving slowly.

In summary, although it is fine to hope or to pray for a cure for diabetes, for now the most important goal is to keep oneself in the best sugar control possible. This will help to prevent other complications, so that if a cure does become possible, the person will be able to benefit from such a miracle.

PREVENTION OF TYPE 1 DIABETES

After knowing about diabetes for approximately 4,000 years, the first two large-scale prevention trials began in the 1990s to try to prevent type 1 diabetes. Both of these were possible because reliable methods to determine who was in the process of developing diabetes became available. Even if neither of the initial two approaches succeeds, the mechanism is now set up to test other agents in the future that show promise. As a result, it is likely that diabetes will someday be able to be prevented.

The method currently being used in the trials for the prediction of type 1 diabetes involves doing two antibody tests, the islet cell antibody (ICA) and the insulin autoantibody (IAA). (Two other antibodies have been shown useful, the GAD-antibody and the ICA-512 antibody, but neither were fully developed when the trials began.) In addition to the antibody tests, the trials require an intravenous glucose tolerance test (IV-GTT). This is currently the best test to determine if insulin can still be released in normal amounts. An oral glucose tolerance test (OGTT) is also done to prevent subjects from entering the trial who already have type 1 diabetes. A summary of the tests is shown in the Table.

The first of the two trials began in Europe, under the direction of Dr. Edwin Gale of the U.K., using a B-vitamin called nicotinamide. It is called **ENDIT** for European Nicotinamide Diabetes Intervention Trial. The study has all subjects entered, is double-blinded, and should provide information as to whether the disease-onset can be delayed or prevented by the year 2003.

The second major prevention trial is the **Diabetes Prevention Trial-Type 1 (DPT-1)** which is taking place in the U.S. under the direction of Dr. Jay Skyler of Miami, FL and a steering committee of 19 scientists. **DPT-1** is studying whether type 1 diabetes can be prevented with insulin injections (high-risk trial) or insulin capsules (intermediate-risk trial). Parents, siblings, or offspring (ages 3-45 years) and cousins, aunts, uncles, nephews, nieces, or half-siblings (ages 3-20 years) who have a relative who started insulin shots by age 40 years can be screened. People are still badly needed for this trial. People have a responsibility to help if they hope to have such studies continue so that future generations may someday be protected from developing diabetes. Call 1-800-425-8361 to find out the nearest site for the free screening.

For the "high-risk" injection study (see Table), subjects must have a greater than 50% likelihood of developing diabetes in the next five years. They are either carefully observed or they receive low-dose Ultralente insulin twice daily plus four days of IV insulin once yearly. For the "intermediate-risk" (25-50% likelihood of developing diabetes in the next five years) subjects are given an oral capsule of either insulin or placebo taken once daily. All subjects in both trials are followed closely to look for the early development of diabetes.

In summary, it is an exciting time to be involved in diabetes research. Methods of non- or minimally invasive glucose monitoring have just become available. Pancreas or islet transplantations are technically feasible, but less dangerous medications or methods to prevent rejection are needed. Studies which will someday lead to the prevention of type 1 diabetes are now under way. The future for people and families with type 1 diabetes is indeed looking brighter.

CLINICAL ADVANCES IN THE MORBIDITY AND MORTALITY OF DIABETES

The good news!

It has been our impression for some time that the mortality from type 1 diabetes has declined. An article in the March, 1999 journal, *Diabetes Care*, notes, "The prognosis of patients with type 1 diabetes has improved considerably during the last 50 years, as shown in epidemiological studies from Europe and the U.S. **The main reason for this improvement in the prognosis is that the risk of developing diabetic nephropathy has decreased dramatically and that patients on their way to developing diabetic nephropathy are diagnosed in the microalbuminuric stage and treated with ACE-inhibitors or other antihypertensive agents.**"

The bad news!

The bad news is that families often do not take the responsibility to bring in the two overnight urines for the microalbumin measurements. (Our clinic has also become so busy that the health care providers cannot always remember to ask you to do this.) If you/your child has had diabetes for at least three years and reached puberty (usually 11-13 years of age), the two overnight urines should be collected every 12 months. Families must take some responsibility in helping to get these important tests done each year.

One change has occurred in the method of collection (see directions at the end of Chapter 21). Because our laboratory was so congested with jugs of urine, we are now asking families to measure the total volume of each of the two overnight collections at home and to just bring in a small portion of each sample to the clinic in a clean container. Urine is sterile and it will not hurt to do the measurements using any cooking measuring cup. Or, if people wish, they can pick up measuring containers and tubes at the time of their routine clinic visit. It is fine to bring in the aliquots of the two overnight samples without asking your health care provider if it has been 12 months since last checked. Remember to label the tubes and to fill out the form at the back of Chapter 21 with the times and volumes.

In summary, mortality from type 1 diabetes has gone down mainly because of a reduction in kidney disease. Kidney disease is declining because of:
i. better glucose control
ii. better blood pressure control
iii. fewer people with diabetes are smoking
iv. earlier detection of kidney damage by the **microalbumin test** so that the early damage can be reversed before it becomes permanent

We need each family to help in accomplishing all four of these!!! Then the news will all be good!!! Remember that data from Scandinavia indicates that if people with diabetes do not develop diabetic kidney damage, they can live as long as any person who does not have diabetes.

Table
The Diabetes Prevention Trial: Type 1 (DPT-1)

1. Screening: Islet cell antibody (ICA) test

60-80,000 first degree relatives (3-45 years old) or second degree relatives (3-20 years old) of people who started insulin shots prior to age 40 years will need to be screened. People can call 1-800-425-8361 to find out the nearest place to go to obtain the free ICA screen.

2. Staging: Intravenous glucose tolerance test (IV-GTT) x 2

Insulin autoantibody (IAA) x 2

HLA 0602 protective gene

Mixed meal (Sustacal®) test

Oral glucose tolerance test (OGTT) to make sure not already diabetic

3. Treatment: The treatment arm of the DPT is divided into two parts:

i. The Parenteral IV/Injection Insulin Trial

The participants have a greater than 50% chance of developing diabetes in the next five years. They must have:

--A positive ICA (islet cell antibody) test on two occasions

--Insulin production on two IV-GTTs below the tenth percentile of normal

--No protective genes (HLA-DQ 0602)

--A normal oral glucose tolerance test

The parenteral trial involves four days of IV insulin therapy once yearly and two injections of low-dose Ultralente insulin daily. Three-hundred forty subjects are being admitted to the trial.

ii. The Oral Insulin Trial

The participants have a 25-50% chance of developing diabetes in the next five years. They must have:

--A positive ICA test (x2) and a positive IAA (insulin autoantibody) test (x2)

--Normal insulin production on two IV-GTTs

--No protective genes (HLA-DQ 0602)

--A normal oral glucose tolerance test

The oral insulin trial is double-blinded so that participants will receive either 7.5 mg of insulin once daily or a placebo. The insulin does not have any hypoglycemic effect, as it is broken down into peptides by the stomach acid. Four-hundred-fifty subjects are being admitted to the trial.

DEFINITIONS

Alginate: Protein from seaweed used to cover islets so that white blood cells cannot get to them.

Bionic Pancreas: An artificial device that would turn off or turn on insulin output as indicated by glucose levels.

DPT-1: Diabetes Prevention Trial-Type 1. The first large trial in the U.S. to determine if type 1 diabetes can be prevented.

ENDIT: European Nicotinamide Diabetes Intervention Trial. The first large trial in Europe to test if diabetes can be prevented.

Encapsulated Islets: Islets covered with a material (such as alginate from seaweed) to prevent white blood cells from being able to get to the islet.

FDA: Food and Drug Administration. Their section on Clinical Chemistry and Toxicology Devices must vote to allow approval of new devices, such as a non-invasive blood glucose meter.

GlucoWatch: A non-invasive watch-like device, made by the Cygnus Company, which measures extracellular glucose levels as an index of blood glucose values.

Immunosuppression: Using medications to suppress the immune system, generally given so that transplanted organs will not be rejected.

MiniMed Continuous Glucose Monitoring System (CGMS): A system in which a small probe is inserted under the skin to read extracellular glucose levels every five minutes over a three-day period.

Non-invasive glucose (sugar) testing: Being able to measure glucose (sugar) levels without requiring blood to be drawn.

Subcutaneous: Under the skin (but not in a blood vessel).

QUESTIONS (Q) AND ANSWERS (A) FROM NEWSNOTES

Q. When is a cure coming?

A. I am asked this question almost daily in clinic. I do not know the answer, other than to say that progress seems to be coming slowly.

Q. Which do you think will come first, a safe cure or the ability to prevent diabetes?

A. A cure is, of course, already possible if one is willing to take the potentially dangerous medicines. As of now, if enough people are willing to help with the screening and enter studies such as DPT-1, I would guess that we will be able to prevent diabetes in the next generation before we can safely cure it in the current generation.

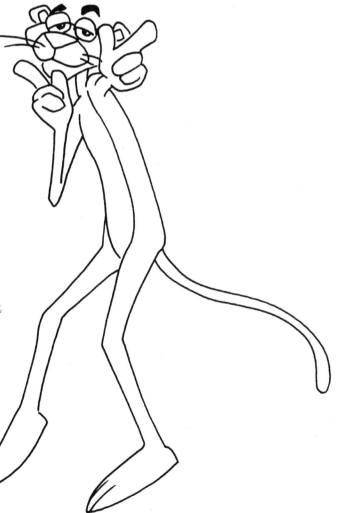

APPENDIX I

GLUCOSE CONVERSION BETWEEN
mg/dl and mmol/L

This is the second edition of this book to include all blood glucose levels in both mg/dl and mmol/L. As parts of the world use one system and other parts the other system, this will allow the book to now be used by both. An easy way to make the conversion from mmol/L to mg/dl is to multiply by 18 (or to divide if changing in the opposite direction). The table below may also help.

mg/dl		mmol/L	mg/dl		mmol/L	mg/dl		mmol/L
10	=	.55	190	=	10.5	370	=	20.55
15	=	.83	195	=	10.8	375	=	20.8
20	=	1.10	200	=	11.1	380	=	21.1
25	=	1.40	205	=	11.3	385	=	21.35
30	=	1.70	210	=	11.6	390	=	21.65
35	=	1.95	215	=	11.9	395	=	21.9
40	=	2.25	220	=	12.2	400	=	22.2
45	=	2.50	225	=	12.5	425	=	23.6
50	=	2.75	230	=	12.75	450	=	25.0
55	=	3.00	235	=	13.0	475	=	26.35
60	=	3.25	240	=	13.3	500	=	27.75
65	=	3.60	245	=	13.6	525	=	29.15
70	=	3.90	250	=	13.9	550	=	30.5
75	=	4.15	255	=	14.15	575	=	31.9
80	=	4.45	260	=	14.5	600	=	33.3
85	=	4.70	265	=	14.7	625	=	34.7
90	=	5.00	270	=	15.0	650	=	36.1
95	=	5.25	275	=	15.25	675	=	37.5
100	=	5.50	280	=	15.55	700	=	38.85
105	=	5.80	285	=	15.8			
110	=	6.10	290	=	16.1			
115	=	6.40	295	=	16.35			
120	=	6.65	300	=	16.65			
125	=	7.00	305	=	16.9			
130	=	7.25	310	=	17.2			
135	=	7.50	315	=	17.5			
140	=	7.75	320	=	17.75			
145	=	8.00	325	=	18.0			
150	=	8.30	330	=	18.3			
155	=	8.50	335	=	18.6			
160	=	8.90	340	=	18.9			
165	=	9.15	345	=	19.15			
170	=	9.50	350	=	19.4			
175	=	9.75	355	=	19.7			
180	=	10.0	360	=	20.0			
185	=	10.25	365	=	20.25			

APPENDIX II: ID TAGS

1. Medi-Check

Medi-Check International Foundation, Inc.
800 Lee Street
Des Plaines, Illinois 60016
847-299-0620

Please print or type

Name (First Name First)

1 2 3 4 5 6 7 8 9 10 11 12 13 14 15 16 17 18 19 20 21

Street Address

City   **State**   **Zip**

Area Code   **Phone**   **Age**

Religion (optional)

Notify in Emergency   **Name (First Name First)**

Area Code   **Phone**

Physician's Name (First Name First)

Area Code   **Phone**

Please send (check box)

❏ **Neck Tag**
❏ **Wallet Card**
❏ **Bracelet**

Medi-Check relies on its income through donations.
Please help if you can with your enclosure.

( ) $35 ( ) $30 ( ) $25 ( ) Other _____

It is suggested that a *minimum* donation of $20.00 or
more be offered for each neck tag, wallet card or bracelet.

For office use only

Date received
_____

Date shipped
_____

Code
A B C D E F G H I
J K L M N O P Q R
S T U V W X Y Z

3/91

251

NOTE: IN FILLING OUT THE MEDICAL INFORMATION FORM BELOW, WE SUGGEST THAT YOU CONSULT YOUR DOCTOR.

1. MEDICAL INFORMATION (Please print or type):

Present medical problems _____

_____

_____

2. Medic Alert

To enroll by phone with credit card call 1-800-432-5378 anytime. Please have the following ready:
  1. Member number
  2. Credit card number and expiration date
  3. Medical information
  4. Name, telephone number and address of persons/physician/pharmacy to contact in an emergency
  5. Bracelet size (when ordering bracelet)

To order by mail: Complete this form and mail with a check or money order to Medic Alert, Designer Department, 2323 Colorado Ave., Turlock, CA 95382. Or fax this form to: 209-669-2450.

Please print or type clearly. A separate application is needed for each person.

i. Are you or have you been a Medic Alert Member ☐ No ☐ Yes
If yes, enter member number _____

ii. Personal Information:

Last Name _____ First _____ Middle _____

Sex ☐ M ☐ F   Social Security Number _____

Mailing address _____ City _____ State ___ Zip _____

Phone _____ Date of Birth (m/d/y) _____

3. Emergency Contacts: Person, Physician, Pharmacy to contact

  Person _____ Phone _____ Address _____

  Physician _____ Phone _____ Address _____

  Pharmacy _____ Phone _____ Address _____

4. Medical Information to be engraved on Emblem: Vital medical conditions and allergies. Allow one space between words. Emblem engraving space is limited. For help, call 1-800-432-5378. Medical professionals are on staff.

_____

_____

5. To be added to your computerized medical file, these vital medical facts: Additional medical conditions, allergies and medications. Dosage data not needed.

_____

_____

6. Membership Benefits: New members receive first-year membership including establishing and maintaining your computerized medical file with personal ID number, record summary, custom-engraved emblem and chain, 24-Hour Emergency Response Center, unlimited free record updates, and member publications. Annual membership renewal after first year only $15.

7. Emblem Selection (mention code 9920):

Two-Tone Executive Emblem with Sterling Silver Figaro Bracelet (small)................**$80.00**

Sterling Silver Braided Polished Pendant with Sterling Silver French Rope Chain............**$80.00**

Sterling Silver Traditional Braided Emblem (large) with Executive Bracelet...............**$80.00**

October 1995—Prices subject to change without notice. Allow 4 weeks for delivery.

Emblem total from above: $ _____

8. Charitable Contribution (Medic Alert is a nonprofit organization that depends on fees and contributions to support a 24-Hour Emergency Response Center.) $ _____

9. Total Amount Enclosed $ _____

10. Method of Payment:

❏ Check   ❏ MasterCard   ❏ VISA   ❏ Discover   ❏ Money Order
No other cards accepted.

No COD's. Payment must accompany order. Send to:
Medic Alert, 2323 Colorado Ave., Turlock, CA 95382

Card Number _____-_____-_____-_____

Expiration Date: _____

Signature for Card Authorization: _____

IMPORTANT: When you receive your personalized Medic Alert emblem and the copy of your emergency medical file, please check both carefully for accuracy and call Medic Alert to report any errors. Also, please be sure to notify Medic Alert (1-800-432-5378) <u>whenever</u> your medical, address, or family physician information changes. Medic Alert believes that the information in your medical file is confidential and should only be released to protect or save a member's life. By accepting membership in Medic Alert, you do authorize Medic Alert to release information in emergencies or to healthcare personnel whom you authorize. We welcome you as a new member and will do our very best to serve you well.

11. Signature of Member   Date _____

_____

3. Dog tags
(Please type or print clearly)

Line 1

Line 2

Line 3

Line 4

Line 5

Two each Genuine Dog Tags and Neck
Chain Set $7.50
Shipping and Handling $2.00
Optional Silencers 2 each $2.00
Total Enclosed $____

Return Address:

_____

_____

_____

Money Order to:
Dog Tags,
P.O. Box 1337
Casper, WY 82602

4. American Medical Identifications

Bracelet - check selection

Stainless Steel ☐ $ 18.95
Sterling Silver ☐ $ 39.95
10K Gold-filled ☐ $ 49.95
10K Gold ☐ $189.95
Bracelet Size: ☐ Sm ☐ Med ☐ Lg
or Specify Inches _____

Necklace - check selection

Stainless Steel ☐ $ 18.95
Sterling Silver ☐ $ 39.95
10K Gold-filled ☐ $ 49.95
10K Gold ☐ $189.95

Medallion - check selection

10K Gold ☐ $ 79.95
14K Gold ☐ $ 99.95

Limit engraving to 5 lines for medallion
Preschool sizes available on all items—indicate age in months:

_____Engraving Information

Name to be engraved: _____

Present medical problem(s): _____

_____

Medications (to be engraved): _____

_____

Allergic to: _____

_____

Other information: _____

_____

Mail identification tag to:

Name: _____

Address: _____

City: _____ State: _____ Zip: _____

Credit card and number:

_____

Exp. Date: _____ Daytime phone: _____

Mail orders

Send completed order form with check, credit card number or money order to:
American Medical Identifications, Inc.
P.O. Box 925512
Houston, TX 77292

Fax orders: Send completed order via fax to 713-695-7358.
*Add $3.00 S&H for orders up to $60.00. For orders over $60.00, add $5.00.

*Texas residents add 8.25% for sales tax.
*One or two week delivery on most orders.

For additional information, call 1-800-363-5985 or visit website at www.MED-ID.COM

APPENDIX III

SHOPPING LIST AND APPROXIMATE COST OF DIABETES SUPPLIES

Supplies	Cost in Dollars

Equipment for Injections

Insulin - Pure Pork or Human	22.00
Regular	
NPH	
Lente	
Semi Lente	
Ultra Lente	27.00
Humalog	
Alcohol Sponges (Box of 100)	2.50
BD Lo Dose Insulin Syringes (Box of 100)	16.50
Or	
Monoject 1cc Insulin Syringes (Box of 100)	16.50

Equipment for Urine Testing

Ketodiastix #100	22.00
Ketodiastix #50	16.00
Ketostix #100	16.00
Ketostix #50	10.00
Ketostix #20 (foil wrapped)	7.00
Chemstrip uGK #100	13.00
Chemstrip K #25	7.00

Equipment for Blood Glucose Testing

Finger stick device	10.00-25.00
Lancets (Box of 200)	11.00
One Touch Strips #50	30.00
Precision Strips	30.00
Blood Glucose Monitor (with memory)	70.00-140.00
Chemstrip BG #50	30.00

Miscellaneous Supplies

Insta-Glucose	4.00
"Pink Panther" Book	
(Understanding Insulin-Dependent Diabetes)	15.00
BD Glucose Tablets	2.50
Identification bracelet or necklace	2.50-20.00
Glucagon	40.00

Questions to Ask Healthcare Providers:

INDEX

PUBLICATIONS

Additional copies of *Understanding Insulin-Dependent Diabetes* may be purchased for $15.00 (price includes shipping and handling), from The Guild of the Children's Diabetes Foundation at Denver:

Make checks payable to:
The Guild-CDF at Denver

Mailing address
The Guild of the
Children's Diabetes Foundation
777 Grant Street
Suite 302
Denver, CO 80203

All orders must be paid in full before delivery. Books are mailed Ground UPS. Allow one to three weeks for delivery.

Canadian and Foreign Purchasers: Please include sufficient funds to equal U.S. currency exchange rates.

The following are also available:

BOOKS

A Coloring Book About Diabetes, a coloring book for children to create a better understanding of diabetes. Also available in Spanish.

Kids Cupboard, Chock Full of Treats for All Ages, a cookbook for diabetics and health conscious nibblers.

For current prices and additional information, please call:
(303)863-1200 or (800)695-2873.

PUBLICATIONS

Additional copies of *Understanding Insulin-Dependent Diabetes* may be purchased for $15.00 (price includes shipping and handling), from The Guild of the Children's Diabetes Foundation at Denver:

Make checks payable to:
The Guild-CDF at Denver

Mailing address
The Guild of the
Children's Diabetes Foundation
777 Grant Street
Suite 302
Denver, CO 80203

All orders must be paid in full before delivery. Books are mailed Ground UPS. Allow one to three weeks for delivery.

Canadian and Foreign Purchasers: Please include sufficient funds to equal U.S. currency exchange rates.

The following are also available:

BOOKS

A Coloring Book About Diabetes, a coloring book for children to create a better understanding of diabetes. Also available in Spanish.

Kids Cupboard, Chock Full of Treats for All Ages, a cookbook for diabetics and health conscious nibblers.

For current prices and additional information, please call:
(303)863-1200 or (800)695-2873.